Lung Cancer: Advances in Diagnosis and Treatment

Lung Cancer: Advances in Diagnosis and Treatment

Editor: Robin Downey

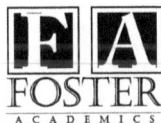

FOSTER
ACADEMICS

www.fosteracademics.com

www.fosteracademics.com

FOSTER
ACADEMICS

Cataloging-in-Publication Data

Lung cancer : advances in diagnosis and treatment / edited by Robin Downey.
    p. cm.
Includes bibliographical references and index.
ISBN 978-1-63242-875-2
1. Lungs--Cancer. 2. Lungs--Cancer--Diagnosis. 3. Lungs--Cancer--Treatment. I. Downey, Robin.
RC280.L8 L86 2020
616.994 24--dc23

© Foster Academics, 2020

Foster Academics,
118-35 Queens Blvd., Suite 400,
Forest Hills, NY 11375, USA

ISBN 978-1-63242-875-2 (Hardback)

Contents

Permissions

List of Contributors

Index

Preface

It is often said that books are a boon to mankind. They document every progress and pass on the knowledge from one generation to the other. They play a crucial role in our lives. Thus I was both excited and nervous while editing this book. I was pleased by the thought of being able to make a mark but I was also nervous to do it right because the future of students depends upon it. Hence, I took a few months to research further into the discipline, revise my knowledge and also explore some more aspects. Post this process, I begun with the editing of this book.

Lung cancer is a malignant tumor of the lung that is characterized by uncontrolled growth of cells in lung tissues. When the cancer metastasizes, it can spread beyond the lung into nearby tissues and parts of the body. It presents symptoms such as shortness of breath, weight loss, coughing and chest pains. The majority of cases of lung cancer are caused due to long-term tobacco smoking. It can be detected through computed tomography scans and chest radiographs. The diagnosis is confirmed with a biopsy. The treatment and prognosis of the cancer depends on the type of cancer, its stage and the performance status of the patient. Most lung cancers are not curable. However, treatment strategies such as chemotherapy, radiotherapy and surgery may be used for the management of lung cancer. This book is compiled in such a manner, that it will provide in-depth knowledge about the diagnosis and treatment of lung cancer. It is a valuable compilation of topics, ranging from the basic to the most complex advancements in oncology. It aims to serve as a resource guide for students and experts alike and contribute to the growth of the discipline.

I thank my publisher with all my heart for considering me worthy of this unparalleled opportunity and for showing unwavering faith in my skills. I would also like to thank the editorial team who worked closely with me at every step and contributed immensely towards the successful completion of this book. Last but not the least, I wish to thank my friends and colleagues for their support.

Editor

NSCLC molecular testing in Central and Eastern European countries

Ales Ryska[1*], Peter Berzinec[2], Luka Brcic[3,4], Tanja Cufer[5], Rafal Dziadziuszko[6], Maya Gottfried[7], Ilona Kovalszky[8], Włodzimierz Olszewski[9], Buge Oz[10], Lukas Plank[11] and Jozsef Timar[8]

Abstract

Background: The introduction of targeted treatments for subsets of non-small cell lung cancer (NSCLC) has highlighted the importance of accurate molecular diagnosis to determine if an actionable genetic alteration is present. Few data are available for Central and Eastern Europe (CEE) on mutation rates, testing rates, and compliance with testing guidelines.

Methods: A questionnaire about molecular testing and NSCLC management was distributed to relevant specialists in nine CEE countries, and pathologists were asked to provide the results of *EGFR* and *ALK* testing over a 1-year period.

Results: A very high proportion of lung cancer cases are confirmed histologically/cytologically (75–100%), and molecular testing of NSCLC samples has been established in all evaluated CEE countries in 2014. Most countries follow national or international guidelines on which patients to test for *EGFR* mutations and *ALK* rearrangements. In most centers at that time, testing was undertaken on request of the clinician rather than on the preferred reflex basis. Immunohistochemistry, followed by fluorescent in situ hybridization confirmation of positive cases, has been widely adopted for *ALK* testing in the region. Limited reimbursement is a significant barrier to molecular testing in the region and a disincentive to reflex testing. Multidisciplinary tumor boards are established in most of the countries and centers, with 75–100% of cases being discussed at a multidisciplinary tumor board at specialized centers.

Conclusions: Molecular testing is established throughout the CEE region, but improved and unbiased reimbursement remains a major challenge for the future. Increasing the number of patients reviewed by multidisciplinary boards outside of major centers and access to targeted therapy based on the result of molecular testing are other major challenges.

Keywords: Non-small cell lung cancer, *EGFR* mutations, *ALK* rearrangements, Molecular testing, Central eastern European region

Background

Globally, for several decades, lung cancer has been the most common cancer and the leading cause of cancer deaths. The situation is particularly serious in Central and Eastern European (CEE) countries, which have the highest age-standardized incidence rates in men around the world [1]. Incidence rates in women are generally lower than in men, but are increasing in many countries worldwide. There are some geographical differences in incidence, reflecting in part the different historical

exposure to tobacco smoking [1]. The diagnosis is often not made until late in the course of the disease and, as a result, only a minority of patients are cured and the ratio of mortality-to-incidence is very high. Almost 70% of patients have locally advanced or metastatic disease at initial diagnosis [2].

Nowadays, only about 15% of lung cancer cases are small cell lung cancer, with the majority of lung cancer cases classified as non-small cell lung cancer (NSCLC). When the diagnosis is made based on a small biopsy or cytology sample, besides the three common types of NSCLC (squamous cell carcinoma, adenocarcinoma, and non-small cell carcinoma not otherwise specified [NOS]) several additional subtypes can be defined by morphology,

* Correspondence: ryskaale@gmail.com
[1]The Fingerland Department of Pathology, Charles University Faculty of Medicine and University Hospital, Hradec Králové, Czech Republic
Full list of author information is available at the end of the article

immunohistochemistry (IHC), and molecular pathology [2, 3]. Although most lung cancers are attributable to tobacco smoking, approximately 10–15% of cases in Western countries occur in lifelong never-smokers and these are almost exclusively adenocarcinomas [4].

The study of molecular biology of NSCLC has had a major impact on diagnosis and treatment of this disease [5–7]. The work of the Lung Cancer Mutation Consortium and other groups has shown that driver mutations or other oncogene alterations are present in more than half of all adenocarcinomas [8]. The discovery of targetable genetic alterations, such as activating mutations of the epidermal growth factor receptor (EGFR) and anaplastic lymphoma kinase (ALK) rearrangements, has led to the implementation of precision therapy for certain subtypes of lung cancer based on appropriate patient selection [9]. Clinical trials have shown significantly longer progression-free survival in patients with EGFR mutations who are treated with EGFR tyrosine kinase inhibitors (TKIs) compared with chemotherapy [10]. Similarly, ALK TKI treatment of patients with ALK-rearranged tumors prolongs progression-free survival compared with first-line chemotherapy [11]. Patients with a druggable molecular alteration who are treated with a corresponding targeted treatment benefit from significantly higher response rates and longer progression-free survival, although an improvement in overall survival with targeted agents has not been shown by the majority of randomized clinical trials [8]. There are probably multiple reasons for the lack of overall survival advantage seen in clinical trials, one of the most important reasons is a high number of patients crossing over to targeted agents after failure of treatment in the chemotherapy arms.

This move towards biomarker-based treatment approaches has highlighted the importance of accurate molecular diagnosis. In addition to classical morphologic classification, molecular analysis of tumor samples is essential to determine if a druggable oncogenic alteration is present. Consequently, the pathologist is now a key member of the multidisciplinary lung cancer team [12].

Identification of the challenges for personalized lung cancer treatment within the CEE region might facilitate molecular diagnostics and improve patient care. Information about molecular testing practices for NSCLC in the CEE region is relatively limited. The INSIGHT study has provided some information on EGFR mutation rates, testing, and compliance with testing guidelines in several Central European countries [13]. However, only very few data from this region are available on ALK testing. Our study was designed to collect information on both EGFR and ALK testing from a large number of CEE countries.

Methods

A Working Group of oncologists, pulmonologists, and pathologists from the CEE region was established to

obtain more information on NSCLC molecular testing in their countries and to raise awareness of the current issues around personalized medicine for lung cancer.

As a first step, a questionnaire (Additional file 1) with 37 questions addressing issues of molecular testing and NSCLC management was distributed in the second quarter of 2014 to 59 specialists (epidemiologists, oncologists, pulmonologists, and pathologists) from nine CEE countries. In June 2015, pathologists were also asked to provide details of the results of EGFR and ALK testing over a 1-year period.

Results
Respondents
There were a total of the 42 responses from nine countries; the number of responders by country are shown in Table 1 (data were not available for some questions; see Additional file 1 for the questionnaire).

Lung cancer types
Table 2 shows the proportion of lung cancer cases that are confirmed morphologically in each country.

Figure 1 shows the breakdown of lung cancer types for selected countries. Adenocarcinoma is the most common type in all countries except Bulgaria, whereas small cell lung cancer represented between 10% and 20% of cases in all countries.

EGFR testing
Most countries have national guidelines or follow European guidelines on EGFR mutation testing [2]. European guidelines are followed in Bulgaria, Croatia, Israel, Slovakia, Slovenia, and Turkey. Bulgaria, Czech Republic, Hungary, Israel, Poland, and Slovakia also have national guidelines, whereas some centers in Poland follow local guidelines. Some Turkish centers follow American College of Pathologists guidelines [12].

Most centers reported that adenocarcinomas and NSCLC-NOS were tested for activating EGFR mutations. In some countries (Bulgaria, Czech Republic, Israel, Slovakia, Slovenia, and Turkey), large cell and squamous

Table 1 Countries participating and number of responders

Bulgaria	2
Croatia	4
Czech Republic	4
Hungary	8
Israel	3
Poland	7
Slovakia	7
Slovenia	3
Turkey	4

Table 2 Lung cancer cases morphologically confirmed

Country (number of responses)	Proportion of cases, %
Bulgaria	75*
Croatia	100*
Czech Republic	85[†]
Israel	100*
Slovakia	83*
Slovenia	92*

*Registry data; [†]Best estimate

cell tumors may be tested in selected cases (mostly on request from the treating physician). In most countries, only advanced tumors (stage IIIb and IV) were generally tested for *EGFR* mutations. In the Czech Republic, Slovakia, and Slovenia, as well as in certain individual centers in other countries, other stages were also tested for research purposes.

In most centers, *EGFR* mutation testing was undertaken when requested by the clinician, usually the oncologist treating the patient. In the Czech Republic, Slovakia, and Slovenia, and some centers in Croatia, testing was reflex (i.e. the pathologist automatically tested all tumors that met the criteria). In Hungary, it is policy to test for *KRAS* mutations first, and the presence of a *KRAS* mutation is an exclusion criterion for *EGFR/ ALK* testing. In Turkey, *EGFR/ALK* testing is not performed in *KRAS* mutation-positive tumors, although *KRAS* testing is not routine.

In many countries (Croatia, Czech Republic, Hungary, Israel, Slovakia, and Slovenia), at least 65% of eligible tumors were actually tested for *EGFR* mutations in 2014. However, a significant proportion of samples (5–25%)

were inadequate for testing, usually because the sample was too small or did not contain enough tumor cells.

Usually, more than one method was used in each country for *EGFR* mutation testing. Real-time polymerase chain reaction (PCR) was used in all countries, direct sequencing in five countries, and other methods were used in addition in only two countries.

The incidence of specific *EGFR* mutations in selected centers in 2014 is shown in Table 3; the frequency of *EGFR*-mutated tumors ranged from 6.7 to 15.2%. These numbers cannot be compared because of the different inclusion criteria for testing.

ALK testing

ALK testing is available in all countries except Bulgaria. Most countries have national guidelines or follow European guidelines on which subtypes to test for *ALK* rearrangements. European guidelines [2] are followed in Croatia, Slovenia, and Turkey, whereas Czech Republic, Hungary, Israel, Poland, and Slovakia follow national guidelines. In all centers, adenocarcinomas and NSCLC-NOS were tested, usually on request from the treating clinician. As for *EGFR* testing, reflex *ALK* testing for all eligible patients was implemented in the Czech Republic, Slovakia, and Slovenia.

In most countries, as for *EGFR* testing, only advanced tumors (stage IIIb and IV) were tested for *ALK* rearrangements. At some centers in Croatia, Czech Republic, Slovakia, and Slovenia, other stages were also tested for research purposes. The presence of a known *EGFR* mutation was an exclusion criterion for *ALK* testing in all countries. In addition, in countries where some or all samples are tested for *KRAS* mutations (Turkey,

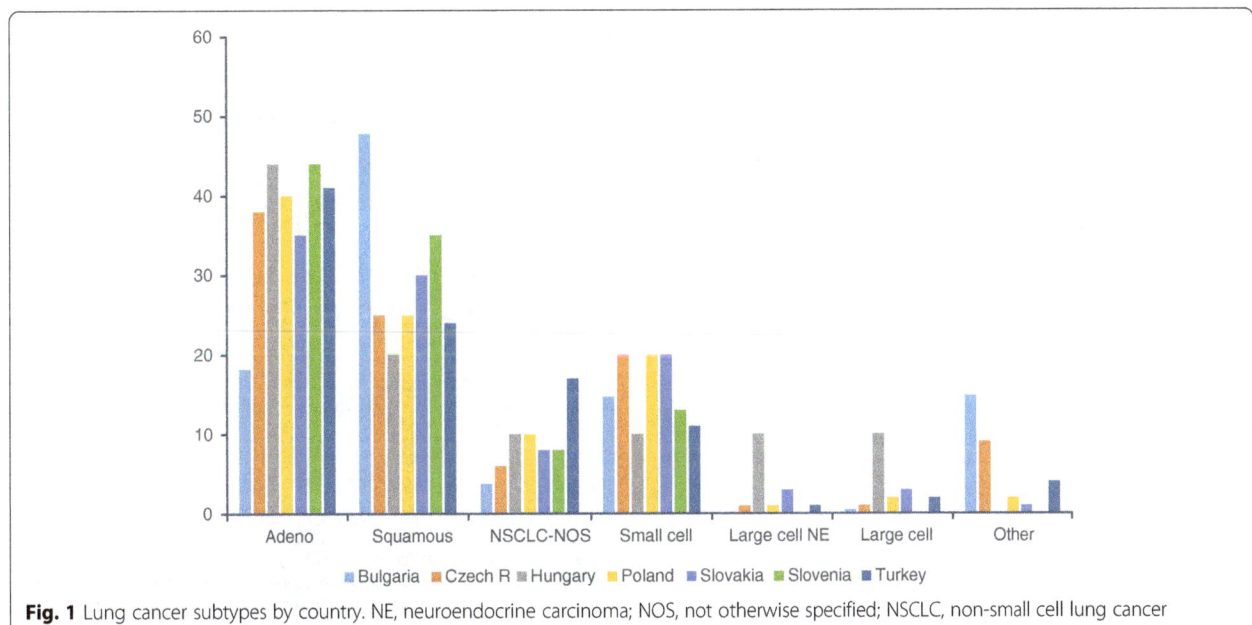

Fig. 1 Lung cancer subtypes by country. NE, neuroendocrine carcinoma; NOS, not otherwise specified; NSCLC, non-small cell lung cancer

Table 3 Results of *EGFR* testing in selected centers in 2014[a]

	EGFR, n (%)					Non-diagnostic
	WT	Mut exon 18	Mut exon 19	Mut exon 20	Mut exon 21	
Croatia (Zagreb)	561 (85.9)	8 (1.2)	46 (7)	8 (1.2)	30 (4.6)	11
Czech (Prague)	154 (90.6)	4 (2.4)	6 (3.5)	2 (1.2)	4 (2.2)	15
Czech (Hradec Kralove)	234 (90.0)	0	15 (5.8)	2 (0.8)	9 (3.5)	6
Hungary (Budapest, Timár)	350 (85.6)	4 (1.0)	22 (5.4)	14 (3.9)	19 (4.6)	57
Hungary (Budapest, Toth)	251 (93.3)	0	9 (3.3)	1 (0.4)	8 (3.1)	2
Hungary (Budapest, Kovalszky)	500 (88.5)	6 (1.1)	27 (4.8)	0	32 (5.7)	–
Hungary (Debrecen)	760 (89.6)	0[†]	61 (7.2)	0[†]	27 (3.2)	13
Hungary (Pécs)	112 (86.8)	0	10 (7.8)	0	7 (5.4)	–
Hungary (Szeged)	617 (92.6)	4 (0.6)	27 (4.1)	2 (0.3)	16 (2.4)	71
Slovakia	361 (87.6)	1 (0.2)	30 (7)	2 (0.5)	16 (3.8)	–
Slovenia	464 (86)	5 (0.9)	39 (7.2)	8 (1.5)	25 (4.6)	57
Turkey (Cerrahpaşa)	714 (87.9)	17 (2.1)	52 (6.4)	3 (0.4)	26 (3.2)	38

EGFR epidermal growth factor receptor, *WT* wild-type
[a]Note that these numbers cannot be compared directly because of the different criteria for selection of samples to test
[†]Exons 18 and 20 not tested

Slovenia, Hungary, and Poland), the presence of a *KRAS* mutation is also an exclusion criterion. For *ALK* testing, IHC followed by fluorescent in situ hybridization (FISH) and/or FISH alone were used in all countries. In Israel, other methods, including next-generation DNA sequencing, were also used (Table 4).

The incidence of *ALK* rearrangements determined in selected centers in 2014 is shown in Table 5. The substantial differences in the frequency, which ranged from 1.6% to 12%, are most probably due to different testing approaches, excluding *KRAS*- and *EGFR*-positive cases from *ALK* testing or not.

Testing for other mutations
Tumor samples were tested routinely for *KRAS* mutations in Hungary and Slovenia; some samples were tested in Turkey and Poland. *ROS1* testing was routine in Slovenia and was undertaken on request in Slovakia.

Reimbursement for molecular testing
There are several different sources of funding for *EGFR* and *ALK* testing in the region. In the Czech Republic, Hungary, Israel, Poland, Slovakia, Slovenia, and Turkey, testing is partly or fully reimbursed by the national

Table 4 *ALK* testing methods

Croatia (Zagreb)	IHC (IHC followed by FISH)
Czech (Hradec Kralove)	IHC, IHC followed by FISH
Czech (Prague)	IHC, IHC followed by FISH, FISH
Hungary (Budapest, Timár)	FISH
Hungary (Budapest, Toth)	FISH
Hungary (Budapest, Kovalszky)	FISH, other
Hungary (Debrecen)	FISH
Hungary (Pécs)	IHC followed by FISH
Hungary (Szeged)	FISH
Israel	IHC, IHC followed by FISH, FISH, sequencing
Poland (Warsaw)	FISH
Slovakia	IHC followed by FISH; FISH
Slovenia	IHC followed by FISH
Turkey (Cerrahpaşa)	IHC followed by FISH

FISH fluorescent in situ hybridization, *IHC* immunohistochemistry

Table 5 Results of *ALK* testing in selected centers in 2014[a]

	ALK, n (%)		Non-diagnostic
	WT	Rearrangement	
Croatia	161 (93.1)	12 (6.9)	28
Czech (Prague)	55 (96.5)	2 (3.5)	10
Czech (Hradec Kralove)	260 (95.2)	13 (4.8)	2
Hungary (Budapest, Timár)	332 (94.9)	18 (5.1)	0
Hungary (Budapest, Toth)	122 (98.4)	2 (1.6)	4
Hungary (Budapest, Kovalszky)	415 (95.6)	19 (4.4)	0
Hungary (Debrecen)	226 (91.5)	21 (8.5)	35
Hungary (Pécs)	55 (94.8)	3 (5.2)	2
Slovakia	375 (88)	51 (12)	0
Slovenia	199 (96.5)	7 (3.5)	0
Turkey (Cerrahpaşa)	764 (95.6)	35 (4.4)	14

ALK anaplastic lymphoma kinase, *WT* wild-type
[a]Note that these numbers cannot be compared directly because of the different criteria for selection of samples to test; in some centers only samples negative for *KRAS* and *EGFR* mutations were tested for *ALK* translocations

health authority/national health insurance. Private insurance covers some testing in Israel and Turkey.

The pharmaceutical industry supported some testing in Hungary, Poland, and Slovenia, and was the only source of financial support for testing in Bulgaria (*EGFR* only) and Croatia (*EGFR* and *ALK*). The industry did not finance testing in Czech Republic, Israel, Slovakia, or Turkey. However, in the personal experience of the authors, although the molecular testing is stated to be fully reimbursed, this is not the case in practice. Often, there are various forms of budget capping with a limitation on the number of tests performed (e.g. based on the number of samples tested in the previous period). This policy is a disincentive to reflex testing. In Hungary, for example, only 30% of tests were reimbursed.

Multidisciplinary approach

Multidisciplinary lung cancer teams/tumor boards are established in all countries; however, these are often only functioning fully as part of routine clinical practice at specialized lung cancer treatment centers. In Hungary, Poland, and Slovenia, it is mandatory for all cases to be discussed by a multidisciplinary tumor board. In Turkey, it is obligatory for selected cases. When multidisciplinary teams/tumor boards are operational, a pathologist is usually a member.

The proportion of NSCLC cases actually discussed at a multidisciplinary tumor board is 75–100% at most specialist centers; however, there is wide variation and can be as low as 20% in some hospitals. There was a trend towards a higher proportion of cases being discussed at multidisciplinary tumor boards at respondents' own centers compared with their estimates for the country as a whole. Data on how many patients with druggable EGFR or ALK alterations get access to targeted drugs were not collected, however according to the personal experience of the authors, access to EGFR and/or ALK TKIs is often limited, mainly due to local reimbursement policy restrictions.

Discussion

The survey confirmed that a very high proportion of lung cancer cases are verified by histology or cytology (75–100%) in CEE countries and that, in most countries, the data can be derived from the established cancer registries. Adenocarcinoma is the most common type in all countries except Bulgaria, whereas 10–20% of cases were small cell lung cancer in all countries, which is consistent with global data [14]. The high incidence of squamous cell carcinoma in Bulgaria may reflect the high levels of smoking, relatively late introduction of filtered cigarettes, and pollution levels [15].

It is encouraging that molecular testing of NSCLC samples has been established in all CEE countries evaluated in 2014, and that most countries follow national or international guidelines on which patients to test for *EGFR* mutations and *ALK* rearrangements. However, in most centers, *EGFR* and *ALK* testing was undertaken on request of the clinician, rather than automatically for eligible samples (reflex testing), an approach which can lead to delays in availability of test results and in the initiation of targeted treatment. There is an increasing focus on shortening the turnaround time for test results, and incorporation of reflex testing at the level of the pathologist can help to avoid such delays [16].

The results showed that a significant proportion of samples were unsuitable for testing for various reasons. Various initiatives, including better communications as well as educational initiatives directed at physicians who collect tissue samples, may improve the situation and help to ensure that samples are of sufficient size and quality for molecular testing [16].

The results of molecular testing presented here (Tables 3 and 5) provide interesting insights into the frequency of *EGFR* mutations and *ALK* rearrangements in the region. Yet only very limited general conclusions can be drawn on the overall frequency of *EGFR* mutations and *ALK* translocations because of the differences between centers in testing policy, selection of samples for testing based on clinical factors (i.e. not all samples were tested) and sequential testing at some centers resulting in *ALK* testing being performed only on EGFR- and KRAS-negative samples. Consistent with published data, most *EGFR* mutations reported were in exons 19 and 21 [17, 18]. Information was not requested on *KRAS* mutation rate, which would have been particular relevant for Hungary where testing was routine. However, a recent paper reported that the incidence of *KRAS* mutations was 28.6% in 532 consecutive Caucasian patients tested at Semmelweis University [19].

The results show that IHC, followed by FISH confirmation in positive cases, had been widely adopted for *ALK* testing in the region in 2014. FISH testing was still regarded as the gold standard for *ALK* testing; however, this method is relatively costly, time-consuming, and technically difficult to perform for routine use, which has led to extensive evaluation of IHC as an alternative used for screening purposes [20–22]. Data published after our survey showed that both D5F3 and 5A4 antibodies are able to detect *ALK* rearrangements reliably and are equally well suited for routine diagnostic use [23]. Several studies have shown good concordance between the results of IHC and FISH for *ALK* testing [24–27]. Indeed, some investigators have shown that IHC can be useful in cases with atypical or borderline FISH results [26, 28].

Acceptance by the United States Food and Drug Administration (FDA) of the Ventana ALK D5F3 IHC as a companion test to identify patients for crizotinib treatment provides additional support for the routine use of

IHC. The test provides a fast and accurate method to identify ALK protein expression, with a binary scoring system, and has been validated clinically by retrospective testing of tissue samples from patients screened for inclusion in crizotinib clinical trials [29]. These promising data encourage some centers to use IHC as a primary method replacing FISH. Immunohistochemistry can readily be applied to tissue samples, cell blocks prepared from effusions and Papanicolaou-stained cytologic slides [22, 27].

The European consensus recommended that all non-squamous NSCLC tumors in patients with advanced/recurrent disease be tested for *EGFR* mutations and *ALK* translocations. Selected squamous tumors (from patients with minimal or remote smoking history) should be strongly considered for testing. Sequential testing is not recommended and parallel testing of multiple mutations on the same sample is becoming the standard [2]. More recent European recommendations are consistent with these statements. Sanger sequencing, pyrosequencing, and next-generation sequencing are recommended for *EGFR* testing and validated tests including FISH and IHC may be used for ALK testing [30]. Real-time PCR is also widely used. National guidelines, where they exist, are broadly consistent with these recommendations; in Hungary, *KRAS* testing is performed before testing for other genetic alterations.

With the increasing number of molecular markers that need to be examined for optimal selection of targeted treatment, the cost of up-to-date molecular testing is rapidly growing. The financial burden of testing the entire cohort of eligible patients can, in fact, reach the cost of the treatment of several individual patients identified by the testing, namely in tumors driven by rare mutations [31]. Thus, routine use of modern approaches, such as next-generation sequencing resulting in dramatic reduction of testing costs, is eagerly awaited.

It should be noted that the data discussed here reflect the status quo in 2014, and molecular testing is evolving fast with changes in testing methods being implemented. The growing use of IHC for *ALK* testing has already been discussed. In addition, many laboratories in Europe are now adopting next-generation sequencing that can be applied to formalin-fixed paraffin-embedded tissue in routine diagnostic practice. This allows for the detection of many genetic alterations and oncogene targets in parallel, providing the opportunity for fast and deep characterization of tumors as well as for the potential for other targeted therapies [32].

Adherence to the best practices in molecular testing is crucial to ensure accurate diagnoses and appropriate clinical decisions [30, 33]. Quality control is essential to ensure consistent and reliable molecular diagnostic results and to facilitate comparison of results from different laboratories. External quality assessment (EQA) programs have been established for both *EGFR* and *ALK*

testing [33, 34]. The vast majority of the laboratories contributing to this study already participate in EQA programs. Many laboratories in the region participate in the European Society of Pathology Lung External Quality Assessment Scheme [19]. As the results of molecular testing directly influence the management of individual patients, EQA is essential to guarantee optimal quality of testing. Therefore, each laboratory should prove successful participation in the appropriate EQA program to be included to the network of testing centers [35].

Multidisciplinary tumor boards play a key role in optimizing the diagnosis and treatment of lung cancer [30]. With rapid progress in the molecular profiling of NSCLC and its increasing complexity, it is essential that the tumor boards include specially trained molecular pathologists, as well as molecular biologists, among the tumor board members when discussing the best possible treatment for each individual patient with NSCLC. Although it is positive that all countries studied have implemented lung cancer tumor boards, these are more likely to be operational only in specialized lung cancer treatment centers.

Conclusions

Non-small cell lung cancer molecular testing is established in all CEE countries participating in this study. The responses show that all countries follow guidelines regarding *EGFR* and *ALK* testing, with most countries testing only advanced stages of adenocarcinomas, NSCLC-NOS, and NSCLC when an adenocarcinoma component cannot be excluded. Most countries are still undertaking testing on request and not implementing the preferred reflex policy.

Limited reimbursement is a significant barrier to molecular testing in the region and a disincentive to reflex testing. The authors recommend that testing should be independently funded.

The results show that ensuring adequate NSCLC samples and enabling wide access of eligible patients to molecular testing are key issues for the future. Increasing the number of patients reviewed by multidisciplinary boards and the access of patients with druggable molecular alterations to targeted drugs are other major challenges.

Abbreviations
ALK: Anaplastic lymphoma kinase; CEE: Central and Eastern European; EGFR: Epidermal growth factor receptor; EQA: External quality assessment; FDA: Food and Drug Administration; FISH: Fluorescent in situ hybridization; IHC: Immunohistochemistry; NOS: Not otherwise specified; NSCLC: Non-small cell lung cancer; PCR: Polymerase chain reaction; TKI: Tyrosine kinase inhibitor

Acknowledgments
This work was presented in part at the 16th World Conference on Lung Cancer, 2015. Abstract P3.04-045.

Funding
This work was supported by an unrestricted educational grant from Pfizer; the unrestricted grant supported the work of the medical writer. The funding body had no role in the design of the study or the collection, analysis, and interpretation of data or the writing of the manuscript.
All authors report receiving financial support from Pfizer for advisory roles and nonfinancial support from SuccinctChoice Medical Communications related to the work under consideration.
Medical writing support, provided by Christine Drewienkiewicz of SuccinctChoice Medical Communications, was funded by Pfizer.

Authors' contributions
AR, PB, TC, RD, MG, WO, BO, LP and JT designed the study and the questionnaire. AR, PB, LB, TC, RD, MG, IK, WO, BO, LP and JT contributed to data collection for their countries and participated in review and revision of the manuscript. All aforementioned authors read and approve the final manuscript.

Competing interests
AR reports receiving grants and personal fees from AstraZeneca and MSD, honoraria for advisory board participation AstraZeneca, MSD, Novartis, Boehringer Ingelheim and personal fees and honoraria for advisory board participation and lectures from BMS, outside the submitted work. PB reports receiving honoraria from AstraZeneca, Boehringer Ingelheim, Pfizer, MSD, and Roche, and has participated at advisory boards for Boehringer Ingelheim, Pfizer, and MSD. LB reports receiving personal fees from Roche, AstraZeneca, Pfizer, Boehringer Ingelheim, outside the submitted work. TC reports receiving consulting fees from Pfizer, Boehringer Ingelheim, BMS outside the submitted work. RD reports personal fees from Pfizer, Roche, AstraZeneca, Boehringer Ingelheim, Novartis, outside the submitted work. MG reports receiving consulting fees from Pfizer, Boehringer Ingelheim, BMS, MSD. IK reports receiving personal fees from Pfizer (participation in 2015 advisory board preparing the manuscript) related to the work under consideration. WO reports receiving honoraria or consulting fees from MSD, Boehringer Ingelheim, Pfizer and Abbott outside the submitted work. OB reports receiving consulting fees from Pfizer, Boehringer Ingelheim, BMS and MSD outside the submitted work. LP reports receiving grants from Slovak Research and Development Agency, Pfizer Slovakia, Ministry of Health Slovakia related to the work under consideration and grants from Novartis Slovakia, Takeda Slovakia, and AstraZeneca Slovakia outside the submitted work. JT reports receiving personal fees from BMS, Lilly, Pfizer, Roche, and Boehringer Ingelheim outside the submitted work. All authors report receiving financial support from Pfizer and non-financial support from SuccinctChoice Medical Communications (funded by Pfizer) related to the work under consideration.

Author details
[1]The Fingerland Department of Pathology, Charles University Faculty of Medicine and University Hospital, Hradec Králové, Czech Republic. [2]Department of Oncology, Specialised Hospital of St Zoerardus Zobor, Nitra, Slovakia. [3]Institute of Pathology, Medical University of Graz, Graz, Austria. [4]Institute of Pathology, University of Zagreb School of Medicine, Zagreb, Croatia. [5]Medical Faculty Ljubljana, University Clinic Golnik, Golnik, Slovenia. [6]Medical University of Gdansk, Gdansk, Poland. [7]Meir Medical Center, Kfar Saba, Israel. [8]1st Institute of Pathology and Experimental Cancer Research, Semmelweis University, Budapest, Hungary. [9]Institute of Oncology, Warsaw, Poland. [10]Cerrahpasa Medical Faculty, Istanbul, Turkey. [11]Department of Pathology, Comenius University, Jessenius Medical Faculty and University Hospital, Martin, Slovakia.

References
1. GLOBOCAN. 2012 v1.0, cancer incidence and mortality worldwide: IARC CancerBase no. 11. Lyon: International Agency for Research on Cancer; 2013. http://globocan.iarc.fr
2. Kerr KM, Bubendorf L, Edelman MJ, Marchetti A, Mok T, Novello S, O'Byrne K, Stahel R, Peters S, Felip E. Second ESMO consensus conference on lung cancer: pathology and molecular biomarkers for non-small-cell lung cancer. Ann Oncol. 2014;25(9):1681–90.
3. Travis WD, Brambilla E, Noguchi M, Nicholson AG, Geisinger KR, Yatabe Y, Beer DG, Powell CA, Riely GJ, Van Schil PE, et al. International Association for the Study of Lung Cancer/American Thoracic Society/European Respiratory Society international multidisciplinary classification of lung Adenocarcinoma. J Thorac Oncol. 2011;6(2n):244–85.
4. Couraud S, Zalcman G, Milleron B, Morin F, Souquet PJ. Lung cancer in never smokers – a review. Eur J Cancer. 2012;48(9):1299–311.
5. Black RC, Khurshid H. NSCLC: an update of driver mutations, their role in pathogenesis and clinical significance. R I Med J (2013). 2015;98(10):25–8.
6. Dacic S. Molecular genetic testing for lung adenocarcinomas: a practical approach to clinically relevant mutations and translocations. J Clin Pathol. 2013;66(10):870–4.
7. Popper HH, Ryska A, Timar J, Olszewski W. Molecular testing in lung cancer in the era of precision medicine. Transl Lung Cancer Res. 2014;3(5):291–300.
8. Kris MG, Johnson BE, Berry LD, Kwiatkowski DJ, Iafrate AJ, Wistuba II, Varella-Garcia M, Franklin WA, Aronson SL, Su PF, et al. Using multiplexed assays of oncogenic drivers in lung cancers to select targeted drugs. JAMA. 2014;311(19):1998–2006.
9. Besse B, Adjei A, Baas P, Meldgaard P, Nicolson M, Paz-Ares L, Reck M, Smit EF, Syrigos K, Stahel R, et al. 2nd ESMO consensus conference on lung cancer: non-small-cell lung cancer first-line/second and further lines of treatment in advanced disease. Ann Oncol. 2014;25(8):1475–84.
10. Zhang WQ, Li T, Li H. Efficacy of EGFR tyrosine kinase inhibitors in non-small-cell lung cancer patients with/without EGFR-mutation: evidence based on recent phase III randomized trials. Med Sci Monit. 2014;20:2666–76.
11. Solomon BJ, Mok T, Kim DW, Wu YL, Nakagawa K, Mekhail T, Felip E, Cappuzzo F, Paolini J, Usari T, et al. First-line crizotinib versus chemotherapy in ALK-positive lung cancer. N Engl J Med. 2014;371(23):2167–77.
12. Lindeman NI, Cagle PT, Beasley MB, Chitale DA, Dacic S, Giaccone G, Jenkins RB, Kwiatkowski DJ, Saldivar JS, Squire J, et al. Molecular testing guideline for selection of lung cancer patients for EGFR and ALK tyrosine kinase inhibitors: guideline from the College of American Pathologists, International Association for the Study of Lung Cancer, and Association for Molecular Pathology. J Mol Diagn. 2013;15(4):415–53.
13. Ramlau R, Cufer T, Berzinec P, Dziadziuszko R, Olszewski W, Popper H, Bajcic P, Dusek L, Zbozinkova Z, Pirker R. Epidermal growth factor receptor mutation-positive non-small-cell lung cancer in the real-world setting in Central Europe: the INSIGHT study. J Thorac Oncol. 2015;10(9):1370–4.
14. Wahbah M, Boroumand N, Castro C, El-Zeky F, Eltorky M. Changing trends in the distribution of the histologic types of lung cancer: a review of 4,439 cases. Ann Diagn Pathol. 2007;11(2):89–96.
15. van Dorn A. Bulgaria lags behind Europe in pollution and smoking targets. Lancet Respir Med. 2014;2(3):182–3.
16. Lim C, Tsao MS, Le LW, Shepherd FA, Feld R, Burkes RL, Liu G, Kamel-Reid S, Hwang D, Tanguay J, et al. Biomarker testing and time to treatment decision in patients with advanced nonsmall-cell lung cancer. Ann Oncol. 2015;26(7):1415–21.
17. Li AR, Chitale D, Riely GJ, Pao W, Miller VA, Zakowski MF, Rusch V, Kris MG, Ladanyi M. EGFR mutations in lung adenocarcinomas: clinical testing experience and relationship to EGFR gene copy number and immunohistochemical expression. J Mol Diagn. 2008;10(3):242–8.
18. Shikhrakab H, Elamin YY, O'Brien C, Gately K, Finn S, O'Byrne K, Osman N. Epidermal growth factor receptor (EGFR) mutation testing, from bench to practice: a single institute experience. Ir Med J. 2014;107(7):201–4.
19. Lohinai Z, Klikovits T, Moldvay J, Ostoros G, Raso E, Timar J, Fabian K, Kovalszky I, Kenessey I, Aigner C, et al. KRAS-mutation incidence and prognostic value are metastatic site-specific in lung adenocarcinoma: poor prognosis in patients with KRAS mutation and bone metastasis. Sci Rep. 2017;7:39721.
20. Pekar-Zlotin M, Hirsch FR, Soussan-Gutman L, Ilouze M, Dvir A, Boyle T, Wynes M, Miller VA, Lipson D, Palmer GA, et al. Fluorescence in situ hybridization, immunohistochemistry, and next-generation sequencing for detection of EML4-ALK rearrangement in lung cancer. Oncologist. 2015;20(3):316–22.

21. Zwaenepoel K, Van Dongen A, Lambin S, Weyn C, Pauwels P. Detection of ALK expression in non-small-cell lung cancer with ALK gene rearrangements – comparison of multiple immunohistochemical methods. Histopathology. 2014;65(4):539–48.

22. Savic S, Bode B, Diebold J, Tosoni I, Barascud A, Baschiera B, Grilli B, Herzog M, Obermann E, Bubendorf L. Detection of ALK-positive non-small-cell lung cancers on cytological specimens: high accuracy of immunocytochemistry with the 5A4 clone. J Thorac Oncol. 2013;8(8):1004–11.

23. Savic S, Diebold J, Zimmermann AK, Jochum W, Baschiera B, Grieshaber S, Tornillo L, Bisig B, Kerr K, Bubendorf L. Screening for ALK in non-small cell lung carcinomas: 5A4 and D5F3 antibodies perform equally well, but combined use with FISH is recommended. Lung Cancer. 2015;89(2):104–9.

24. von Laffert M, Warth A, Penzel R, Schirmacher P, Kerr KM, Elmberger G, Schildhaus HU, Buttner R, Lopez-Rios F, Reu S, et al. Multicenter immunohistochemical ALK-testing of non-small-cell lung cancer shows high concordance after harmonization of techniques and interpretation criteria. J Thorac Oncol. 2014;9(11):1685–92.

25. Park HS, Lee JK, Kim DW, Kulig K, Kim TM, Lee SH, Jeon YK, Chung DH, Heo DS. Immunohistochemical screening for anaplastic lymphoma kinase (ALK) rearrangement in advanced non-small cell lung cancer patients. Lung Cancer. 2012;77(2):288–92.

26. Houang M, Toon CW, Clarkson A, Sioson L, Watson N, Farzin M, Selinger CI, Chou A, Morey AL, Cooper WA, et al. Reflex ALK immunohistochemistry is feasible and highly specific for ALK gene rearrangements in lung cancer. Pathology. 2014;46(5):383–8.

27. Wang W, Tang Y, Li J, Jiang L, Jiang Y, Su X. Detection of ALK rearrangements in malignant pleural effusion cell blocks from patients with advanced non-small cell lung cancer: a comparison of Ventana immunohistochemistry and fluorescence in situ hybridization. Cancer Cytopathol. 2015;123(2):117–22.

28. von Laffert M, Stenzinger A, Hummel M, Weichert W, Lenze D, Warth A, Penzel R, Herbst H, Kellner U, Jurmeister P, et al. ALK-FISH borderline cases in non-small cell lung cancer: implications for diagnostics and clinical decision making. Lung Cancer. 2015;90(3):465–71.

29. VENTANA ALK (D5F3) CDx Assay - P140025. https://www.accessdata.fda.gov/cdrh_docs/pdf14/p140025b.pdf. Accessed 25 Jan 2018.

30. Dietel M, Bubendorf L, Dingemans AM, Dooms C, Elmberger G, Garcia RC, Kerr KM, Lim E, Lopez-Rios F, Thunnissen E, et al. Diagnostic procedures for non-small-cell lung cancer (NSCLC): recommendations of the European expert group. Thorax. 2016;71(2):177–84.

31. Atherly AJ, Camidge DR. The cost-effectiveness of screening lung cancer patients for targeted drug sensitivity markers. Br J Cancer. 2012;106(6):1100–6.

32. Dietel M, Johrens K, Laffert MV, Hummel M, Blaker H, Pfitzner BM, Lehmann A, Denkert C, Darb-Esfahani S, Lenze D, et al. A 2015 update on predictive molecular pathology and its role in targeted cancer therapy: a review focussing on clinical relevance. Cancer Gene Ther. 2015;22(9):417–30.

33. von Laffert M, Penzel R, Schirmacher P, Warth A, Lenze D, Hummel M, Dietel M. Multicenter ALK testing in non-small-cell lung cancer: results of a round robin test. J Thorac Oncol. 2014;9(10):1464–9.

34. Patton S, Normanno N, Blackhall F, Murray S, Kerr KM, Dietel M, Filipits M, Benlloch S, Popat S, Stahel R, et al. Assessing standardization of molecular testing for non-small-cell lung cancer: results of a worldwide external quality assessment (EQA) scheme for EGFR mutation testing. Br J Cancer. 2014;111(2):413–20.

35. van Krieken JH, Siebers AG, Normanno N. European consensus conference for external quality assessment in molecular pathology. Ann Oncol. 2013;24(8):1958–63.

2

Small cell and non small cell lung cancer form metastasis on cellular 4D lung model

Dhruva K. Mishra[1], Ross A. Miller[2], Kristi A. Pence[3] and Min P. Kim[1,3]*

Abstract

Background: Metastasis is the main cause of death for lung cancer patients. The ex vivo 4D acellular lung model has been shown to mimic this metastatic process. However, the main concern is the model's lack of cellular components of the tumor's microenvironment. In this study, we aim to determine if the intact lung microenvironment will still allow lung cancer metastasis to form.

Methods: We harvested a heart-lung block from a rat and placed it in a bioreactor after cannulating the pulmonary artery, trachea and tying the right main bronchus for 10–15 days without any tumor cells as a control group or with NSCLC (A549, H1299 or H460), SCLC (H69, H446 or SHP77) or breast cancer cell lines (MCF7 or MDAMB231) through the trachea. We performed lobectomy, H&E staining and IHC for human mitochondria to determine the primary tumor's growth and formation of metastatic lesions. In addition, we isolated circulating tumor cells (CTC) from the model seeded with GFP tagged cells.

Results: In the control group, no gross tumor nodules were found, H&E staining showed hyperplastic cells and IHC showed no staining for human mitochondria. All of the models seeded with cancer cell lines formed gross primary tumor nodules that had microscopic characteristics of human cancer cells on H&E staining with IHC showing staining for human mitochondria. CTC were isolated for those cells labeled with GFP and they were viable in culture. Finally, all cell lines formed metastatic lesions with cells stained for human mitochondria.

Conclusion: The cellular ex vivo 4D model shows that human cancer cells can form a primary tumor, CTC and metastatic lesions in an intact cellular environment. This study suggests that the natural matrix scaffold is the only necessary component to drive metastatic progression and that cellular components play a role in modulating tumor progression.

Keywords: 4D cellular model, Lung Cancer, Breast cancer

Background

Stage IV, the point in tumor progression in which cancer spreads beyond the primary site and regional lymph nodes and is found in other organs, is the cancer stage that most often leads to patient mortality [1]. The tumor's microenvironment plays a critical role in tumor growth and the development of metastasis where the interaction between tumor cells and the associated stroma and cellular components modulates the tumor's progression and patient prognosis. Recently, the acellular 4D lung model has successfully mimicked the development of metastasis [2]. It is named the 4D model because of its perfusion of tumor nodules that allows it to change over time and grow in the 3D space. Findings from the 4D model suggest that the only component of tumor microenvironment that is important to show tumor progression is an intact natural matrix [2].

The acellular 4D lung model is created by removing all of the cells from a rat heart and lung block [3, 4]. This natural lung matrix maintains its three-dimensional architecture, including perfusable vascular beds and preserved airways. The matrix is composed of collagen, proteoglycans, and elastic fibers that preserve the architecture of airways and capillaries. A unique feature of the matrix

* Correspondence: mpkim@houstonmethodist.org
[1]Department of Surgery, Houston Methodist Hospital Research Institute, Houston, TX, USA
[3]Division of Thoracic Surgery, Department of Surgery, Weill Cornell Medical College, Houston Methodist Hospital, 6550 Fannin Street, Suite 1661, Houston, TX 77030, USA
Full list of author information is available at the end of the article

is that this composition is preserved among species in the distal airways [5]. Furthermore, the basement membranes of the alveolar septa are preserved after decellularization in this model [3]. The acellular 4D lung model shows that when tumor cells are placed into the trachea, they form perusable nodules in the lung matrix [6]. Moreover, the model allows tumor cells to secrete proteins that are more similar those found in lung cancer patients than the same tumor cells grown on a petri dish [7]. The acellular 4D lung model mimics metastasis, with the placement of all tumor cells in the left lung lobes and perfusion of the model in the bioreactor through the pulmonary artery. In order for the tumor cells to enter the right lung, the cells would need to leave the epithelial space in the left side, enter the vasculature, and enter the other epithelial space on the right side. Over time, this process occurred as metastatic lesions formed in the right lung and grew over time in the 4D model [2]. There are significant differences in the spatial organization of the tumor cells where the primary tumor grew in a pattern along the airway and the metastatic lesion formed in a distribution that is consistent with cancer distributed along the vasculature. The model's unique vascular channel allowed dead cells as well as live circulating tumor cells (CTC) to enter the vasculature. The CTC showed differences in behavior and gene expression compared to those cells initially placed in the model. The CTC took longer to attach to the petri dish than the parental cells placed in the model and they stayed alive in supernatant with decreased expression of integrin beta 4 (ITGB4) [8]. In addition, CTCs were resistant to chemotherapy [9]. There is no difference in the number of live CTC from the 4D model when they are placed in the petri dish, with or without Cisplatin, while the same dose for the parental cells (2D) placed in the model showed a significant reduction of live cells [9]. Previous studies also show that the CTC form metastatic lesions in the 4D model [2].

A major drawback of this acellular 4D model has been the lack of cellular components that are found in a patient's tumor microenvironment. These studies suggest that the natural matrix architecture is the only component necessary for complex perfusable nodules to form, the creation of CTC, and ultimately metastatic lesion formation. However, one could argue that this phenomenon is simply due to the artificial creation of an acellular environment. Thus, in this study, we show that the ex vivo 4D lung model can mimic the metastatic process in a normal cellular environment. We postulate that non-small cell and small cell lung cancer cell lines as well as breast cancer cell lines will grow in the model and form a primary tumor, CTC, and metastatic lesions.

Methods

All of the animal experiments were carried out in accordance with all applicable laws, regulations, guidelines, and policies governing the use of laboratory animal in research. The Institutional Animal Care and Use Committee (IUCAC) at the Houston Methodist Research Institute approved the protocols for animal experiments.

Rat lung isolation

We harvested the lung–heart block from 4 to 6 week old male Sprague-Dawley rats as previously described [6]. Briefly, we euthanized Sprague-Dawley rats with ketamine (100 mg/mL) and xylazine (10 mg/mL) and performed bilateral thoracotomy to open the thoracic cavity. We injected 2 mL of heparin (1000 units/mL, Sagent Pharmaceuticals, IL, USA) into the right ventricle of heart, removed the rib cage and injected 20 mL of heparinized Phosphate Buffered Saline (12.5 Units/mL) in the right ventricle after placing an 18-gauge needle (McMaster Carr, USA) in the left ventricle as a vent. The superior vena cava and inferior vena cava were cut and the lungs were flushed again with 20 mL of heparinized PBS. Next, we divided the trachea at the level of the thyroid, the branches of the aorta at the arch, and the descending aorta at the level of the hemiazygos vein. The heart-lung block was then separated from the esophagus and the rest of the rat body. We performed ventriculotomy to expose the right and left ventricles and placed a custom-made prefilled 18-gauge stainless steel needle (McMaster Carr, USA) through the right ventricle into the main pulmonary artery. This was secured with a 2–0 silk tie (Ethicon, San Angelo, TX, USA). We also placed a female luer bulkhead (Cole-Parmer, IL, USA) in the left ventricle and secured it with a 2–0 silk tie. We flushed the pulmonary artery cannula with heparinized PBS and placed it in a container containing heparinized PBS.

Cell culture

Human cancer cell lines A549, H1299, H460, H69, H446, SHP-77, MCF7, and MDAMB231 were obtained from ATCC (Manassas, VA, USA). These cell lines were grown in BD T175 cell culture flasks in RPMI 1640 medium (Hyclone, UT, USA) supplemented with 10% fetal bovine serum (Gibco, USA) and antibiotics (100 IU/mL penicillin, 100 mg/mL streptomycin, and 0.25 mg/mL amphotericin; Gibco, USA) at 37°C in 5% CO_2. Once the cells were 85% confluent, they were washed with PBS and subjected to trypsinization using 0.25% trypsin (Gibco, USA) to collect the cells from flasks. The cells were washed with medium and finally suspended in 50 mL of complete culture medium. Approximately 15 million cells were used to seed the lung matrix.

Bioreactor for the cellular 4D lung

A simplified small closed-system bioreactor was set up in an incubator for the lung cell culture (Fig. 1a). We used a custom-designed 500-mL glass bottle with three holes in

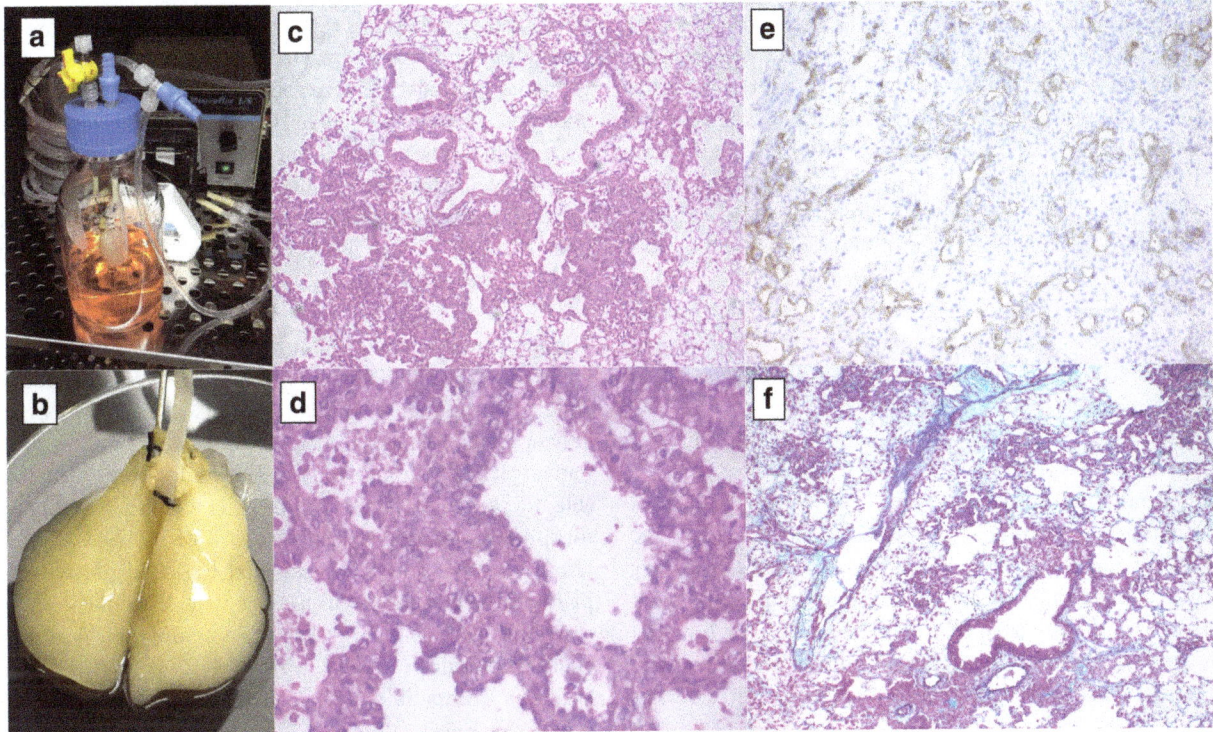

Fig. 1 Cellular ex vivo 4D lung model in a bioreactor without any tumor cells (control). Bioreactor showing connection from the lung to oxygenator and pump in cell culture incubator (**a**). The lung after 15 days in the bioreactor is intact (**b**). H&E staining shows intact alveoli, bronchus and vasculature (**c**) with some apoptotic cells. CD34 staining shows the endothelial lining in intact vasculature (**e**) and Movat pentachrome staining represents the components of extracellular matrix (**f**)

the cap fitted with a female luer thread-style panel (Cole-Parmer, USA): one for the pulmonary artery cannula, one for the trachea cannula, and one for the circulation of medium from the bottle. To obtain a controlled flow through the pulmonary artery, the cap was connected to a 3-way stopcock (Smith Medical, Dublin, OH, USA). The bottle was filled with 200 mL of complete medium that was circulated through the oxygenator tubing to prevent air bubbles.

Before seeding the human lung cancer cells into the lung matrix, the trachea was cannulated using an 18-gauge needle, and the scaffold was fixed to the bioreactor bottle in a hanging position. To modify it for the metastasis model, we tied the right main bronchus with a silk tie that was left there for the entire experiment and placed it in the bioreactor. The cells diluted in 50 mL complete media were seeded into the left lung lobes through the tracheal cannula via a sterile syringe fed by gravity. We perfused the scaffold at a flow rate of 6 mL/min. The culture medium in the bottle was changed every day to ensure the nutrients were optimal for cell growth, and the CTC were spun down and counted. We grew the cells on the matrix for 10–15 days. The lung matrix was carefully removed from the bioreactor bottle, maintaining sterile conditions, and a lobectomy performed

under a culture hood by tying the anatomic lobe with a 2–0 silk tie and resecting it on different days.

Impact of cellular lung on tumor growth on 2D

We plated 500,000 GFP labeled of A549, H460 and H1299 cells in 6-well plate, with different lung lobes from cellular and acellular rat lungs in cell culture incubator. After 48 h, cells were trypsinized and GFP positive cells were counted using fluorescence activated cell sorting (FACS) with same gating parameters (HMRI NIR Ariall, USA). All the cells were plated from same stock of cells on same day to avoid any bias with the GFP intensity. We determined the percentage of cells that that GFP+ cells in each sample. We compared the groups using student t-test and used $p < 0.05$ as significant.

Histology and immunohistochemistry

After lobectomy, the lung tissues were placed in 10% paraformaldehyde and shipped to the Pathology Core Laboratory at The Methodist Hospital Research Institute for further processing. Briefly, the tissues were fixed in 10% formalin overnight, processed, and embedded in paraffin. Hematoxylin and eosin (H&E) staining and immunohistochemistry were performed for human mitochondria to identify human cancer regions. The embedded tissues were cut into 4-µm slides and dewaxed; antigen retrieval was performed with antigen-unmasking solution (H-3300; Vector Laboratories, Burlingame, CA) in a steamer for 20 min. Slides were cooled for 20 min at room temperature, washed in PBS, and stained with H&E, Movat Pentachrome (American MasterTech Scientific, CA, USA), Human Anti-mitochondria (Abcam, MA, USA), CD34 and other markers following the standard protocol [10]. Expert board-certified pathologists examined stained slides, and images were captured using a microscope (EVOS, Fisher Scientific, USA). The metastatic lesions per high power field were determined by averaging the number of human mitochondria positive tumor cells per high power field (40X) of 10 areas.

Results
Cellular rat lung model
The cellular ex vivo lung was intact in the bioreactor for up to 15 days (Fig. 1b). The control tissue's histology shows a marginally intact matrix and lung with some apoptotic and non-viable cells (Fig. 1c and d). The lung tissue showed the lung with bronchovascular bundles, alveolar tissue and overlying pleural tissue. The peribronchiolar

tissue areas have collections of histiocytes resembling non-necrotizing granulomas (Fig. 1c and d). The alveoli are degenerating and many non-viable cells are seen along with scattered intra-alveolar macrophages. IHC of human mitochondria showed no positive staining, as there were no human cells seeded. Furthermore, staining the lung with Movat pentachrome highlights the matrix architecture showing the presence of collagen, proteoglycans and elastin (Fig. 1f). The immunohistochemistry of CD34 showed its presence in vessels (Fig. 1e).

Primary tumor in the cellular model
After 10–15 days of incubation, in the presence of cellular components, human NSCLC, SCLC, and breast cancer cells formed microscopic tumor nodules on a native rat lung though no gross nodules were visualized (Fig. 2a, e and i). These tumor cells showed a distinctive morphology unique to cell type. All of the NSCLC cells (A549, H1299, and H460) formed the solid pattern of a primary tumor in a bronchocentric distribution, but they differ in histology based on subtype. A549, an adenocarcinoma cell line, formed a focal acinar pattern and was compatible with human lung adenocarcinoma

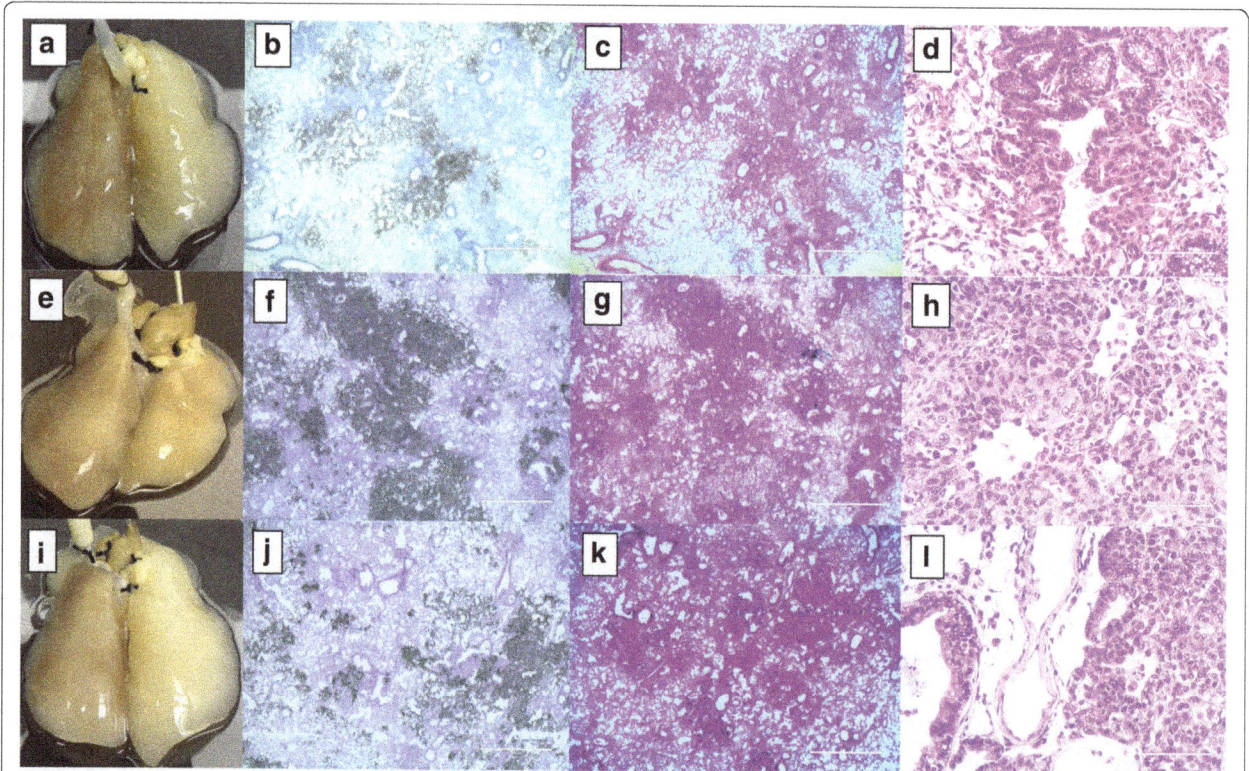

Fig. 2 Non small cell lung cancer (NSCLC) cells on the cellular 4D lung model. Primary tumors were formed in a bronchocentric fashion on the cellular lung upon A549 (**a–d**), H1299 (**e–h**) and H460 (**i–l**) cell seeding though the trachea. Human mitochondrial IHC staining clearly shows the presence of a tumor formed by human lung cancer cells in a rat lung after 12 days of culture in a bioreactor. Low and high power H&E staining indicates the presence of a microscopic tumor with distinctive histology based on type of cell placed in the model. A549 cells formed a focal acinar pattern with enlarged nuclei and scattered atypical mitotic cells (**c** and **d**). H1299 cells formed a solid tumor and resemble poorly differentiated cells with scattered atypical mitosis (**g** and **h**). H460 cells formed a solid tumor with vague glandular formation (**k** and **l**)

(Fig. 2b, c and d). The tumor cells were enlarged epithelioid cells with enlarged nuclei containing prominent nucleoli and scattered atypical mitotic cells (Fig. 2d). The Anti-Human mitochondrial stain highlights the cytoplasmic stain in tumor cells, but not the peribroncholar histocyte aggregates (Fig. 2b). H1299 cell lines also formed primary tumors with a solid growth pattern (Fig. 2f, g and h) and resemble poorly differentiated NSCLC. The cells resembled enlarged epithelioid, large central nuclei with large centrally placed nucleoli. Some of the nuclei are vesicular with scattered atypical mitosis, but this is not a definitive characteristic of squamous or adenocarcinoma (Fig. 2g and h). H460 cell lines also formed tumors on the cellular model with brocho/bronchiolar centric distribution (Fig. 2j, k and l). These tumor cells showed a solid pattern of tumor growth with vague glandular formation and a similar pattern to adenocarcinoma (Fig. 2k and l). Tumor cells appear similar to A549 cells in the cellular model.

In addition to NSCLC cell lines, we placed small cell lung carcinoma (SCLC) cell lines (H69, H446, SHP77) on the 4D cellular lung model (Fig. 3a, e and i). H69 cell lines showed the primary tumor in the broncho/bronchiolar centric space (Fig. 3b, c and d) with a peculiar pattern of high-grade basaloid malignancy, relatively scant cytoplasm,

dark-hyperchromatic nucei, lack of nucleoli, abundant mitosis, and karyorrhectic debris in the background. The tumor was arranged in a nest and there was a vague rosette/acinar appearance (Fig. 3c and d). H446 cells grew on the cellular model and formed a collection of tumors in a bronchiolar centric distribution and intra-alveolar (Fig. 3f, g and h). Cytomorphologic features were typical of small cell carcinoma similar to H69 features. SHP77 cells also formed the primary tumor on the cellular model and appeared more like poorly differentiated carcinoma within alveolar spaces (Fig. 3j, k and l). The tumor cells have large nuclei with some cells having nucleoli. Numerous mitotic cells with associated karyorrhetic debris were also visible (Fig. 3k and l).

Breast cancer cell lines (MCF7 and MDAMB231) also colonized on the cellular 4D lung model and formed microscopic tumor nodules (Fig. 4a and e). An ER/PR positive MCF7 cell formed a primary tumor in the left lobes that resembled a solid gland carcinoma in a broncho-bronchiolar centric distribution (Fig. 4b, c and d). The tumor cells forming the gland were medium to large epithelioid cells with large nuclei, some vesicular and some with prominent nucleoli (Fig. 4c and d). The morphologic features were similar to metastatic high-grade breast carcinoma (ductal). MDAMB231 cells grown on the cellular model formed

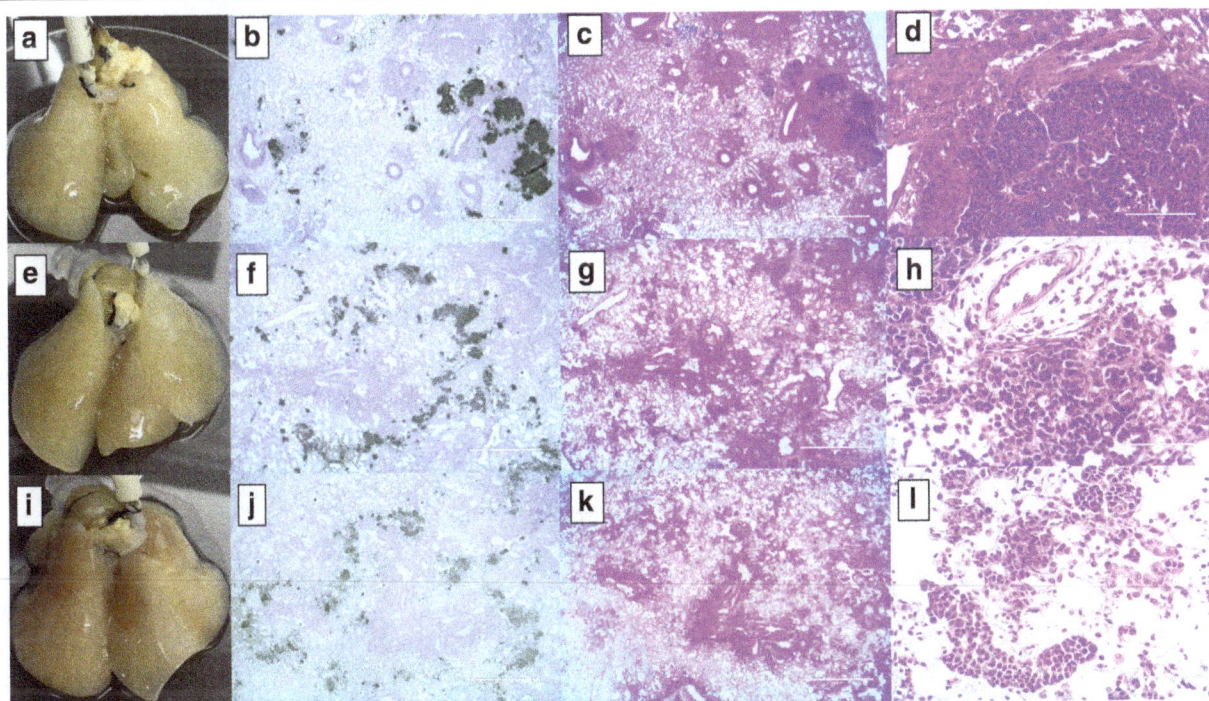

Fig. 3 Small cell cancer (SCLC) cells on the cellular 4D lung model. Primary tumors formed in a bronchocentric fashion on the cellular lung upon H69 (**a–d**), H446 (**e–h**) and SHP77 (**i–l**) cell seeding though no distinct nodules appeared. Human mitochondrial IHC staining clearly shows the presence of a tumor formed by human lung cancer cells in a rat lung after 10 days of culture in a bioreactor. Low and high power H&E staining indicates the presence of microscopic tumor with distinctive histology based on the cell type seeded. H69 cells formed tumors similar to high-grade basaloid malignancy with vague rosette/acinar appearance (**c** and **d**). H446 cells formed a collection of tumors, typical of small cell carcinoma (**g** and **h**). SHP77 cells formed a tumor more like a poorly differentiated carcinoma within alveolar spaces (**k** and **l**)

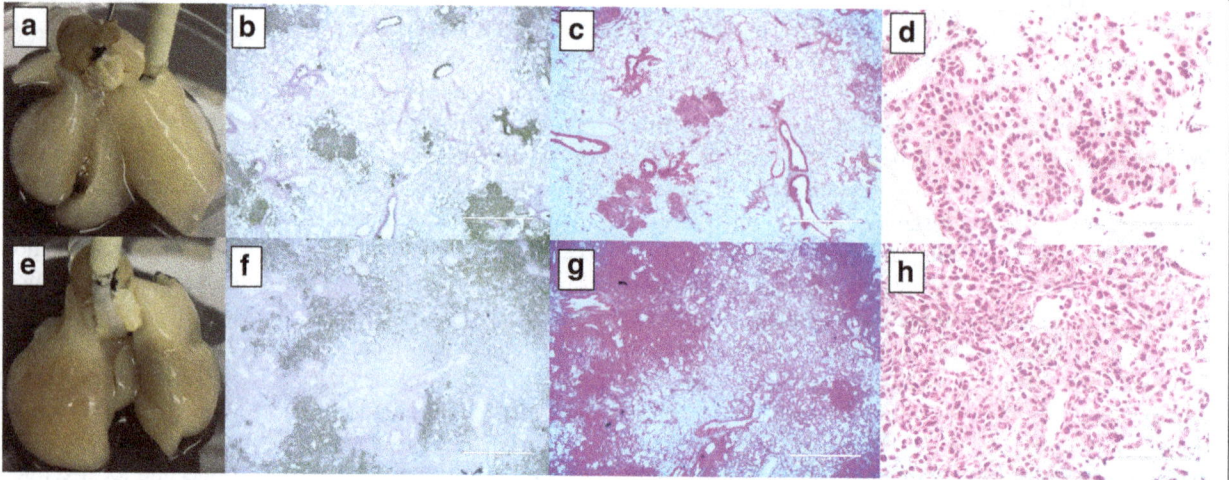

Fig. 4 Breast cancer cell lines on the cellular 4D lung model. Primary tumors were formed in a bronchocentric fashion on cellular lung upon MCF7 (**a**) and MDAMB231 (**e**) cell seeding though no distinct nodules appeared. Human mitochondrial IHC staining clearly shows the presence of a tumor formed by human breast cancer cells in a rat lung after 15 days of culture in a bioreactor. Low and high power H&E staining indicates the presence of a microscopic tumor with distinctive histology based of the cell type seeded. MCF7 cells formed solid gland carcinoma with large epithelioid cells and prominent nucleoli (**c** and **d**). MDAM231 cells formed large confluent primary tumors with poorly differentiated malignant carcinoma having spindle cell morphology (**g** and **h**)

large confluent primary tumors with poorly differentiated malignant carcinoma (Fig. 4f, g and h). There were loosely cohesive cells with rare acinar formation. Most of the malignant cells have spindle cell morphology with atypical mitosis, looking like metaplastic carcinoma (Fig. 4g and h).

Circulating tumor cells

We seeded the cellular model with GFP tagged tumor cells (H1299 and H460). We found GFP positive cells in the circulation and plated them in 96 well plates. These GFP tagged circulatory cells floated and survived in the media for a longer time compared to respective 2D cells. We visualized the viable GFP tagged cells attached to the surface and dividing, under a fluorescent microscope after 7 days (Fig. 5i and j).

Metastasis to contralateral lung

The NSCLC, SCLC and breast cancer cell lines formed metastatic lesions that were positive for human mitochondrial cells in the contralateral lung in a vascular distribution (Fig. 6). Unlike the primary tumor, where most of the tumors grew in bronchial distribution, the metastatic lesions were uniformly distributed in the lung. However, there were differences in the number of cells per HPF based on the cell type. Among NSCLC cells, A549 formed the least amount of metastatic lesions (0.9 ± 0.35 cells per HPF), while H1299, a metastatic cell line, formed the maximum number of metastatic lesions (3.6 ± 1.03 cells per HPF). H460 cells showed 1.6 ± 0.88 cells per HPF (Fig. 6a–d). Among SCLC cell lines, H69 formed the highest number of metastatic lesions (12.9 ± 3.49 cells per HPF) as compared to SHP-77 and H446 (4.4 ± 2.09

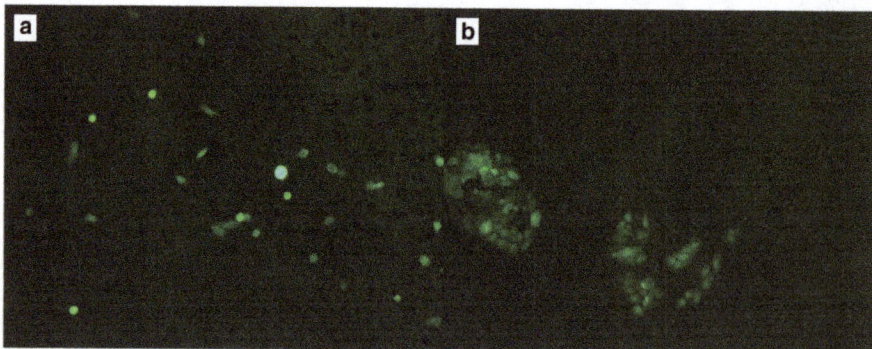

Fig. 5 Circulatory tumor cells. We seeded GFP labeled H1299 or H460 tumor cells on the cellular 4D lung model, collected CTC and plated in 96 well plates. Fluorescent microscopy shows CTC from H1299 (**a**) or H460 (**b**) attached to the plate and actively undergoing mitosis

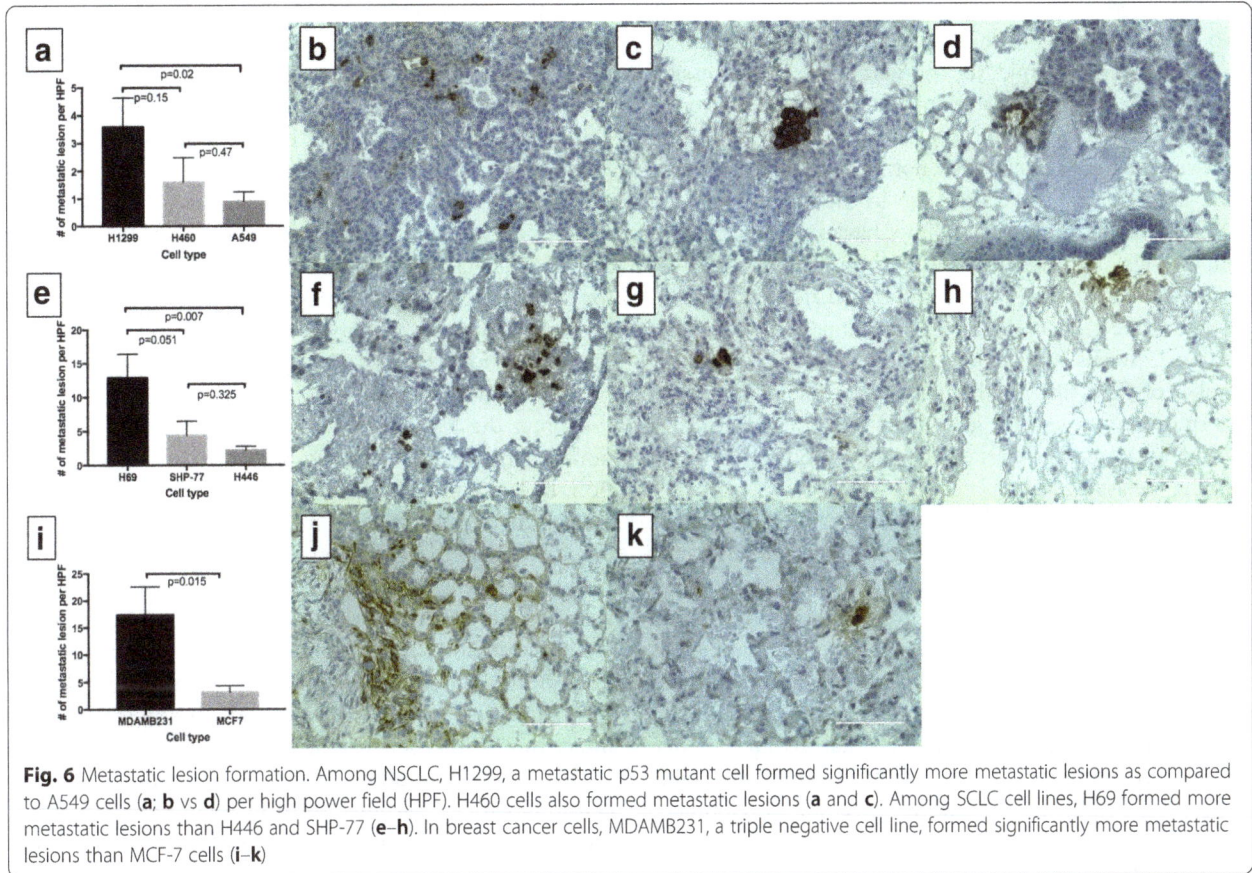

Fig. 6 Metastatic lesion formation. Among NSCLC, H1299, a metastatic p53 mutant cell formed significantly more metastatic lesions as compared to A549 cells (**a**; **b** vs **d**) per high power field (HPF). H460 cells also formed metastatic lesions (**a** and **c**). Among SCLC cell lines, H69 formed more metastatic lesions than H446 and SHP-77 (**e**–**h**). In breast cancer cells, MDAMB231, a triple negative cell line, formed significantly more metastatic lesions than MCF-7 cells (**i**–**k**)

cells per HPF and 2.2 ± 0.57 cells per HPF) (Fig. 6e–h). MDAMB231, a metastatic breast cancer cell line, formed more metastatic lesions than MCF7 cells (3.2 ± 1.15 cells per HPF vs. 17.4 ± 5.18 cells per HPF) (Fig. 6i–k).

Impact of cellular lung on tumor growth
Cellular lung significantly decreased cell growth on 2D of H1299 ($p = 0.01$, Fig. 7a), H460 ($p = 0.03$, Fig. 7b) and A549 ($p = 0.0002$, Fig. 7c) compared to control. In addition,

there was significantly lower number of tumor cells in the presence of cellular lung compared to acellular lung for H1299 ($p = 0.01$) and A549 ($p = 0.0009$). There were significantly less A549 cells with acellular lung compared to control ($p = 0.002$).

Discussion
Tumor models play an important role in understanding tumor progression, metastasis, and cancer therapeutics.

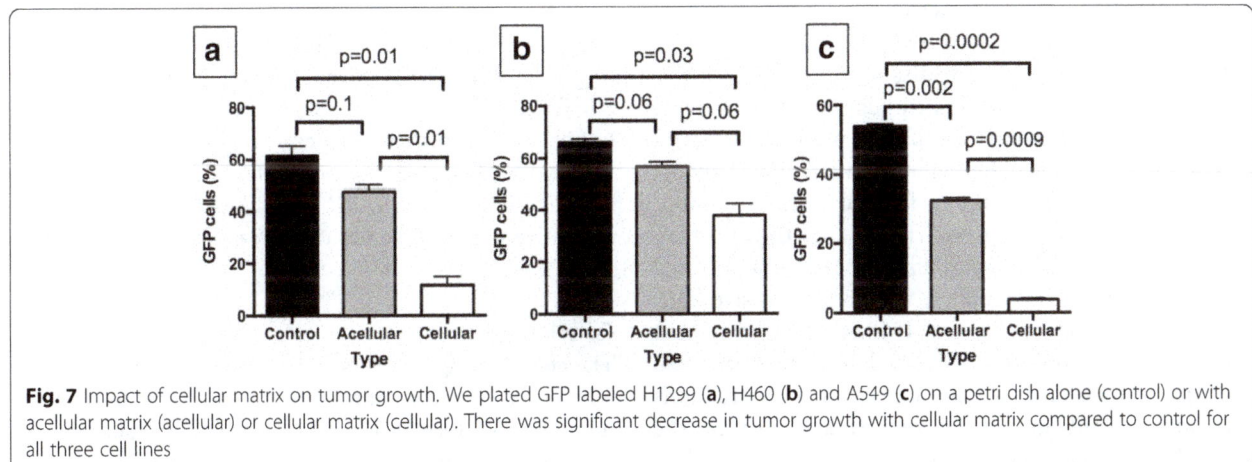

Fig. 7 Impact of cellular matrix on tumor growth. We plated GFP labeled H1299 (**a**), H460 (**b**) and A549 (**c**) on a petri dish alone (control) or with acellular matrix (acellular) or cellular matrix (cellular). There was significant decrease in tumor growth with cellular matrix compared to control for all three cell lines

To date, there are several 2D/3D in vitro, in vivo and ex vivo cancer models in use, but each one has considerable shortcomings to mimic the human cancer progression [11, 12]. We previously developed an acellular ex vivo 4D lung model for cancer metastasis [2]. The model's main criticism was that it lacked the normal lung tissue component, and thus the metastasis seen in the acellular ex vivo 4D model could be an artifact of not having cellular components. Thus, we pursued the creation of the cellular model (Additional file 1). We discovered that like the acellular model, the cellular 4D model can mimic tumor progression in 2 weeks and allows for the isolation of a high number of CTC that are the main driver for metastasis. In this study, we successfully grew both NSCLC and SCLC as well as breast cancer cells in the model with all of them forming metastatic lesions.

The cellular lung matrix model is a complex system that supports the growth of human tumor cells in a natural lung microenvironment. The cellular 4D lung model could provide a better model for cancer studies than existing 3D/2D and acellular lung models due to improved cell-cell interactions, cell-ECM interactions and presence of cell populations and a structure that resembles the in vivo environment. Similar to the acellular 4D lung model, the control native lung (devoid of tumor cells) maintains its matrix architecture and leads to tumor development with nutrient perfusion through the vasculature. The major difference lies in the presence of lung cellular components, which the acellular 4D lung model lacks. In both the acellular and cellular model, the tumor grows in an airway centric fashion due to seeding tumor cells through the trachea. Most of the NSCLC tumor cells showed similar histology and tumor cell morphology in the acellular and cellular lung model. The main difference between the cellular and acellular model was the primary tumor volume. We often visualized gross tumor nodules in the acellular model after 2 days while they were not readily visible on the cellular model. Furthermore, on pathologic examination, the nodules were much smaller in the cellular model than the acellular model. We also observed this difference when tumor cells were co-cultured with cellular lung on a petri dish (2D). Several possibilities might account for this difference. One issue is the limited nutrients for the cancer cells in the cellular model. We placed a similar amount of complete media in the cellular and acellular model but the cellular model has a normal cellular component that leaves fewer nutrients for the primary tumor cells. Another possibility is that the normal lung environment may play a tumor suppressive role. We have shown that normal lung fibroblasts can inhibit tumor progression [10]. Thus, it is possible that cancer coordinates with intercellular interactions that are present in normal tissues and disrupt the normalizing cues from the microenvironment, and in turn, the microenvironment evolves to accommodate the growing tumor [13–15].

Compared to the isolation of CTC from in vivo models [16], the process of isolating the CTC is simpler with the ability to tag tumor cells with GFP and sort them with FACS analysis. The GFP-tagged CTC were viable when they were placed on a petri dish similar to the CTC isolated from the acellular model. Moreover, like cells isolated in the acellular model, the CTC were in the supernatant for several days prior to attaching to the petri dish and showed a different phenotype than the parental cells. This feature supports the concept that these cells are a unique phase of tumor development.

Among the NSCLC, the presence of the cellular component impacts the efficacy of metastatic lesion formation. In the acellular model, despite forming fewer CTC, H460 cells tended to form more metastatic lesions compared to H1299 [2] but in the cellular model, there were more metastasis with H1299 compared to H460. In both models, the A549 cells have the least amount of metastatic lesion formation. This deviating behavior may be due to the difference in kinetics of metastatic tumor formation between the models with the presence of an intact tumor microenvironment.

This model also allows for the rapid growth of small cell lung cancer cell lines to form nodules and eventual metastasis. Most of these SCLC cell lines grow slowly and float (less adherent) in vitro which makes them difficult to study [17]. For most in vitro studies, these cells have to be grown in suspension, which does not mimic the growth in patients with small cell lung cancer. When we placed these cells in our model, they formed a primary tumor, CTC and metastatic lesions within 10–14 days. This rapid growth and tumor progression can provide a much-needed new model in understanding the biology of small cell lung cancer.

Furthermore, we were able to show growth of breast cancer cell lines in this model. Breast cancer is the most common cancer in women and the lung is one of the sites of metastasis. We have successfully grown breast cancer cell lines in the acellular model [18] and now we have been able to grow them in the cellular model. Like the NSCLC and SCLC cell lines, the breast cancer cell lines form a primary tumor and metastatic lesions. The MDAMB231, triple negative cell line showed more metastatic cells in contralateral lung lobes than MCF7 cells. This correlates with the aggressiveness of triple negative breast cancer compared to ER + PR+ breast cancer in patients.

Conclusion

The cellular lung model is an advanced cancer model that mimics the crucial phases of tumor growth—primary tumor, CTC formation and metastatic lesions—in the presence of normal lung tissue. This supports the concept that the natural matrix scaffold is the only component necessary to mimic metastasis and that cellular components modulate the process of metastasis. This ex vivo model can be used to study the complex mechanism of tumor metastasis.

Abbreviations
3D: Three dimensional; 4D: Four dimensional; ATCC: American Type Culture Collection; CTC: Circulating tumor cells; Ex vivo: Out of the living; GFP: Green fluorescent protein; H&E: Haematoxylin and eosin; IACUC: Institutional animal care and use committee; IHC: Immunohistochemistry; ITGB4: Integrin subunit beta 4; IU: International unit; mg: Milligram; mL: Milliliter; NSCLC: Non-small cell lung cancer; PBS: Phosphate-buffered saline; SCLC: Small cell lung cancer

Acknowledgements
We thank Anna Saikin for editing the language of the manuscript.

Funding
Dr. Kim received grant support from the Second John W. Kirklin Research Scholarship, American Association for Thoracic Surgery, Graham Research Foundation, Houston Methodist Specialty Physician Group Grant and Michael M. and Joann H. Cone Research Award. The funding body had no role in the design of the study and collection, analysis, and interpretation of data and in writing the manuscript.

Authors' contributions
DKM, RM, KAP, MPK made substantial contributions to conception and design, or acquisition of data, or analysis and interpretation of data; DKM, RM, KAP, MPK has been involved in drafting the manuscript or revising it critically for important intellectual content; DKM, RM, KAP, MPK has given final approval of the version to be published. Each author should have participated sufficiently in the work to take public responsibility for appropriate portions of the content; and DKM, RM, KAP, MPK agreed to be accountable for all aspects of the work in ensuring that questions related to the accuracy or integrity of any part of the work are appropriately investigated and resolved. DKM, RM, KAP, MPK read and approved the final manuscript.

Competing interests
The authors declare that they have no competing interests in relation to this work.

Author details
[1]Department of Surgery, Houston Methodist Hospital Research Institute, Houston, TX, USA. [2]Department of Pathology and Genomic Medicine, Houston Methodist Hospital, Houston, TX, USA. [3]Division of Thoracic Surgery, Department of Surgery, Weill Cornell Medical College, Houston Methodist Hospital, 6550 Fannin Street, Suite 1661, Houston, TX 77030, USA.

References
1. Siegel R, Naishadham D, Jemal A. Cancer statistics, 2013. CA Cancer J Clin. 2013;63(1):11–30.
2. Mishra DK, Creighton CJ, Zhang Y, Chen F, Thrall MJ, Kim MP. Ex vivo four-dimensional lung cancer model mimics metastasis. Ann Thorac Surg. 2015; 99(4):1149–56.
3. Ott HC, Clippinger B, Conrad C, Schuetz C, Pomerantseva I, Ikonomou L, Kotton D, Vacanti JP. Regeneration and orthotopic transplantation of a bioartificial lung. Nat Med. 2010;16(8):927–33.
4. Petersen TH, Calle EA, Colehour MB, Niklason LE. Matrix composition and mechanics of Decellularized lung scaffolds. Cells Tissues Organs. 2012;195(3): 222–31.
5. Kuttan R, Spall RD, Duhamel RC, Sipes IG, Meezan E, Brendel K. Preparation and composition of alveolar extracellular matrix and incorporated basement membrane. Lung. 1981;159(6):333–45.
6. Mishra DK, Thrall MJ, Baird BN, Ott HC, Blackmon SH, Kurie JM, Kim MP. Human lung cancer cells grown on acellular rat lung matrix create perfusable tumor nodules. Ann Thorac Surg. 2012;93(4):1075–81.
7. Mishra DK, Sakamoto JH, Thrall MJ, Baird BN, Blackmon SH, Ferrari M, Kurie JM, Kim MP. Human lung cancer cells grown in an ex vivo 3D lung model produce matrix metalloproteinases not produced in 2D culture. PLoS One. 2012;7(9):e45308.
8. Mishra DK, Scott KL, Wardwell-Ozgo JM, Thrall MJ, Kim MP. Circulating tumor cells from 4D model have less integrin beta 4 expression. J Surg Res. 2015;193(2):745–53.
9. Vishnoi M, Mishra DK, Thrall MJ, Kurie JM, Kim MP. Circulating tumor cells from a 4-dimensional lung cancer model are resistant to cisplatin. J Thorac Cardiovasc Surg. 2014;148(3):1056–63. discussion 1063-4
10. Mishra DK, Compean SD, Thrall MJ, Liu X, Massarelli E, Kurie JM, Kim MP. Human lung fibroblasts inhibit non-small cell lung Cancer metastasis in ex vivo 4D model. Ann Thorac Surg. 2015;100(4):1167–74. discussion 1174
11. Yang S, Zhang JJ, Huang XY. Mouse models for tumor metastasis. Methods Mol Biol. 2012;928:221–8.
12. McClatchey AI. Modeling metastasis in the mouse. Oncogene. 1999;18(38): 5334–9.
13. Bissell MJ, Hines WC. Why don't we get more cancer? A proposed role of the microenvironment in restraining cancer progression. Nat Med. 2011;17(3):320
14. Egeblad M, Nakasone ES, Werb Z. Tumors as organs: complex tissues that interface with the entire organism. Dev Cell. 2010;18(6):884–901.
15. Joyce JA, Pollard JW. Microenvironmental regulation of metastasis. Nat Rev Cancer. 2009;9(4):239–52.
16. Francia G, Cruz-Munoz W, Man S, Xu P, Kerbel RS. Mouse models of advanced spontaneous metastasis for experimental therapeutics. Nat Rev Cancer. 2011;11(2):135–41.
17. Yuan J, Knorr J, Altmannsberger M, Goeckenjan G, Ahr A, Scharl A, Strebhardt K. Expression of p16 and lack of pRB in primary small cell lung cancer. J Pathol. 1999;189(3):358–62.
18. Pence KA, Mishra DK, Thrall M, Dave B, Kim MP. Breast cancer cells form primary tumors on ex vivo four-dimensional lung model. J Surg Res. 2017; 210:181-187.

3

Effective osimertinib treatment in a patient with discordant T790 M mutation detection between liquid biopsy and tissue biopsy

Isa Mambetsariev[1], Lalit Vora[2], Kim Wai Yu[3] and Ravi Salgia[1*] (iD)

Abstract

Background: We report the successful treatment of the patient with osimertinib 80 mg/day following disease progression and a discordance in the detection of a mechanism of resistance epithelial growth factor receptor (EGFR) T790 M between liquid biopsy and tissue biopsy methods.

Case presentation: A 57-year-old Hispanic male patient initially diagnosed with an EGFR 19 deletion positive lung adenocarcinoma and clinically responded to initial erlotinib treatment. The patient subsequently progressed on erlotinib 150 mg/day and repeat biopsies both tissue and liquid were sent for next-generation sequencing (NGS). A T790 M EGFR mutation was detected in the blood sample using a liquid biopsy technique, but the tissue biopsy failed to show a T790 M mutation in a newly biopsied tissue sample. He was then successfully treated with osimertinib 80 mg/day, has clinically and radiologically responded, and remains on osimertinib treatment after 10 months.

Conclusions: Second-line osimertinib treatment, when administered at 80 mg/day, is both well tolerated and efficacious in a patient with previously erlotinib treated lung adenocarcinoma and a T790 M mutation detected by liquid biopsy.

Keywords: EGFR T790 M-positive NSCLC, Osimertinib, Progression, Liquid biopsy, Dose, Case report

Background

Non-Small Cell Lung Cancer (NSCLC) is a devastating disease and is the leading cause of cancer-related death worldwide. However, the treatment options for NSCLC have evolved dramatically in the last decade and NSCLC has become instrumental in advancing the new age of personalized medicine where standard platinum doublet chemotherapy is substituted by tyrosine kinase inhibitors (TKIs) when patients are tested and diagnosed with actionable mutations. The specificity of the disease and the histological differences in individual cancer types, such as lung adenocarcinoma, no longer dictate the clinical outcome and potential treatment options, but it is really the omic-architecture of individual patients that becomes the driver of treatment for targeted therapy as

well as immunotherapy. The genomic layout of adenocarcinomas is continuously being redefined with a myriad of genetic alterations, such as mutations in EGFR, MET, and BRAF, translocations in ALK and ROS1, detected and present in the TCGA dataset [1]. For example, approximately 10% of patients with NSCLC in the US have tumor involving the epidermal growth factor receptor (EGFR) somatic activating mutations [2]. Exon 19 deletion mutations and single-point substitution mutation L858R in exon 21 are considered "classic" mutations that are sensitive to EGFR TKIs and account for 90% of all EGFR mutations in NSCLC [3, 4]. The presence of these mutations in select NSCLC patients showed dramatic TKI response rates (RRs) of 68% with a mean progression-free survival (PFS) and time to progression of 12 months [5–7].

Based on this evidence, EGFR testing and EGFR TKIs have become a staple of lung cancer clinical treatment and since then the College of American Pathologists, International Association for the Study of Lung Cancer,

* Correspondence: rsalgia@coh.org
[1]Department of Medical Oncology and Therapeutics Research, City of Hope Comprehensive Cancer Center and Beckman Research Institute, 1500 E Duarte Rd, Duarte, CA 91010-3000, USA
Full list of author information is available at the end of the article

and the Association for Molecular Pathology have standardized the testing guidelines for selection of lung cancer patients for EGFR inhibitors as well as the methods of testing, such as real-time polymerase chain reaction (PCR) and next-generation sequencing (NGS) [8]. Nevertheless, almost all patients who initially respond to EGFR inhibitors in NSCLC eventually develop acquired resistance (AR). So far, it is known that a secondary T790 M mutation in exon 20 of the EGFR gene accounts for approximately 50% of cases of AR, alongside other less understood mechanisms of resistance [9]. The FDA has recently approved Osimertinib for the treatment of patients with metastatic T790 M mutation-positive non-small cell lung cancer (NSCLC) based on the evidence of the AURA3 trial where progression-free survival benefit was observed in both progressive NSCLC following first-line EGFR TKI therapy and EGFR T790 M mutation-positive NSCLC identified by the cobas EGFR mutation test [10, 11]. A recent study on the detection of T790 M by Tumor Biopsy versus Noninvasive Blood-based methods showed that the overall T790 M mutation positive rate was approximately 50% consistent with previous biopsy series [12]. In this case report, we present a male patient diagnosed with EGFR positive lung adenocarcinoma that partially responded to erlotinib, but eventually progressed. Upon progression the patient's blood and tissue samples were tested using NGS. The tissue biopsy test failed to detect a T790 M mutation, while the liquid biopsy test successfully showed a T790 M resistance mutation present in the patient's blood. The patient was treated with osimertinib with notable clinical and radiological response. The patient continues to be treated successfully with osimertinib and will remain on osimertinib treatment after 6 months.

Case presentation

A 57 year old Hispanic male who smoked for one year initially presented with lower back pain that eventually progressed to increasing upper back pain. An orthopedic surgeon performed an MRI scan which revealed multiple metastases to the thoracic spine. An initial CT scan revealed a right lung mass and a subsequent bronchoscopy revealed a non-small cell lung cancer consistent with poorly differentiated adenocarcinoma. For first line therapy, he received one cycle of carboplatin and docetaxel which was tolerated well with only mild nausea. He completed four cycles of chemotherapy and a pathology report identified an EGFR exon 19 deletion. The patient started on erlotinib, an EGFR inhibitor, at 150 mg capsule per day taken by mouth without food or on an empty stomach 1 h before or 2 h after food. Patient was also advised to avoid sunlight while on therapy due to skin toxicity. He tolerated it well and had clinically responsive disease as well as a decrease in primary mass from 5 cm to 2.8 cm on CT

scan for over a year until he had started developing worsening back pain and complications caused by papulopustular lesions as well as paronychia and xerosis. He also developed a Klebsiella folliculitis which necessitated discontinuation of the trimethoprim-sulfamethoxazole that he had been taking for the acneiform lesions and a brief course of ciprofloxacin that had led to the resolution of the papulopustular eruption.

He also started to have persistent elevation of carcinoembryonic antigen (CEA) level from 5.4 ng/ml rising steadily to 13.4 ng/ml and eventually rising exponentially to 24.3 ng/ml but continued on erlotinib, dose reduced to 100 mg one capsule per day, due to stable MRI scans. Patient was evaluated for a possible surgery on the spine but was unfortunately not a surgical candidate. A CT of the chest with and without contrast reported significant primary site progression of bilateral varying size small lung nodular lesions, consistent with metastatic. The right infrahilar nodular mass also increased from 2.1 × 1.5 cm to 2.8 × 2.4 cm. Clinically he was progressing and he underwent a fine needle biopsy on the right lung mass and pathology reported moderately differentiated metastatic adenocarcinoma. Tissue was sent for molecular testing via next generation sequencing with CLIA-certified Foundation Medicine multi-gene assay and a blood draw was performed for liquid biopsy utilizing the Guardant 360 platform, which are both comparable to the cobas EGFR tissue test and plasma ctDNA test in the AURA3 trial. While awaiting the results, erlotinib was stopped and he was given one cycle of carboplatin AUC 5 and pemetrexed 500 mg/m2. Soon afterward liquid biopsy report returned and was shown to be positive for a T790 M mutation that is a mechanism of acquired resistance to EGFR tyrosine kinase inhibitor (TKI) therapy. Liquid biopsy utilizing the Guardant 360 platform also detected ten other mutations; EGFR exon 19 deletion, TP53 R196Q mutation, FGFR3 L406R mutation, VHL S65A mutation, RHOA E47K mutation, APC D1512N mutation, NTRK1 T360 T mutation, PDGFRA I497I mutation, FGFR2 E767K mutation, BRCA1 E962K mutation.

Based on the T790 M mutation he was started on osimertinib, at 80 mg tablet per day taken by mouth, and tolerated it well. A few weeks into the osimertinib treatment the tissue biopsy test reported five mutations, CDK4 amplification, MDM2 amplification, FRS2 amplification, GLI1 amplification as well as the EGFR exon 19 deletion and nine variants of unknown significance; EP300 M2372 V, GNAS P345R and P349_I357del, IRF4 A341V, MED12 Q2120_Q2121 > HQQQQQ, MET D1373H, MLL A53V, SMARCA4 A1186_Q1187del, SOX9 A481T, SPTA1 R1077C. However, tissue biopsy test did not detect a T790 M mutation showing discordance between the tissue biopsy and the liquid biopsy. He continued on osimertinib treatment and a Chest CT (Fig. 1) scan ten months into the

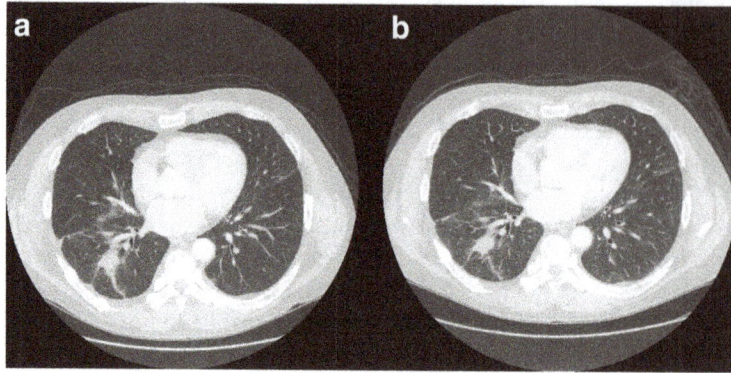

Fig. 1 Chest CT Scans of Patient on Osimertinib Treatment. **a** Chest CT Scan Prior to Osimertinib Treatment. **b** CT Chest w/Abdomen wwo/Pelvis w Contrast Scan Post-Osimertinib Treatment

treatment showed a decrease in the right lower lobe mass and numerous bilateral pulmonary nodules had either significant decrease or resolved. There were also stable widespread osseous metastases. This was noted to be a partial response and it was decided that the patient will continue on osimertinib. He has tolerated osimertinib well with only symptoms of a mild rash and low platelets which quickly stabilized without dose adjustment.

Discussion and conclusions

In this study, the treatment plan for the patient could have been potentially undermined by the NGS technology and lack of standardization of detection methods for EGFR mechanisms of resistance. This shows that tumor heterogeneity plays an important role not only therapeutically but is reliant on clinical efficacy to do what is beneficial for the patient based on the evidence of a blood-based T790 M detection. Our case report reflects not only a molecular switch within the tumor, but also highlights the discordance in one sample and not the other. As can be appreciated, the patient initially had L858R EGFR abnormality and responded to erlotinib. However, upon clinical and radiological progression, the tumor biopsy of the lung lesion still showed the original L858R EGFR abnormality, but did not detect the classic T790 M mutation of acquired resistance. Interestingly, the liquid biopsy revealed the classic T790 M EGFR mutation along with the original EGFR mutation. The

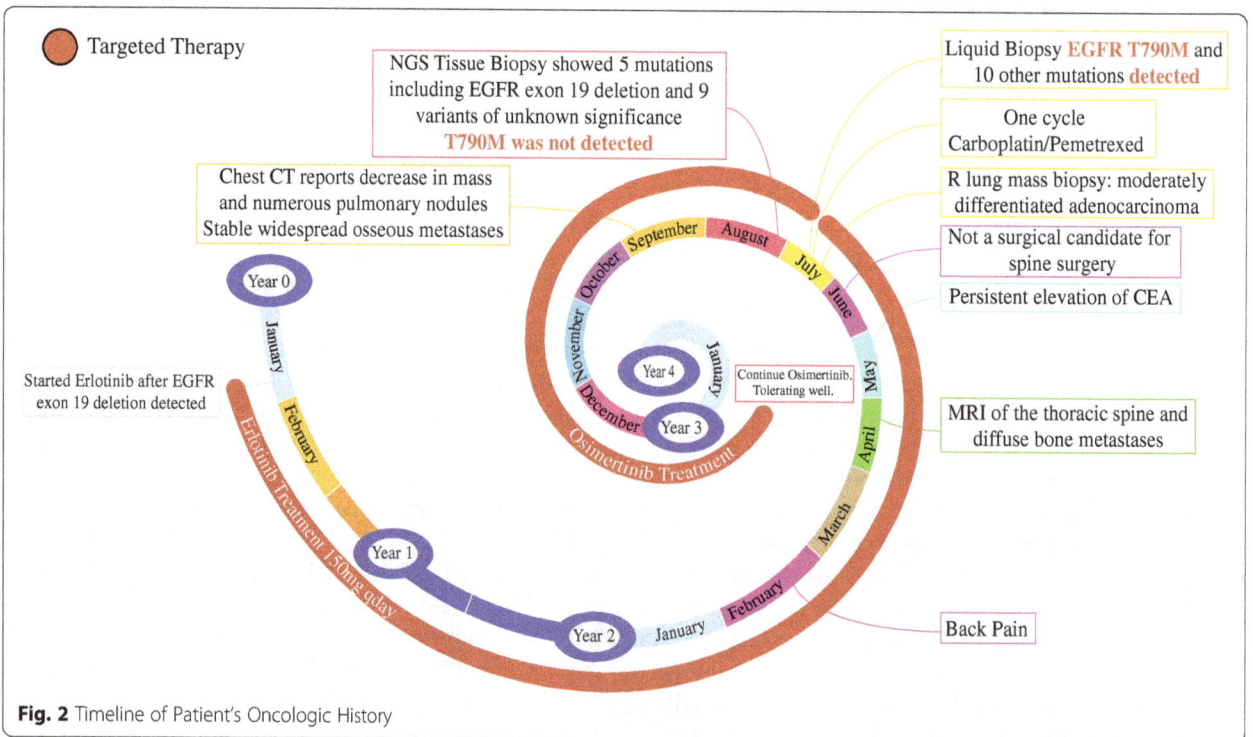

Fig. 2 Timeline of Patient's Oncologic History

absence of a T790 M mutation in tumor tissue may be explained by the limited tissue available from the lung as well as inter- and intra-tumor heterogeneity where the tissue biopsy does not give a full viewpoint of the entire tumor or the genetic heterogeneity of metastatic disease. Meanwhile the detection of a T790 M mutation in the liquid biopsy may be due to the nature of metastatic disease and the diverse circulating tumor DNA population that represents the overall mixed heterogeneity of the disease rather than limited to a small tissue sample from a single site. Based on this, we were able to make intelligent clinical decision to start osimertinib and the patient is responding (thus far, up to 10 months and continuing). Figure 2 summarizes the patient's oncologic history as a timeline.

In the past, we had poorly utilized biomarkers such as CEA and CA125 to determine the response or progression to therapy [13]. More recently, we have begun to determine the role of tumor tissue genomic biomarkers and circulating biomarkers. The molecular diagnostic field has come far over the past few years and the advent of liquid biopsies offers an opportunity to circumvent invasive tissue biopsies at the time of each disease progression. Liquid biopsies offer flexibility and repeatability for the patient that tissue biopsies do not due to high costs, high morbidity, or lack of available tissue. Though the list of currently available approved targeted therapies remains limited, only recently the FDA granted accelerated approval to the EGFR TKI osimertinib for patients with advances T790 M mutation-positive NSCLC based on the evidence of two-single arm studies with RRs between 57–61% [14, 15]. Consequently, in a recent study, we showed that NSCLC patient assessment of targeted therapies using commercially available ctDNA assays had a high concordance of 80% between paired tissue and blood for truncal oncogenic drivers and patients with biomarkers identified in plasma had expected progression free-survival (PFS) [16]. Though there may be no difference in progression-free survival between the liquid-positive and tissue-positive groups, there is still a necessity to consider this as a novel molecular diagnostic tool that requires less intervention and can possibly in the future be widely used to treat tumor heterogeneity over time in advanced stage NSCLC [17]. Therefore, we would recommend that analysis of biomarkers be routinely considered in mechanisms of resistance as well in the initial molecular diagnosis of advanced stage adenocarcinoma of the lung [17]. This case reflects the discordance between tissue and liquid biopsy. As we go forward in decision making, we might have to utilize both diagnostics to arrive at a meaningful clinical decision.

Abbreviations
AR: Acquired resistance; CEA: Carcinoembryonic antigen; CT: Computed tomography; ctDNA: Circulating tumor DNA; EGFR: Epithelial growth factor receptor; MRI: Magnetic resonance imaging; NGS: Next-generation sequencing; NSCLC: Non-small cell lung cancer; PCR: Polymerase chain reaction; PFS: Progression free survival; RR: Response rate; TKI: Tyrosine kinase inhibitor

Acknowledgements
We thank the nursing staff of City of Hope Comprehensive Cancer Center, for their skill and dedication in helping the patient presented in this case report.

Funding
We declare that there has been no funding for this project.

Authors' contributions
IM, LV, KWY and RS participated in patient care, reviewed the literature, prepared the figures, helped to draft and read and approved the final manuscript.

Competing interests
The authors declare that they have no competing interests.

Author details
[1]Department of Medical Oncology and Therapeutics Research, City of Hope Comprehensive Cancer Center and Beckman Research Institute, 1500 E Duarte Rd, Duarte, CA 91010-3000, USA. [2]Department of Diagnostic Radiology, City of Hope Comprehensive Cancer Center and Beckman Research Institute, Duarte, CA 91010, USA. [3]Department of Pharmacy Services, City of Hope Comprehensive Cancer Center and Beckman Research Institute, Duarte, CA 91010, USA.

References
1. Cancer Genome Atlas Research N. Comprehensive molecular profiling of lung adenocarcinoma. Nature. 2014;511(7511):543–50. https://doi.org/10.1038/nature13385. PubMed PMID: 25079552; PMCID: 4231481
2. Lynch TJ, Bell DW, Sordella R, Gurubhagavatula S, Okimoto RA, Brannigan BW, Harris PL, Haserlat SM, Supko JG, Haluska FG, Louis DN, Christiani DC, Settleman J, Haber DA. Activating mutations in the epidermal growth factor receptor underlying responsiveness of non-small-cell lung cancer to gefitinib. N Engl J Med. 2004;350(21):2129–39. https://doi.org/10.1056/NEJMoa040938. PubMed PMID: 15118073
3. Gazdar AF. Activating and resistance mutations of EGFR in non-small-cell lung cancer: role in clinical response to EGFR tyrosine kinase inhibitors. Oncogene. 2009;28(Suppl 1):S24–31. https://doi.org/10.1038/onc.2009.198. PubMed PMID: 19680293; PMCID: 2849651
4. Ladanyi M, Pao W. Lung adenocarcinoma: guiding EGFR-targeted therapy and beyond. Mod Pathol. 2008;21(Suppl 2):S16–22. https://doi.org/10.1038/modpathol.3801018. PubMed PMID: 18437168
5. Shepherd FA, Rodrigues Pereira J, Ciuleanu T, Tan EH, Hirsh V, Thongprasert S, Campos D, Maoleekoonpiroj S, Smylie M, Martins R, van Kooten M, Dediu M, Findlay B, Tu D, Johnston D, Bezjak A, Clark G, Santabarbara P, Seymour L, National Cancer Institute of Canada Clinical Trials G. Erlotinib in previously treated non-small-cell lung cancer. N Engl J Med. 2005;353(2):123–32. https://doi.org/10.1056/NEJMoa050753. PubMed PMID: 16014882
6. Stinchcombe TE, Socinski MA. Gefitinib in advanced non-small cell lung cancer: does it deserve a second chance? Oncologist. 2008;13(9):933–44. https://doi.org/10.1634/theoncologist.2008-0019. PubMed PMID: 18784157
7. Thatcher N, Chang A, Parikh P, Rodrigues Pereira J, Ciuleanu T, von Pawel J, Thongprasert S, Tan EH, Pemberton K, Archer V, Carroll K. Gefitinib plus best supportive care in previously treated patients with refractory advanced non-small-cell lung cancer: results from a randomised, placebo-controlled, multicentre study (Iressa survival evaluation in lung Cancer). Lancet. 2005;366(9496):1527–37. https://doi.org/10.1016/S0140-6736(05)67625-8. PubMed PMID: 16257339
8. Lindeman NI, Cagle PT, Beasley MB, Chitale DA, Dacic S, Giaccone G, Jenkins RB, Kwiatkowski DJ, Saldivar JS, Squire J, Thunnissen E, Ladanyi M. Molecular testing guideline for selection of lung cancer patients for EGFR and ALK

tyrosine kinase inhibitors: guideline from the College of American Pathologists, International Association for the Study of Lung Cancer, and Association for Molecular Pathology. J Thorac Oncol. 2013;8(7):823–59. https://doi.org/10.1097/JTO.0b013e318290868f. PubMed PMID: 23552377; PMCID: 4159960

9.   Stewart EL, Tan SZ, Liu G, Tsao MS. Known and putative mechanisms of resistance to EGFR targeted therapies in NSCLC patients with EGFR mutations-a review. Translational lung cancer research. 2015;4(1):67–81. https://doi.org/10.3978/j.issn.2218-6751.2014.11.06. PubMed PMID: 25806347; PMCID: 4367712

10. Bland J, Altman D. Multiple significance tests: the Bonferroni method. BMJ. 1995;310:170.

11. Mok TS, Wu YL, Ahn MJ, Garassino MC, Kim HR, Ramalingam SS, Shepherd FA, He Y, Akamatsu H, Theelen WS, Lee CK, Sebastian M, Templeton A, Mann H, Marotti M, Ghiorghiu S, Papadimitrakopoulou VA, Investigators A. Osimertinib or platinum-Pemetrexed in EGFR T790M-positive lung Cancer. N Engl J Med. 2017;376(7):629–40. https://doi.org/10.1056/NEJMoa1612674. PubMed PMID: 27959700

12. Sundaresan TK, Sequist LV, Heymach JV, Riely GJ, Janne PA, Koch WH, Sullivan JP, Fox DB, Maher R, Muzikansky A, Webb A, Tran HT, Giri U, Fleisher M, Yu HA, Wei W, Johnson BE, Barber TA, Walsh JR, Engelman JA, Stott SL, Kapur R, Maheswaran S, Toner M, Haber DA. Detection of T790M, the acquired resistance EGFR mutation, by tumor biopsy versus noninvasive blood-based analyses. Clin Cancer Res. 2016;22(5):1103–10. https://doi.org/10.1158/1078-0432.CCR-15-1031. PubMed PMID: 26446944; PMCID: 4775471

13. Rubin BP, Skarin AT, Pisick E, Rizk M, Salgia R. Use of cytokeratins 7 and 20 in determining the origin of metastatic carcinoma of unknown primary, with special emphasis on lung cancer. Eur J Cancer Prev. 2001;10(1):77–82. PubMed PMID: 11263595

14. Yang JC, Wu YL, Schuler M, Sebastian M, Popat S, Yamamoto N, Zhou C, Hu CP, O'Byrne K, Feng J, Lu S, Huang Y, Geater SL, Lee KY, Tsai CM, Gorbunova V, Hirsh V, Bennouna J, Orlov S, Mok T, Boyer M, Su WC, Lee KH, Kato T, Massey D, Shahidi M, Zazulina V, Sequist LV. Afatinib versus cisplatin-based chemotherapy for EGFR mutation-positive lung adenocarcinoma (LUX-lung 3 and LUX-lung 6): analysis of overall survival data from two randomised, phase 3 trials. The Lancet Oncology. 2015;16(2):141–51. https://doi.org/10.1016/S1470-2045(14)71173-8. PubMed PMID: 25589191

15. Yang J, Ramalingam SS, Janne PA, Cantarini M, Mitsudomi T. LBA2_PR: Osimertinib (AZD9291) in pre-treated pts with T790M-positive advanced NSCLC: updated phase 1 (P1) and pooled phase 2 (P2) results. J Thorac Oncol. 2016;11(4 Suppl):S152–3. https://doi.org/10.1016/S1556-0864(16)30325-2. PubMed PMID: 27198353

16. Villaflor V, Won B, Nagy R, Banks K, Lanman RB, Talasaz A, Salgia R. Biopsy-free circulating tumor DNA assay identifies actionable mutations in lung cancer. Oncotarget. 2016;7(41):66880–91. https://doi.org/10.18632/oncotarget.11801. PubMed PMID: 27602770

17. Ito K, Suzuki Y, Saiki H, Sakaguchi T, Hayashi K, Nishii Y, Watanabe F, Hataji O. Utility of liquid biopsy by improved PNA-LNA PCR clamp method for detecting EGFR mutation at initial diagnosis of non-small-cell lung Cancer: observational study of 190 consecutive cases in clinical practice. Clinical lung cancer. 2018;19(2):181–90. https://doi.org/10.1016/j.cllc.2017.10.017. PubMed PMID: 29174086

4

Outcomes of Pemetrexed-based chemotherapies in *HER2*-mutant lung cancers

Yan Wang[1†], Shijia Zhang[1,3†], Fengying Wu[1], Jing Zhao[1], Xuefei Li[2], Chao Zhao[2], Shengxiang Ren[1*] and Caicun Zhou[1]

Abstract

Background: *HER2* mutation has been found to be an oncogenic driver gene in non-small cell lung cancers(NSCLC) and HER2-directed therapies have shown promising results in this unique population, while little is known about its association with outcomes of chemotherapy. The aim of this study was to investigate the efficacy of first line chemotherapy in patients with advanced *HER2*-mutant lung adenocarcinomas.

Methods: Patients with advanced NSCLC(N = 1714) initially underwent testing for *EGFR, KRAS, BRAF* mutations and *ALK, ROS1* rearrangements, and negative cases were then assessed for *HER2* mutations using the method of amplification refractory mutation system(ARMS). The efficacy of first line pemetrexed-based chemotherapy was investigated in patients with *HER2*-mutant and those with *EGFR*-mutant, *ALK/ROS1*-rearranged and *KRAS*-mutant advanced adenocarcinomas.

Results: *HER2* mutations were detected in 29 of 572(5.1%) specimens from a selected population of *EGFR/KRAS/BRAF/ALK/ROS1* negative patients. All of them are adenocarcinomas. Among patients with *HER2*-mutant lung cancers, 25 received pemetrexed-based first line chemotherapy. The objective response rate(ORR) was 36.0%. Their median progression free survival(PFS) was 5.1 months, which was similar with that of *KRAS*-mutant group (n = 40,5.0 months, p = 0.971), numerically shorter than that of *EGFR*-mutant group(n = 74, 6.5 months, p = 0.247) and statistically significantly shorter than that of *ALK/ROS1*-rearranged group (n = 39,9.2 months, p = 0.004). Furthermore, *HER2* variants subgroup analysis showed that PFS was inferior in A775_G776insYVMA group compared with other variants (4.2 vs 7.2 months, p = 0.085).

Conclusions: Patients with advanced *HER2*-mutant lung adenocarcinomas showed an inferior outcome of first line pemetrexed-based chemotherapy compared to those with *ALK/ROS1* rearrangements, which strengthen the need for effective HER2-targeted drugs in clinical practice.

Keywords: *HER2* mutation, Lung adenocarcinoma, Pemetrexed

Background

Human epidermal growth factor receptor2(*HER2*) positivity is well-studied in breast cancer, while much less defined in lung cancer. Although anti-HER2 monoclonal antibody such as trastuzumab has been proven effective in breast cancer and gastric cancer [1, 2], the clinical trials [3, 4] of lung cancer including patients treated with trastuzumab combined with chemotherapy failed to demonstrate benefit in survival in HER2 IHC positive patients. Besides that, pan-HER TKI dacomitinib also showed no response in patients with HER2 amplifications in a phase II trial [5].

Apart from HER2 over-expression and amplification, *HER2* gene mutation is a distinct entity in lung carcinogenesis with an incidence of 4.8% among *EGFR* wild-type lung adenocarcinoma resection samples [6]. Drugs that

* Correspondence: harry_ren@126.com
†Equal contributors
[1]Department of Medical Oncology, Shanghai Pulmonary Hospital, Tongji University School of Medicine, Tongji University Medical School Cancer Institute, No. 507 Zheng Min Road, Shanghai 200433, People's Republic of China
Full list of author information is available at the end of the article

target *HER2* gene mutations are currently being investigated. The National Comprehensive Cancer Network (NCCN) recommend trastuzumab or afatinib as potential therapy options for non-small cell lung cancers(NSCLC) patients with *HER2* mutations. Several phase I/II trials [5, 7–9] is now investigating the efficacy of other irreversible pan-HER receptor family inhibitors, such as dacomitinib, neratinib and pyrotinib. Currently, *HER2* mutation is emerging as a promising druggable target, while the optimal choice of targeted therapy remains poorly defined.

Chemotherapy is still the standard first-line regimen for patients with advanced NSCLC who are improper for targeted therapy. Among them, pemetrexed-based regimen has showed superior efficacy with less side effects and was recommended preferentially for patients with adenocarcinomas [10, 11]. *ALK/ROS1/RET* positive patients showed a superior progression free survival(PFS) after pemetrexed-based therapy than patients with *KRAS* mutations [12–16]. While the effects of *HER2* mutation on the outcomes of pemetrexed-based chemotherapy is still unknown in patients with advanced NSCLC.

Aim to investigate the efficacy of pemetrexed-based chemotherapy in patients with *HER2*-mutant lung adenocarcinomas, we conducted this retrospective study in Chinese patients with 1714 advanced NSCLC. In addition, we also observed the clinicopathologic and molecular features of *HER2* mutations in patients with advanced NSCLC.

Methods
Patients population
Patients with advanced NSCLC (stage IIIB/IV) and performed *EGFR, ALK, ROS1, BRAF* and *KRAS* testing at Shanghai Pulmonary Hospital, Tongji University School of Medicine, Shanghai, China from January 2015 to September 2016 were included into this study. *HER2* mutations testing were performed in all these 5 genes pan-negative patients. Their clinical data were collected including age, gender, smoking status, tumor histology, performance status (PS) and the outcomes of anti-cancer therapies. Patients with *HER2, EGFR* or *KRAS* mutation or *ALK* or *ROS1* rearrangement and received first-line pemetrexed-based chemotherapy (pemetrexed monotherapy or combination therapy with platinum) were eligible for analysis. A history of radiotherapy, first-line targeted therapy, or immune-directed therapy was exclusionary.

Molecular testing
HER2 mutation testing was performed using the method of amplification refractory mutation system(ARMS) by ADx HER2 Mutation Detection Kit (Amoy Diagnostics, Xiamen, China). Samples positive for *HER2* mutations were confirmed by DNA sequencing using primers with the following sequences: 5'GCC ATG GCT GTG GTT

TGT GAT AGG3' (forward) and 5'ATC CTA GCC CCT TGT GGA CAT AGG3', which amplified a 342-bp fragment in exon20 of the *HER2* gene. The details can be referred to our previous study [6].

Similarly, *EGFR, BRAF* and *KRAS* mutation were performed using EGFR, BRAF V600 and KRAS Mutations Detection Kit (Amoy Diagnostics, Xiamen, China) respectively by ARMS method. *ALK* and *ROS1* rearrangement testing were performed using AmoyDx EML4-ALK and ROS1 Fusions Detection Kit (Amoy Diagnostics, Xiamen, China) respectively by the method of reverse transcriptase polymerase chain reaction(RT-PCR). The details were described in our previous articles [13, 17–19].

Statistical analysis
Tumor response was evaluated every 2 cycles of chemotherapy according to response evaluation criteria in solid tumors (version 1.1). PFS was defined as the time interval from the first day of treatment to documented disease progression or death of any cause. All of the statistical tests were performed using the SPSS 19.0. Chi-square test or Fisher's exact test was used to examine the clinicopathologic association of HER2 mutations and response rate comparison. Age differences were compared using the t test for independent samples or the one-way analysis of variance. The Kaplan–Meier method was used to estimate the PFS and the log-rank test was used to analyze PFS between the different groups. Results were considered significantly different if the *p* value was less than 0.05 in a two-way analysis.

Results
Patients' characteristics
From January 2015 to September 2016, a total of 1714 patients with advanced NSCLC underwent testing for *EGFR, KRAS, BRAF, ALK* and *ROS1*.The results showed that there were 809 patients(47.2%) with *EGFR* mutations,149(7.8%) with *KRAS* mutations,19(1.1%) with *BRAF* mutations,106(6.2%) with *ALK* rearrangements, 43(2.5%) with *ROS1* rearrangements, and 16 patients (0. 9%) with multiple positive results. In addition, 572 pan-negative patients also have tested their *HER2* status by ARMS and 29 (29/572,5.1%) were identified as *HER2* mutation positive (Fig 1).

HER2-mutant lung cancer patients had a median age of 58 (range 44–77 years) and mutations were more common in females (p<0.001),non-smokers (*p* = 0.034) and adenocarcinomas (*p* = 0.002)(Table 1). Twenty-four of 29 patients had available samples for sequencing and had the details variants of *HER2* mutation including 14 with exon20 A775_G776insYVMA, 3with P780_Y781insGSP, 3with G776 > VC, 2with G776 > IC, 1with G776 > LC, and 1with G776C (Additional file 1: Figure S1).

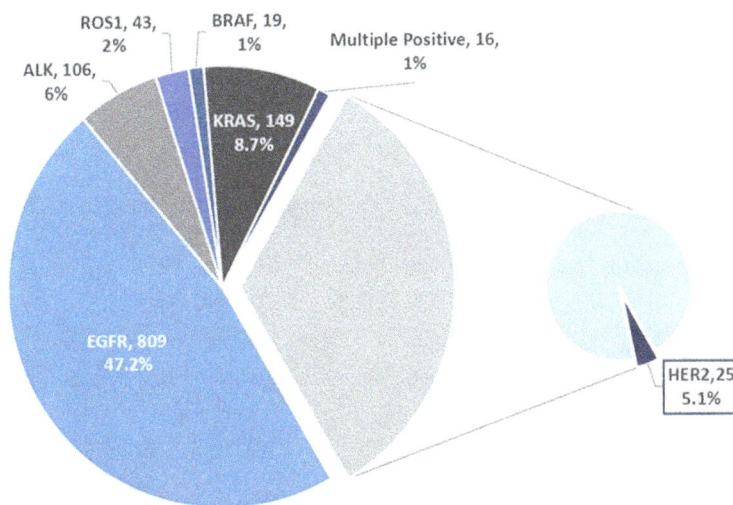

Fig. 1 Mutations-testing results of 1714 patients with advanced non-small cell lung cancers.(multiple positive results 7EGFR&ALK, 1EGFR&ROS1, 2EGFR&KRAS, 2EGFR&BRAF, 2ALK&KRAS, 1ROS1&KRAS, 1EGFR&ROS1&KRAS)

Outcomes of chemotherapy: Comparison among oncogenic mutations groups

Patients received first-line pemetrexed-based chemotherapy were eligible for analysis($n = 25$,14 combined with carboplatin, 7 combined with cisplatin and 4 monotherapy). Since most patients with druggable mutations chose TKI as a first-line treatment, only 74 of 809 *EGFR*-mutant patients and 39 of 149 *ALK/ROS1*-rearranged patients were included. While there were a relatively large number of patients with *KRAS* mutation, the first 40 of *KRAS* identified were selected for this study.

The baseline characteristics of patients with *HER2*-mutant were compared with patients with *EGFR*-mutant,

Table 1 Clinical characteristics of patients with HER2-mutant lung cancers

Clinical characteristics	Total ($n = 572$)	HER2 negative ($n = 543$)	HER2 positive ($n = 29$)	P value
Age, years (median,range)	64(27–92)	64(27–92)	58(44–77)	0.017
< 65	305(53.3%)	283(52.1%)	22(75.9%)	
≥ 65	267(46.7%)	260(47.9%)	7(24.1%)	
Gender				
Male	430(75.2%)	417(76.8%)	13(44.8%)	<0.001
Female	142(24.8%)	126(23.2%)	16(55.2%)	
Smoking status				
Non-smoker	305(53.3%)	284(52.3%)	21(72.4%)	0.034
Smoker	267(46.7%)	259(47.7%)	8(27.6%)	
Histology				
Adenocarcinoma	429(75%)	400(74.0%)	29(100%)	0.002
Non-Adenocarcinoma	143(25%)	117(21.3%)	0	

ALK/ROS1-rearranged, and *KRAS*-mutant lung cancers as summarized in Table 2. *HER2*, *EGFR*, *KRAS* mutations and *ALK*, *ROS1* rearrangements did not co-occur with each other in individual patient samples. *KRAS* mutations were more frequently detected in patients with more than 65 years old, male and smokers. And comparison revealed no significant differences in terms of PS score ($p = 0.269$), monotherapy versus combination therapy ($p = 0.570$), maintenance therapy versus non-maintenance therapy($p = 0.175$).

The response was evaluated in all 178 patients. Both the objective response rate(ORR) and the disease control rate (DCR) were not significantly different among four groups (Table 3). However, PFS was significantly different among all groups. Patients in the *HER2*-mutant group had a median PFS of 5.1 months (95% confidence interval [CI], 4.90–5.30) (95% CI 4.90–5.30), which was numerically shorter than that of the *EGFR*-mutant group (6.5 months, 95% CI 4.48–8.52, $p = 0.247$) and significantly shorter than that of the *ALK/ROS1*-rearranged (9.2 months, 95% CI 6.41–11.99, $p = 0.004$). Similarly, in *KRAS*-mutant lung cancers, PFS (5.0 months, 95% CI 3.67–6.33) was inferior compared with *EGFR*-mutant (6.5 months, $p = 0.242$) and *ALK/ROS1*-rearranged (9.2 months, $p = 0.007$) lung cancers. PFS was not significantly different between the *HER2*-mutant and the *KRAS*-mutant lung cancers groups (5.1 vs 5.0 months, $p = 0.971$) (Fig.2a).

Outcomes of chemotherapy: Comparison among HER2 variants subgroups

Twenty patients of the 25 patients receiving first-line pemetrexed-based chemotherapy had known HER2 variants (Additional file 1: Figure S1). According to the frequency of the variants, they were divided into the

Table 2 Baseline characteristics of patients treated with pemetrexed-containing chemotherapy

Clinical characteristics	HER2	EGFR	ALK/ROS1	KRAS	P value
N	25	74	39	40	
Age, years (median,range)	55(44–77)	58(27–80)	54(37–77)	64.5(33–80)	0.002
< 65	21(84.0%)	55(74.3%)	28(71.8%)	20(50.0%)	
≥ 65	4(16.0%)	19(25.7%)	11(28.2%)	20(50.0%)	
Gender					
Male	12(48.0%)	37(50.0%)	20(51.3%)	33(82.5%)	0.004
Female	13(52.0%)	37(50.0%)	19(48.7%)	7(17.5%)	
Smoking status					
Non-smoker	18(72.0%)	56(75.7%)	29(74.4%)	15(37.5%)	<0.001
Smoker	7(28.0%)	18(24.3%)	10(25.6%)	25(62.5%)	
PS					
0–1	22(88.0%)	68(91.9%)	36(92.3%)	32(80.0%)	0.269
≥ 2	3(12.0%)	6(8.1%)	3(7.7%%)	8(20.0%)	
Therapy					
Monotherapy	4(16.0%)	9(12.2%)	3(7.7%)	9(22.5%)	0.570
Plus carboplatin	14(56.0%)	42(56.8%)	24(61.5%)	23(57.5%)	
Plus cisplatin	7(28.0%)	23(31.1%)	12(30.8%)	8(20.0%)	
Maintenance therapy	7(28.0%)	18(24.3%)	13(33.3%)	5(12.5%)	0.175
No maintenance	18(72.0%)	56(75.7%)	26(66.7%)	35(87.5%)	

exon20 A775_G776insYVMA group ($n = 13$) and the other variants group ($n = 7$, 3with P780_Y781insGSP, 2with G776 > IC, 1with G776 > LC, and 1with G776C). PFS has a trend to be inferior in the YVMA group, even though no statistically significant difference existed between the 2 groups (4.2 vs 7.2 months, $p = 0.085$) (Fig 2b).

Discussion

As far as we know, this study is the first study to compare the efficacy of pemetrexed-based chemotherapy between *HER2*-mutant and groups of *EGFR*-mutant, *ALK/ROS1*-rearranged and *KRAS*-mutant lung adenocarcinoma. We found that patients with *HER2*-mutant lung cancers had a PFS of 5.1 months that was similar with *KRAS*-mutant (5.0 months, $p = 0.971$) lung cancers, and numerically shorter than *EGFR*-mutant (6.5 months, $p = 0.247$) and significantly shorter than *ALK/ROS1*-rearranged (9.2 months, $p = 0.004$) lung cancers, showing

Table 3 The objective response rate(ORR)and the disease control rate (DCR) of patients treated with pemetrexed-based therapy in four groups

	HER2	EGFR	ALK/ROS1	KRAS	P value
n	25	74	39	40	
ORR%	36.0	33.8	41.3	35.0	0.896
DCR%	92.0	78.4	87.2	72.5	0.139

that *HER2*-mutant lung cancer patients may have poor outcomes with chemotherapy, which strengthen the importance of developing HER2-targeted drugs in this population. We also investigate the clinicopathologic features in patients with advanced *HER2*-mutant lung adenocarcinomas and found that *HER2* mutations were more common in younger patients, females, non-smokers and adenocarcinomas.

Different from HER2 over-expression and amplification, *HER2* mutations was found to be a distinct entity in patients with NSCLC [20]. *HER2* mutations are found in about 1%–2% of NSCLC [20–22]. In this study, the incidence of *HER2* mutations was 5.1% in *EGFR/KRAS/BRAF/ALK/ROS1* negative patients, indicating that *HER2* mutations will be enriched in the population without other driver gene mutations. Consistent with our study, a study from the Memorial Sloan Kettering Cancer Center (MSKCC) group [23] showed that in a selected population with *EGFR/KRAS/ALK* negative, the incidence of *HER2* mutations can reach up to 6%. In the early stage resection samples, our previous study [6] showed that the presence of HER2 mutations was not correlated with gender, age, or smoking status. However, another retrospective study [24] of resection samples obtained at Fudan University Shanghai Cancer Center found that the incidence of HER2 mutations can reach up to 5.94% in non-smoking patients with lung adenocarcinoma. Similarly, in biopsied samples from advanced

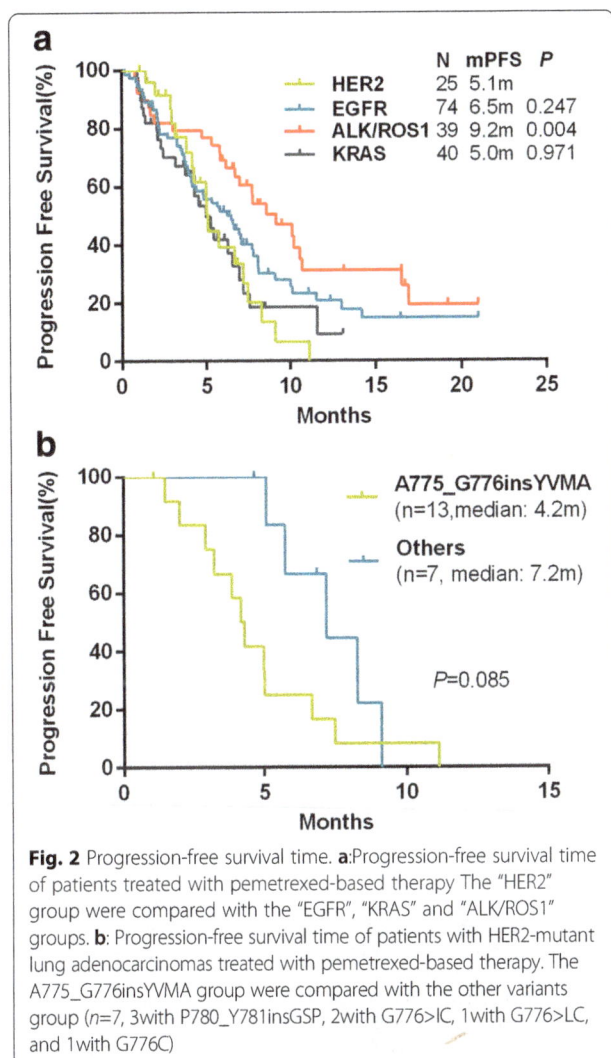

Fig. 2 Progression-free survival time. **a**:Progression-free survival time of patients treated with pemetrexed-based therapy The "HER2" group were compared with the "EGFR", "KRAS" and "ALK/ROS1" groups. **b**: Progression-free survival time of patients with HER2-mutant lung adenocarcinomas treated with pemetrexed-based therapy. The A775_G776insYVMA group were compared with the other variants group (n=7, 3with P780_Y781insGSP, 2with G776>IC, 1with G776>LC, and 1with G776C)

NSCLC, our study showed that *HER2* mutations were more common in non-smokers and lung adenocarcinomas. But *HER2* mutations were also frequently detected in younger patients and females in our study. Furthermore, exon20 A775_G776insYVMA was the most frequently alteration.

In the era of targeted therapy, several oncogenic driver mutations were found not only could predict the efficacy of targeted therapy, but also associated with superior outcome of first line pemetrexed chemotherapy, such as *ALK*, *ROS1* and *RET* [12–16]. Thus, we further investigate the association of *HER2* mutation with the efficacy of pemetrexed-based chemotherapy in patients with advanced lung adenocarcinomas. We found that patients with *HER2*-mutant lung cancers had a PFS of 5.1 months. Similar to this study, in the EUHER2 study [25] of patients with *HER2*-mutant lung cancers, ORR and PFS with chemotherapy were 43.5% and 6 months in first-line and 10% and 4.3 months in second-line therapies. Our study also showed that *HER2*-mutant lung

cancers had a similar PFS of pemetrexed-based chemotherapy with *KRAS*-mutant lung cancers (5.0 months), which was inferior compared with *EGFR*-mutant(6.5 months) and *ALK/ROS1*-rearranged (9.2 months), indicating that *HER2* mutation might predict a poor efficacy of pemetrexed-based chemotherapy, just like *KRAS* mutation. Although pemetrexed-based chemotherapy had the longest duration among chemotherapies(pemetrexed/taxane/gemcitabine/vinorelbine/etoposide±platinum) for patients with *HER2* mutations according to Eng et al's study [26] and Gow et al's study [27], outcomes of pemetrexed for *HER2* were poor compared to other oncogene subgroups,such as *ALK* and *ROS1*. Furthermore, we further divide *HER2* mutations into the exon20 A775_G776insYVMA group and the other variants group and it was the first time that we found that patients with YVMA insertion were associated with an inferior PFS (4.2 vs 7.2 months, $p = 0.085$).

Currently, NCCN guideline recommend trastuzumab and afatinib as the targeted therapeutic options for patients with advanced *HER2*-mutant NSCLC. While, in EUHER2 study [25], afatinib showed a modest response of 18.2% and median PFS of 3.9 months even though this drug has showed response in all 3 assessable patients with *HER2*-mutant adenocarcinoma in a preliminary study [28]. Meanwhile, several other studies [5, 7, 8] investigated the efficacy of other irreversible pan-HER receptor family inhibitors, dacomitinib, neratinib, or neratinib combining with mTOR inhibitors in advanced NSCLC patients harboring *HER2* mutations and showed a moderate response of 12%–21%. Although these ORR or PFS are much diminished compared with those of TKIs directed at other targets in NSCLC, HER2-targeted drugs is still promising. A phase II study recently investigated a novel EGFR/HER2 inhibitor, pyrotinib, in heavily pre-treated patients with *HER2*-mutant adenocarcinomas and found a promising results with RR of 54.5%(6/11) and median PFS of 6.2 months [9]. Large number cohort study is still needed to validate the efficacy of pyrotinib in this setting.

Our study does have several limitations. First, it was a retrospective study with limited patients number($n = 25$), while this study presented the real world nature in Chinese population. Second, *HER2* mutation testing was performed using the method of ARMS, thus some rare mutations might be missed in our population. Next generation sequencing (NGS), which allows for simultaneous testing for multiple mutations using one platform and one sample, is emerging as an important method for identification of gene mutations in NSCLC, but single-gene sequencing is still more widely used. Thirdly, a substantial part of the patients with *HER2* mutations also participant into the previous clinical trial of HER2-targeted drugs [9], thus the overall survival might be heavily influenced by the subsequent therapy.

Conclusions

In conclusion, *HER2* mutations were more frequent happened in younger patients, females, non-smokers and adenocarcinomas of advanced NSCLC. Patients with *HER2*-mutant lung adenocarcinomas, especially YVMA insertion, showed poor response to pemetrexed-based chemotherapy. Thus, developing HER2-targeted drugs to improve their poor prognosis is urgently needed for this population.

Abbreviations
ARMS: Amplification refractory mutation system; HER2: Human epidermal growth factor receptor2; NCCN: The National Comprehensive Cancer Network.; NSCLC: Non-small cell lung cancers; ORR: The objective response rate; PFS: Progression free survival; RT-PCR: Reverse transcriptase polymerase chain reaction

Acknowledgments
This study was supported in part by grants from projects of the Science and Technology Commission of Shanghai Municipality (No.16411964600), and Shanghai Municipal Education Commission (No.16SG18).

Funding
The funding body had no role in the design of the study and collection, analysis, and interpretation of data and in writing the manuscript

Authors' contributions
YW and SZ contributed equally in preparing and conducting this research. FW, JZ, XL and CZ provided the patient information and followed the patient survival data. SR and CZ designed and coordinated the research in the whole process. All authors read and approved the final manuscript.

Competing interests
No potential conflicts of interest were disclosed.

Author details
[1]Department of Medical Oncology, Shanghai Pulmonary Hospital, Tongji University School of Medicine, Tongji University Medical School Cancer Institute, No. 507 Zheng Min Road, Shanghai 200433, People's Republic of China. [2]Department of Lung Cancer and Immunology, Shanghai Pulmonary Hospital, Tongji University School of Medicine, Shanghai, People's Republic of China. [3]Department of Respiratory Medicine, Huaihe Hospital, Henan University, Kaifeng, People's Republic of China.

References
1. Plosker GL, Keam SJ. Spotlight on Trastuzumab in the management of HER2-positive metastatic and early-stage breast cancer. BioDrugs. 2006;20(4):259–62.
2. Bang YJ, Van Cutsem E, Feyereislova A, Chung HC, Shen L, Sawaki A, et al. Trastuzumab in combination with chemotherapy versus chemotherapy alone for treatment of HER2-positive advanced gastric or gastro-oesophageal junction cancer (ToGA): a phase 3, open-label, randomised controlled trial. Lancet. 2010;376:687–97.
3. Gatzemeier U, Groth G, Butts C, Van Zandwijk N, Shepherd F, Ardizzoni A, et al. Randomized phase II trial of gemcitabine-cisplatin with or without trastuzumab in HER2-positive non-small-cell lung cancer. Ann Oncol. 2004; 15:19–27.
4. Krug LM, Miller VA, Patel J, Crapanzano J, Azzoli CG, Gomez J, et al. Randomized phase II study of weekly docetaxel plus trastuzumab versus weekly paclitaxel plus trastuzumab in patients with previously untreated advanced nonsmall cell lung carcinoma. Cancer. 2005;104:2149–55.
5. Kris MG, Camidge DR, Giaccone G, Hida T, Li BT, O'Connell J, et al. Targeting HER2 aberrations as actionable drivers in lung cancers: phase II trial of the pan-HER tyrosine kinase inhibitor dacomitinib in patients with HER2-mutant or amplified tumors. Ann of Oncol. 2015;26:1421–7.
6. Li X, Zhao C, Su C, Ren S, Chen X, Zhou C. Epidemiological study of HER-2 mutations among EGFR wild-type lung adenocarcinoma patients in China. BMC Cancer. 2016;16:828.
7. Gandhi L, Bahleda R, Tolaney SM, Kwak EL, Cleary JM, Pandya SS, et al. I Phase study of neratinib in combination with temsirolimus in patients with human epidermal growth factor receptor 2-dependent and other solid tumors. J Clin Oncol 2014;32(January (2)):68–75.
8. Besse B, Soria J-C, Yao B. Neratinib with or without temsirolimus in patients with non-small cell lung cancer carrying HER2 somatic mutations: an international randomized phase II study. ESMO Cong 2014. Abstract LBA39 PR.
9. Ren S, Gao G, Wu F, Su C, Chen X, He Y, et al. Preliminary Results of a Phase II Study about the Efficacy and Safety of Pyrotinib in Patients with HER2 Mutant Advanced NSCLC. WCLC 2016.Abstract MA 0403.
10. Scagliotti GV, Parikh P, von Pawel J, Biesma B, Vansteenkiste J, Manegold C, et al. Phase III study comparing cisplatin plus gemcitabine with cisplatin plus Pemetrexed in chemotherapy-naive patients with advanced-stage non-small-cell lung Cancer. J Clin Oncol. 2008;26(21):3543–51.
11. Kim K, Oh I, Kim K, Jang T, Choi Y, Kim Y, et al. A randomized phase iii study of docetaxel plus cisplatin versus pemetrexed plus cisplatin in first line non-squamous non-small cell lung cancer (NSQ-NSCLC). Ann Oncol (2014) 25 (suppl 4; abstr LBA41_PR).
12. Lee JO, Kim TM, Lee SH, Kim DW, Kim S, Jeon YK, et al. Anaplastic lymphoma kinase translocation: a predictive biomarker of Pemetrexed in patients with non-small cell lung Cancer. J Thorac Oncol. 2011 Sep; 6(9):1474–80.
13. Ren S, Chen X, Kuang P, Zheng L, Su C, Li J, et al. Association of EGFR mutation or ALK rearrangement with expression of DNA repair and synthesis genes innever-smoker women with pulmonary adenocarcinoma. Cancer. 2012;118:5588–94.
14. Chen YF, Hsieh MS, Wu SG, Chang YL, Yu CJ, Yang JC, et al. Efficacy of Pemetrexed-based chemotherapy in patents with ROS1 fusion-positive lung adenocarcinoma compared with in patients harboring other driver mutations in east Asian populations. J Thorac Oncol. 2016;11(7):1140–52.
15. Zhang L, Jiang T, Zhao C, Li W, Li X, Zhao S, et al. Efficacy of crizotinib and pemetrexed-based chemotherapy in Chinese NSCLC patients with ROS1 rearrangement. Oncotarget. 2016 Nov 15;7(46):75145–54.
16. Drilon A, Bergagnini I, Delasos L, Sabari J, Woo KM, Plodkowski A, et al. Clinical outcomes with pemetrexed-based systemic therapies in RET-rearranged lung cancers. Ann Oncol. 2016;27:1286–91.
17. Ren S, Kuang P, Zheng L, Su C, Li J, Li B, et al. Analysis of driver mutations in femalenon-smoker Asian patients with pulmonary adenocarcinoma. Cell Biochem Biophys. 2012;64:155–60.
18. Wang Y, Zhang J, Gao G, Li X, Zhao C, He Y, et al. EML4-ALK fusion detected by RT-PCR confers similar response to crizotinib as detected by FISH in patients with advanced NSCLC. J Thorac Oncol. 2015;10:1546–52.
19. Wang Y, Liu Y, Zhao C, Li X, Wu C, Hou L, et al. Feasibility of cytological specimens for ALK fusion detection in patients with advanced NSCLC using the method of RT-PCR. Lung Cancer. 2016;94:28–34.
20. Li BT, Ross DS, Aisner DL, Chaft JE, Hsu M, Kako SL, et al. HER2 amplification and HER2 mutation are distinct molecular targets in lung cancers. J Thorac Oncol. 2016 Mar;11(3):414–9.
21. Mazières J, Peters S, Lepage B, Cortot AB, Barlesi F, Beau-Faller M, et al. Lung cancer that harbors an HER2 mutation: epidemiologic characteristics and therapeutic perspectives. J Clin Oncol. 2013;31(16):1997–2003.
22. Barlesi F, Mazieres J, Merlio JP, Debieuvre D, Mosser J, Lena H, et al. Routine molecular profiling of patients with advanced non-small-cell lung cancer: results of a 1-year nationwide programme of the French cooperative thoracic intergroup (IFCT). Lancet. 2016 Apr 2;387(10026):1415–26.
23. Arcila ME, Chaft JE, Nafa K, Roy-Chowdhuri S, Lau C, Zaidinski M, et al. Prevalence, clinicopathologic associations, and molecular spectrum of

ERBB2 (HER2) tyrosine kinase mutations in lung adenocarcinomas. Clin Cancer Res 2012;18(September (18)):4910–4918.

24. Li C, Fang R, Sun Y, Han X, Li F, Gao B, et al. Spectrum of oncogenic driver mutations in lung adenocarcinomas from east Asian never smokers. PLoS One. 2011;6:e28204.

25. Mazières J, Barlesi F, Filleron T, Besse B, Monnet I, Beau-Faller M, et al. Lung cancer patients with HER2 mutations treated with chemotherapy and HER2-targeted drugs: results from the European EUHER2 cohort. Ann Oncol. 2016 Feb;27(2):281–6.

26. Eng J, Hsu M, Chaft JE, Kris MG, Arcila ME, Li BT. Outcomes of chemotherapies and HER2 directed therapies in advanced HER2-mutant lung cancers. Lung Cancer. 2016;99:53–6.

27. Gow CH, Chang HT, Lim CK, Liu CY, Chen JS, Shih JY. Comparable clinical outcomes in patients with HER2-mutant and EGFR-mutant lung adenocarcinomas. Genes Chromosomes Cancer. 2017 May;56(5):373–81.

28. De Grève J, Teugels E, Geers C, Decoster L, Galdermans D, De Mey J, et al. Clinical activity of afatinib (BIBW 2992) in patients with lung adenocarcinoma with mutations in the kinase domain of HER2/neu. Lung Cancer 2012;76(April (1)): 123–127.

5

Evaluation of efficacy and safety for Brucea javanica oil emulsion in the control of the malignant pleural effusions via thoracic perfusion

Dai Fuhong[†], Gao Xiang[1*†], Li Haiying[2], Wang Jiangye[1], Gao Xueming[1] and Chai Wenxiao[1]

Abstract

Background: Brucea javanica oil emulsion (BJOE) is traditional Chinese medicine with implicated anti-tumor activity, which has been used for treating lung cancer in China. The aim of this investigation was to evaluate the effects and safety of intrapleural injection of BJOE in treating malignant pleural effusion (MPE).

Methods: The randomised controlled trials (RCTs) on the effects and safety of BJOE in treating MPE were searched from electronic medical database including MEDLINE, SCI, EMBASE, Cochrance Library and CNKI. A total of 14 RCTs with 1085 patients were involved in this meta-analysis.

Results: The overall response rate (ORR) of traditional chemotherapy drugs plus BJOE was higher than that of traditional chemotherapy drugs alone ($p = 0.001$; odds ratio = 1.39). Meanwhile, the combination of BJOE and traditional chemotherapy drugs improved the quality of life (QOL) of patients with MPE ($p < 0.001$; odds ratio = 1.56) compared with traditional chemotherapy drugs alone. Moreover, the participation of BJOE reduced the myelotoxicity and digestive reactions caused by traditional chemotherapy drugs ($p < 0.05$).

Conclusions: The efficacy and safety of traditional chemotherapy drugs plus BJOE was superior to traditional chemotherapy drugs alone via intrapleural injection in controlling MPE, which suggested that BJOE can be used to treat MPE.

Keywords: Brucea javanica oil emulsion, BJOE, Malignant pleural effusion, MPE, Meta-analysis, Efficacy, Safety

Background

Malignant pleural effusion (MPE) is a common complication of many malignancies, which denotes an advanced malignant disease process. Most of the MPE are metastatic involvement of the pleura from primary malignancy at lung, breast, and other body sites apart from lymphomas [1]. Clinical practice has found that most lung cancer patients will always be associated with MPE, and lead to lower QOL, and ultimately reduce the life expectancy. Therefore, the treatment of MPE caused more attention of doctors [2]. The present treatments of MPE include the drainage of pleural effusion, intrapleural chemotherapy and systemic chemotherapy. Unfortunately, not all patients with MPE can benefit from quasi chemotherapy and treatment [3]. During the last decade there has been significant progress in unravelling the pathophysiology of MPE, as well as its diagnostics, imaging, and management [4]. Despite its frequent occurrence, current knowledge of MPE remains limited and controversy surrounds almost every aspect in its diagnosis and management [5]. At present, some new drugs studied in China have a certain effect on MPE. These drugs seem to exhibit antitumor activity and low toxicity, they have been used to control MPE [2, 3, 6].

Traditional Chinese Medicines (TCMs) have become increasingly popular in the treatment of cancer in China. Brucea javanica oil emulsion (BJOE) is one of TCMs products, which takes Brucea Jen petroleum ether extracts as raw material and purified soybean lecithin as emulsifier [7]. BJOE (also named yadanzi oil in China) is an extract

* Correspondence: gaoxiangyffs68@aliyun.com
[†]Equal contributors
[1]Department of Interventional Medicine, Gansu Provincial Hospital, 204 Dong gang West Road, Lanzhou 730000, China
Full list of author information is available at the end of the article

of the ripe fruit of the simaroubaceae plant Brucea javanica (L.) Merr., which was first recorded in the Supplement to Compendium of Materia Medica. Brucea javanica oil (BJO) contains oleic acid, linoleic acid, stearic acid, palmitic acid, arachidonic acid, and other unsaturated fatty acids [8], which mainly produced in the People's Republic of China's coastal tropical and subtropical regions such as Hainan, Guangdong, Guangxi, Yunnan, and other places [9]. The fruit of Brucea javanica has been used for the treatment of various types of cancer in China for centuries. Dozens of single compounds have been isolated and identified from *B. javanica*, which have demonstrated relatively high activities and broad antitumor spectrums in vitro [10]. Previous investigations indicates that BJOE can enhance the chemotherapeutic effect on non-mall cell lung cancer (NSCLC) patients, improve the QOL and reduce adverse effects of platinum-contained chemotherapeutics and thus it is worth referring in clinic [11]. In addition, BJOE combined with chemotherapy could be considered as a safe and effective regimen in treating patients with advanced gastric cancer according to previous study [12].

So far, many investigations have specially disclosed the clinical effectiveness and safety of traditional chemotherapy drugs plus BJOE versus traditional chemotherapy drugs alone in controlling MPE via intrapleural injection. Whether or not BJOE has the potential therapeutic and/or adjuvant therapeutic application in the treatment of human MPE is conflicting. Thus, we performed a systematic literature review to assess the clinical benefit and safety of BJOE combined therapy in controlling MPE.

Methods
Identification of literature
We searched and identified relevant RCTs from the databases of MEDLINE/PubMed, EMBASE, Cochrance Library, Web of Science, and CNKI database (from January 2000 to April 2017). The key words applied in the search were as followed: "malignant pleural effusion", "MPE", "Brucea javanica oil emulsion", "BJOE injection", "BJOEI," "BJOE," "Yadanzi", and "chemotherapy", "Brucea javanica oil emulsion injection," "Yadanzi injection," and "Ya-dan-zi injection." In addition, if we find that the references of the included studies are closely related to BJOE, we should further search and identify them. The retrieved studies were regarded as potential source and reviewed manually. Moreover, although the published year of these literatures were unlimited, only English and Chinese literatures were involved in this study.

Data variables of studies
The general data that we selected are as follows: (1) the publication date of each randomized controlled trial; (2) the number of patients included in each study and

grouping; (3) the clinical and pathologic features of patients included each study, (4) the patterns of treatment intervention for treating MPE; (5) trials design and implementation. The data on outcomes in present meta-analysis included clinical efficacy, QOL, and adverse effects (AEs) according to World Health Organization (WHO) criteria and Response Evaluation Criteria in Solid Tumors (RECIST). The tumor response included complete response (CR), partial response (PR), stable disease (SD), and progressive disease (PD). The overall response rate (ORR) was defined as CR + PR/ overall cases and disease control rate (DCR) was calculated as CR + PR+ SD /overall cases. Toxicity was graded from 0 to IV in severity on the basis of the WHO Recommendations. This meta-analysis only investigated the incidence of Grade II or above.

Inclusion criteria of the study
Inclusion criteria: (1) study design was confined to RCTs on comparing traditional chemotherapy drugs plus BJOE with chemotherapy drugs alone for treating the MPE; (2) study subjects with MPE must be diagnosed pathologically and (or) cytologically; (3) drugs must be administered by intraluminal injection; (4) outcome measures determined by WHO criteria or RECIST, improvement of QOL evaluated by Karnofsky score (KPS), and AEs assessed by WHO Recommendations for Grading of Acute and Subacute Toxicity must be showed and (6) the sample size of the study must be more than or equal to 60.

Exclusion criteria of the study
The following criteria were used for the literature exclusion: (1) animal experiments, review, and other irrelevant studies; (2) patient also received other medications; (3) non-RCTs studies; (4) no detailed data about ORR, DCR, evaluation of QOL, and AEs or no indicators for them; (5) investigations were supported by drug producers; (6) lack of comparable control group and (7) single-arm study.

Supervision of the implementation process
The test design must meet the following rules: (1) RCTs of traditional chemotherapy drugs plus BJOE versus traditional chemotherapy drugs alone via intrapleural injection for controlling MPE; (2) the dosage of BJOE was determined by the suggestions of producers; (3) dosing interval: once a week; (3) number of times of administration: more than or equal to 2 times; and (3) observations on efficacy and safety: ORR, DCR, QOL, and AEs.

Assessment for quality of RCTs
The criteria of assessment that provided by Cochrane Handbook was employed to evaluate the quality of

included investigations. It contained the following Items: (1) sequence generation; (2) how to carry out blinding; (3) how to carry out allocation concealment; (4) how to perform outcome data selective; (5) a description of intention to treat and (6) other sources. According to the above criterion, the quality of trials was defined into three levels: low risk of bias, unclear risk of bias, and high risk of bias [7].

Statistical methods and analysis

All of the data was calculated by 14.0 (Stata Corporation, TX, USA) software package and Review Manager 5.3 software. The odds ratio (OR) with 95% confidence intervals (CI) was applied to analyze the dichotomous data [6]. By calculating the Z-value of the chi-square test, the statistical p-value < 0.05 was considered to be significantly different. The fixed effect model and the random effect model are commonly used statistical models for meta-analysis. According to the presence or absence of heterogeneity, both were selected to measure the safety and efficacy of BJOE pleural perfusion in the treatment of MPE. The χ^2 statistic and the I^2 statistic tests were used to assess statistical heterogeneity among included studies [3]. A more common way to indicate the degree of heterogeneity is the statistical test, which is often described as the Cochran chi-square test. A p value is often cited as an indicator of the degree of variability in the study. If the P value is less than 0.05, no statistical difference is considered, suggesting that the heterogeneity is small. The I^2 value describes the percentage of variability in point estimates that is due to heterogeneity rather than sampling error, may be readily calculated from most published meta-analyses, and a closed form uncertainty interval is available. If the I^2 value is less than 50%, the heterogeneity of the study is considered acceptable. If no heterogeneity existed, the method of fixed effects model was adopted, or using the random effects model. To assess the impact of a single study on overall statistical performance, we removed each study from the estimated library one by one, to analyze the impact of each study on overall effectiveness [2]. Further, we employed Begg's funnel plot and Egger's test to test the publication bias [7]. The SPSS (version 19.0, Chicago, USA) software was employed to finish the statistics of varying variables. The statistical p-value < 0.05 was considered to be significantly different.

Results

Literature retrieval process

Originally, we conducted the systematic research from online database, and 96 potentially relevant references were yielded. Of them, 25 studies were discarded because the design and implementation of these studies are not eligible for our research analysis. After further screening and eligibility assessment, 29 trials were

excluded because some of them were not RCTs and others did not belong to first-hand research data such as summary of meetings, medical reviews and newsletters. Remaining 42 studies seemed to meet the inclusion criterion, but 28 studies were deleted because of the following reasons: repeated data reporting, animal studies, statistical irregularities and too little sample size. Finally, 14 trials were selected as appropriate for inclusion in this meta-analysis. The flow chart showing the selection process was presented in Fig. 1A.

General characteristics of included studies

The 14 selected trials [13–26] were all RCTs and conducted in China. The qualified 14 studies included a total of 1085 patients, the total number of samples included in the study was from 60 [13, 26] to 123 [16] patients. The volume of pleural effusion of all patients in the amount were all more than 1000 mL and patients' age varied from 25 [17] to 86 [22] years. From these studies, lung cancer and breast cancer were the most common cause of MPE. A detailed database for meta-analysis on general characteristics was listed in Table 1.

Quality of study design

We found that the number of males (569) was more than the females (546) in the BJOE combined group and control group, respectively. The design of 12 studies were that BJOE combined with cisplatin versus cisplatin alone through thoracic perfusion for treating MPE [13–18, 20, 22–26], one study was BJOE combined with bleomycin versus bleomycin alone [21], another was BJOE combined with oxaliplatin versus oxaliplatin alone [19]. The dosages of BJOE via thoracic perfusion and follow-up times for efficacy evaluation had a good consistency, which was shown in Table 2. All studies had a certain tumor diagnosis by pathology or pleural effusion cytology diagnosis, and KPS score of each patient greater than 50 points. Generally, the dosage of BJOE was administered at the range of 40-100 mg per one time and frequency of administration was two times at least, which were given by thoracic perfusion after drainage of pleural effusions. There was no significant difference between the two groups in the general data ($p > 0.05$), indicating that they had good comparability.

The assessment of heterogeneity

Two investigators of us independently reviewed and assessed the quality of each study according to the criteria shaped by the Cochrane Handbook, which was specialized in evaluating the systematic reviews of Interventions (Version 5.0.1) [3]. As shown in Table 3, we found that 8 of the 14 studies (57.1%) showed the low risk of bias [17, 20–26] and that the remaining 6 investigations [13–16, 18, 19] displayed the unclear risk

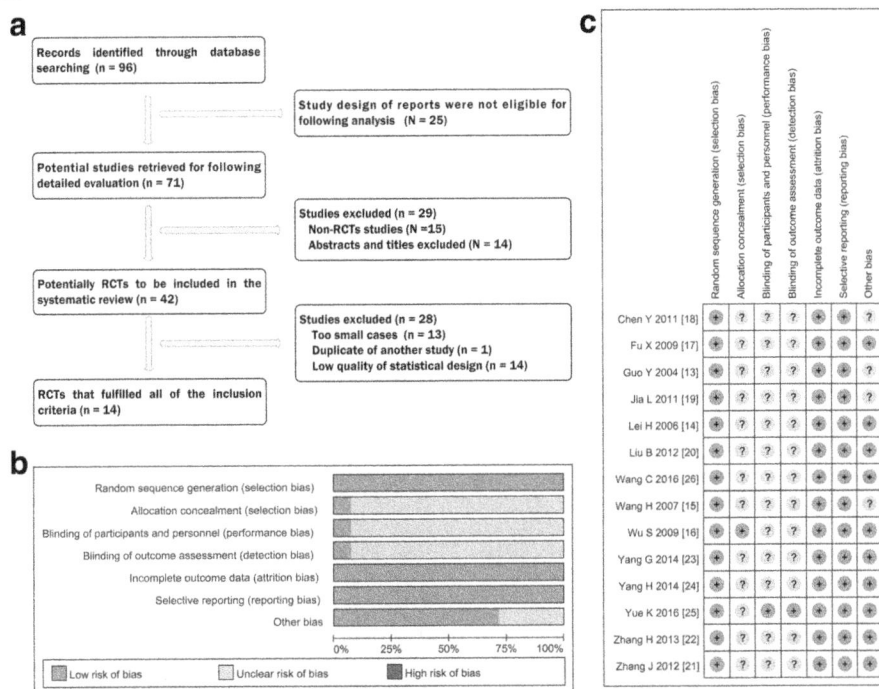

Fig. 1 Selection and assessment of literature. **a** Studies were retrieved from the electronic bibliographic databases such as PubMed, Embase, Cochrane Library, Web of Science and CNKI database. **b** and **c** According to the criteria made by the Cochrane Handbook (Version 5.0.1), no heterogeneity existed in eligible RCTs; Overall, these studies had moderate to higher quality

Table 1 Data analysis of included studies

Study	N	Male	Female	Age (average)	MPE	Histology of Lung cancer				Volume of MPE(N)	Quality of Life	End point
						LAC	LSCC	SCLC	Others			
Guo Y 2004 [13]	60	40	20	59.5	60	–	–	–	–	> 1000 ml	KPS	RR, DCR, AEs
Lei H 2006 [14]	61	–	–	58–79	61	31		9	–	> 1000 ml	KPS	RR, DCR, SI, AEs
Wang H 2007 [15]	70	45	25	26–81	70	42	7	13	8	Large(46) Moderate(24)	KPS	RR, DCR, SI, AEs
Wu S 2009 [16]	123	86	37	39–75	123	–	–	–	–	> 1000 ml	KPS	RR, DCR, AEs
Fu X 2009 [17]	120	82	38	25–78	120	–	–	–	–	Large(88) Moderate(32)	KPS	RR, DCR, AEs
Chen Y 2011 [18]	61	27	34	43–75	61	–	–	–	–	> 1000 ml	KPS	RR, DCR, AEs
Jia L 2011 [19]	70	38	32	39–85	70	–	–	–	–	> 1000 ml	KPS	RR, DCR, SI, AEs
Liu B 2012 [20]	64	31	33	36–77	64	46	13	5	0	Large(36) Moderate(28)	KPS	RR, DCR, SI, AEs
Zhang J 2012 [21]	64	45	19	28–81	64	20	29	12	3	> 1000 ml	KPS	RR, DCR, SI, AEs
Zhang H 2013 [22]	64	52	12	33–86	64	39	11	14	0	> 1000 ml	KPS	RR, DCR, SI, AEs
Yang G 2014 [23]	94	–	–	–	94	–	–	–	–	> 1000 ml	KPS	RR, DCR, SI, AEs
Yang H 2014 [24]	64	42	22	38–72	64	19	24	13	8	> 1000 ml	KPS	RR, DCR, SI, AEs
Yue K 2016 [25]	111	57	53	–	110	–	70	19	21	> 1000 ml	KPS	RR, DCR, SI, AEs
Wang C 2016 [26]	60	34	26	40–74	60	11	17	–	32	> 1000 ml	KPS	RR, DCR, SI, AEs

N number of patients, MPE malignant pleural effusion, LAC lung adenocarcinoma, LSCC lung squamous cell carcinoma, SCLC small cell lung cancer, KPS karnofsky physical status score, RR response rate, DCR disease control rate, SI symptom improvement, AEs adverse effects

Table 2 Assessment method of administration of included studies

Study	Trial group (N)	Control group (N)	Interventions (Groups)		Treatment cycle	Termination of treatment
			Brucea javanica oil emulsion (BJOE) combined with chemotherapeutic agents	Chemotherapeutic agents alone		
Guo Y 2004 [13]	30	30	Cisplatin 150 mg, 1/week BJOE 50 mL, 1/week	Cisplatin 150 mg, 1/W	1 week	> 2 weeks, or pleural effusion disappeared
Lei H 2006 [14]	31	30	Cisplatin 40-60 mg, 1/week BJOE 40-60 mL, 1/week	Cisplatin 40-60 mg, 1/W	1 week	> 1 weeks, or pleural effusion disappeared
Wang H 2007 [15]	35	35	Cisplatin 20-30 mg/m^2, 1/week BJOE 80-100 mL, 1/week	Cisplatin 20-30 mg/m^2, 1/5-7D	1/5-7D	> 2 weeks, or pleural effusion disappeared
Wu S 2009 [16]	68	55	Cisplatin 60 mg, 1/week BJOE 50 mL, 1/week	Cisplatin 60 mg, 1/W	1 week	> 4 weeks, or pleural effusion disappeared
Fu X 2009 [17]	60	60	Cisplatin 40/m^2, 1/week BJOE 100 mL, 1/week	Cisplatin 40/m^2, 1/W	1 week	> 4 weeks, or pleural effusion disappeared
Chen Y 2011 [18]	31	30	Cisplatin 60 mg, 1/week BJOE 60 mL, 1/week	Cisplatin 60 mg, 1/W	1 week	> 4 weeks, or pleural effusion disappeared
Jia L 2011 [19]	35	35	Oxaliplatin 100/m^2, 1/week BJOE 60 mL, 1/week	Oxaliplatin 100/m^2, 1/W	1 week	> 4 weeks, or pleural effusion disappeared
Liu B 2012 [20]	32	32	Cisplatin 40/m^2, 1/week BJOE 100 mL, 1/week	Cisplatin 40/m^2, 1/W	1 week	> 4 weeks, or pleural effusion disappeared
Zhang J 2012 [21]	28	36	Bleomycin 45-60 mg, 1/week BJOE 80-100 mL, 1/week	Bleomycin 45-60 mg, 1/W	1 week	> 2 weeks, or pleural effusion disappeared
Zhang H 2013 [22]	34	30	Cisplatin 40-60 mg, 1/week BJOE 40-50 mL, 1/week	Cisplatin 40-60 mg, 1/W	1 week	> 2 weeks, or pleural effusion disappeared
Yang G 2014 [23]	48	46	Cisplatin 40 mg/m^2, 1/week BJOE 80 mL, 1/week	Cisplatin 40 mg/m^2, 1/W	1 week	> 3 weeks, or pleural effusion disappeared
Yang H 2014 [24]	32	32	Cisplatin 40 mg/m^2, 1/week BJOE 50 mL/m^2, 1/week	Cisplatin 40 mg/m^2, 1/W	1 week	> 4 weeks, or pleural effusion disappeared
Yue K 2016 [25]	60	50	Cisplatin 40 mg/m^2, 1/week BJOE 80-100 mL, 1/week	Cisplatin 80 mg/m^2, 1/W	1 week	> 2 weeks, or pleural effusion disappeared
Wang C 2016 [26]	45	45	Cisplatin 40 mg/m^2, 1/week BJOE 60 mL, 1/week	Cisplatin 40 mg/m^2, 1/7d	7D/cycle, 2 cycles	> 2 cycles, or pleural effusion disappeared

BJOE Brucea javanica oil emulsion, *N* numbers of patients, *D* day, *W* week

of bias (42.9%) (Table 3, Fig. 1B, C). We conducted a heterogeneity analysis of included studies. The results showed that chi-squared was 1.61 (Degrees of freedom = 13; p = 1.000) and that the value of I-squared (variation in OR attributable to heterogeneity) showed as 0.0%. These results indicated that these included RCTs had very good homogeneity. Combining the clinical information of these studies, we believe that these studies have very good comparability. Based on no heterogeneity, we completed the subsequent statistical analysis using the fixed effects model.

Comparison of ORR and DCR between traditional chemotherapy drugs plus BJOE versus traditional chemotherapy drugs alone via intrapleural injection for controlling MPE

As shown in Table 4, all of fourteen RCTs [13–26] in this meta-analysis showed the data on comparison of ORR between traditional chemotherapy drugs plus BJOE versus traditional chemotherapy drugs alone via intrapleural injection for controlling MPE. Via the fixed effects model analysis, we found that odds ratio was 1.39 (95% CI 1.15 to 1.67; Z value = 3.46, p = 0.001), which suggested that

Table 3 Design quality of included trials

Study	Region	Sequence generation	Allocation concealment	Blind	Outcome data	Selective outcome reporting	Other sources of bias	ITT	Risk of bias
Guo Y 2004 [13]	Single center	Random number table (SPSS)	Unclear	Unclear	Yes	No	Unclear	Yes	Unclear risk of bias
Lei H 2006 [14]	Single center	Random number table (SPSS)	Unclear	Unclear	Yes	No	Unclear	Yes	Unclear risk of bias
Wang H 2007 [15]	Single center	Random number table (SPSS)	Clear	Unclear	Yes	No	Unclear	Yes	Unclear risk of bias
Wu S 2009 [16]	Single center	Random number table (SPSS)	Unclear	Unclear	Yes	No	Unclear	Yes	Unclear risk of bias
Fu X 2009 [17]	Single center	Random number table (SPSS)	Unclear	Unclear	Yes	No	Clear	Yes	Low risk of bias
Chen Y 2011 [18]	Single center	Random number table (SPSS)	Unclear	Unclear	Yes	No	Unclear	Yes	Unclear risk of bias
Jia L 2011 [19]	Single center	Random number table (SPSS)	Unclear	Unclear	Yes	No	Unclear	Yes	Unclear risk of bias
Liu B 2012 [20]	Single center	Random number table (SPSS)	Unclear	Unclear	Yes	No	Clear	Yes	Low risk of bias
Zhang J 2012 [21]	Single center	Random number table (SPSS)	Unclear	Unclear	Yes	No	Clear	Yes	Low risk of bias
Zhang H 2013 [22]	Single center	Random number table (SPSS)	Unclear	Unclear	Yes	No	Clear	Yes	Low risk of bias
Yang G 2014 [23]	Multiple center	Random number table (SPSS)	Unclear	Unclear	Yes	No	Clear	Yes	Low risk of bias
Yang H 2014 [24]	Single center	Random number table (SPSS)	Unclear	Unclear	Yes	No	Clear	Yes	Low risk of bias
Yue K 2016 [25]	Single center	Random number table (SPSS)	Unclear	Clear	Yes	No	Clear	Yes	Low risk of bias
Wang C 2016 [26]	Single center	Random number table (SAS)	Unclear	Unclear	Yes	No	Clear	Yes	Low risk of bias

SAS SAS software, *SPSS* SPSS software, *ITT* intention-to-treat

the ORR of traditional chemotherapy drugs plus BJOE was remarkably higher than that of traditional chemotherapy drugs alone (Fig. 2A). In addition, fourteen studies [13–26] showed the data about DCR and displayed that the BJOE combination arms and chemotherapeutic agents single group had the same DCR rate (odds ratio = 1.04, 95% CI 0.888 to 1.23; test for overall effect: Z = 0.44, p = 0.663).

Comparison of QOL between traditional chemotherapy drugs plus BJOE versus traditional chemotherapy drugs alone via intrapleural injection for controlling MPE

As shown in Table 4, a total of 8 trials [14, 15, 17, 20, 21, 23, 25, 26] provided the data on comparing the QOL between the BJOE plus traditional chemotherapy drugs versus traditional chemotherapy drugs alone via intrapleural injection for controlling MPE. The QOL improvement was evaluated by the KPS score of patient. After treatment, the KPS score increased by ≥10 points was defined as improvement of QOL. We found that the improvement rate of BJOE combined perfusion group (262/324, 80.86%) was significantly higher than that of chemotherapy group alone (168/319, 52.66%). The results

of meta-analysis showed that the odds ratio ranged from 1.17 to 1.99 and the pooled odds ratio in this analysis displayed a value of 1.56 (95% CI 1.21 to 2.00; Z = 3.49, p < 0.001), which suggested that BJOE combined with chemotherapeutic agents significantly improved the QOL of patients with MPE, as compared with single chemotherapeutic agents (Fig. 2B).

Composition ratio of AEs on traditional chemotherapy drugs plus BJOE versus traditional chemotherapy drugs alone via intrapleural injection for controlling MPE

Nine [14, 15, 17, 18, 20, 23–25] of 14 studies compared the AEs on traditional chemotherapy drugs plus BJOE versus traditional chemotherapy drugs alone via intrapleural injection for controlling MPE. As shown in Table 5, the most common AEs in combined group and single group were myelotoxicity (71/363, 19.5% versus 141/350, 40.3%), nausea/vomiting (55/392, 14.03% versus 104/386, 28.4%), liver and renal injury (7/124, 5.6% versus 10/124, 8.1%), chest pain (39/299, 13.04% versus 52/299, 17.39%) and fever (30/309, 9.7% versus 45/305, 14.75%).

Table 4 Efficacy of BJOE injection in treating malignant pleural effusion

Study	Study design (N)		Pleural perfusion (N)		Efficacy of therapy								Improvement of SI (N,%)	
			Group 1	Group 2	Group 1				Group 2					
	Group 1	Group 2			CR	PR	SD	PD	CR	PR	SD	PD	Group 1	Group 2
Guo Y 2004 [13]	30	30	BJOE + P	P	11	15	4	0	5	11	14	0	–	–
Lei H 2006 [14]	31	30	BJOE + P	P	11	14	6	0	5	10	15	0	24(77.4)	12(40)
Wang H 2007 [15]	35	35	BJOE + P	P	13	16	6	0	7	13	15	0	32(91.4)	20(57.1)
Wu S 2009 [16]	68	55	BJOE + P	P	39	20	9	0	16	28	11	0	–	–
Fu X 2009 [17]	60	60	BJOE + P	P	22	28	8	2	14	21	18	7	44(73.3)	33(55)
Chen Y 2011 [18]	31	30	BJOE + P	P	12	13	6	0	8	9	13	0	–	–
Jia L 2011 [19]	35	35	BJOE+ L-OHP	L-OHP	10	18	7	0	8	15	12	0	–	–
Liu B 2012 [20]	32	32	BJOE + P	P	18	7	4	3	13	4	9	6	28(75)	24(50)
Zhang J 2012 [21]	28	36	BJOE + BLM	BLM	10	16	2	0	9	17	10	0	25(89.3)	21(58.3)
Zhang H 2013 [22]	34	30	BJOE + P	P	19	10	5	0	11	6	13	0	–	–
Yang G 2014 [23]	48	46	BJOE + P	P	14	26	8	0	4	22	16	4	42(87.5)	24(52.17)
Yang H 2014 [24]	32	32	BJOE + P	P	18	7	4	3	13	4	9	6	–	–
Yue K 2016 [25]	60	50	BJOE + P	P	23	27	10	0	13	14	23	0	43(71.7)	18(36)
Wang C 2016 [26]	30	30	BJOE + P	P	10	14	5	1	8	11	7	4	24(80)	16(53.3)

N cases; *Group 1* BJOE combined with chemotherapeutic agents; *Group 2* Chemotherapeutic agents alone, *BJOE* Brucea javanica oil emulsion; *P* cisplatin, *L-OHP* Oxaliplatin, *BLM* bleomycin, *CR* complete response, *PR* partial response, *SD* stable disease, *PD* progressive disease

Comparison of AEs between traditional chemotherapy drugs plus BJOE versus traditional chemotherapy drugs alone via intrapleural injection for controlling MPE

Nine [14, 15, 17, 18, 20, 23–25] of 14 studie compared the myelotoxicity on traditional chemotherapy drugs plus BJOE versus traditional chemotherapy drugs alone via intrapleural injection for controlling MPE, we found that the incidence rate of myelotoxicity in BJOE combined perfusion group was lower than that of traditional chemotherapy drugs alone group (odds ratio = 0.5, 95% CI 0. 36 to 0.70, $p < 0.001$) (Fig. 3A). Ten [14, 15, 17, 18, 20, 21, 23–25] of 14 studie compared the gastrointestinal reactions, the incidence rate of nausea/vomiting in BJOE combined group also showed a significant decrease compared with traditional chemotherapy drugs alone group (odds ratio = 0.50, 95% CI 0. 35 to 0.72, $p < 0.001$) (Fig. 3B). In addition, three studies compared liver and renal injury (odds ratio = 0.70, 95% CI 0. 25 to 1.91, $p = 0.483$), eight studies compared the incidence of chest pain (odds ratio = 0.70, 95% CI 0. 44 to 1.11, $p = 0.130$), and seven studies compared the incidence of fever (odds ratio = 0.67, 95% CI 0. 41 to 1.10, $p = 0.111$). However, these results suggested that the incidence rate of these AEs did not have differences between both of two projects ($p > 0.05$) (Fig. 4A-C).

Assessment of publication bias and sensitivity analysis

Through removing each study, a further meta-analysis was performed to compare with previous results of meta-analysis to explore whether the deleted study have an certain impact on the overall statistical effect [27]. Sensitivity analysis shows that excluding of any study could not change the overall statistical effect, nor could it affect the final statistical conclusion, with an OR pool oscillating between 1.08 and 1.63 (Fig. 5A). We also drew a funnel plot of included studies and noticed that the included studies are symmetrically distributed on both sides of the funnel (Fig. 5B). In addition, for comparing traditional chemotherapy drugs with chemotherapy drugs plus BJOE for controlling MPE, we performed the Egger's test and the results were as the following: $t = 1.75$ with 13 d.f, $p = 0.105$ (Fig. 5C). We also performed a Begg's test and the test results showed that Std. Dev. of Score was 18.27, p value was 0.112 (Fig. 5D). Come together, the funnel plot, Egger's tests and the Begg's test all suggested that publication biases did not have a significant influence on the results.

Discussion

BJOE is composed of the active ingredients extracted from the ripe fruit of *Sophora flavescens*. The main components are oleic acid and linoleic acid. BJOE is a traditional Chinese medicine. It has been shown that BJOE could directly kill the cancer cells by up-regulating the tumor suppress or genes [7]. Moreover, BJOE has also been found to reverse the tumor cell resistance to chemotherapy and improve the body immunity, without significant AEs [28]. Some experiments show that BJOE is cell cycle non-specific anti-cancer drug, which has an efficacy of killing and inhibition in the G0, G1, S, G2, M phases of tumor cells, and can significantly inhibits DNA synthesis of tumor cells [15, 26, 29]. In addition, previous studies also suggest that the anti-tumor activity of BJOE might be correlated to the mechanism of

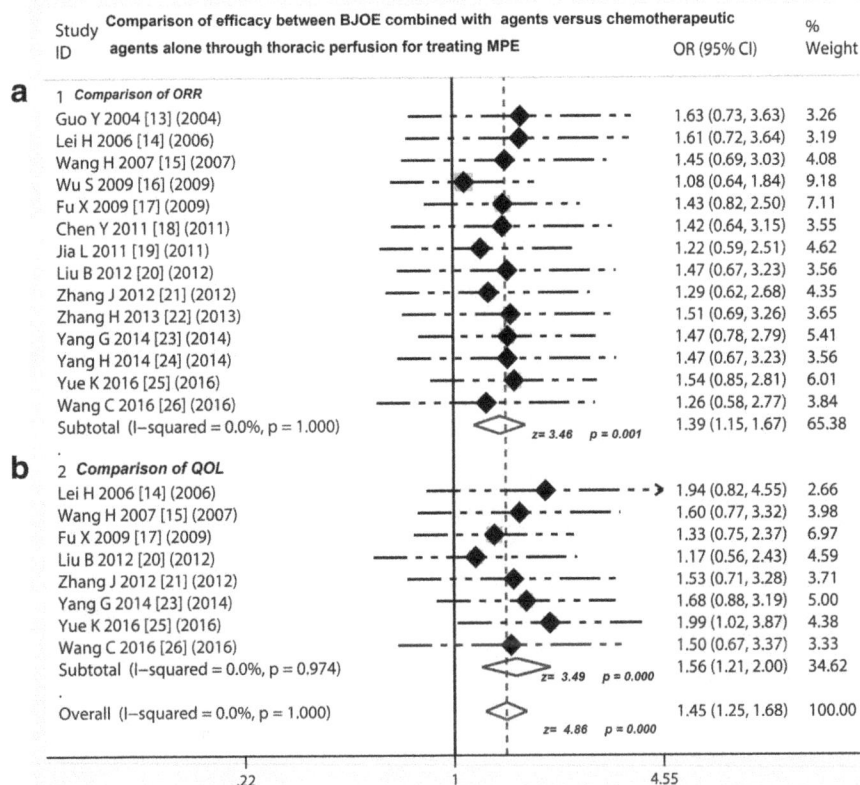

Fig. 2 Efficacy comparison of BJOE combined with another agent versus another agent alone by thoracic perfusion for controlling MPE. **a** Thoracic perfusion of BJOE combined with other agents had a higher ORR compared with other agents alone; **b** Thoracic perfusion of BJOE combined with other agents improved the QOL of patients with MPE compared with other agents alone. BJOE, brucea javanica oil emulsion; ORR, overall response rate; MPE, malignant pleural effusion; OR, odds ratio; QOL, quality of life

Table 5 Comparison of adverse events between BJOE combined with chemotherapeutic agents versus chemotherapeutic agents alone

Study	Myelotoxicity (%)		Nausea/vomiting (%)		Liver and renal injury (%)		Chest pain (%)		Fever (%)	
	Group 1	Group 2	Group 1	Group 2	Group 1	Group 2	Group 1	Group 2	Group 1	Group 2
Lei H 2006 [14]	9(29)	22(73.3)	5(16.1)	12(40)			3(9.7)	5(16.7)	3(9.7)	4(13.3)
Wang H 2007 [15]	9(25.7)	21(60)	2(5.7)	5(14.3)	–	–	1(2.9)	1(2.9)	–	–
Fu X 2009 [17]	15(25)	36(60)	4(6.67)	12(20)	1(1.7)	2(3.3)	3(5)	8(13.3)	3(5)	11(18.33)
Chen Y 2011 [18]	9(29.03)	22(73.33)	5(16.13)	12(40)	–	–	3(9.68)	5(16.67)	3(9.68)	4(13.33)
Jia L 2011 [19]	8(22.86)	9(25.7)	15(42.86)	14(40)	–	–	–	–	–	–
Liu B 2012 [20]	5(15.6)	6(18.8)	5(15.6)	7(21.9)	3(9.4)	4(12.5)	3(9.4)	4(12.5)	5(15.6)	4(12.5)
Zhang J 2012 [21]	–	–	2(7.14)	6(16.6)	–	–	0(0)	3(8.3)	3(10.7)	11(30.6)
Zhang H 2013 [22]	–	–	–	–	–	–	12(35.3)	10(33.3)	–	–
Yang G 2014 [23]	8(16.7)	10(26.7)	2(4.17)	6(13.04)	–	–	14(29.17)	16(34.8)	–	–
Yang H 2014 [24]	5(15.6)	6(18.8)	5(15.6)	7(21.9)	3(9.4)	4(12.5)	–	–	5(15.6)	4(12.5)
Yue K 2016 [25]	3 (5.0)	9 (18)	10(16.7)	23 (46)	–	–	–	–	8 (13.3)	7(14)
	$P < 0.05$		$P < 0.05$		$P > 0.05$		$P > 0.05$		$P > 0.05$	

Values are given as number of patients (%).*Group 1* Brucea javanica oil emulsion (BJOE) combined with chemotherapeutic agents; *Group 2* Chemotherapeutic agents alone

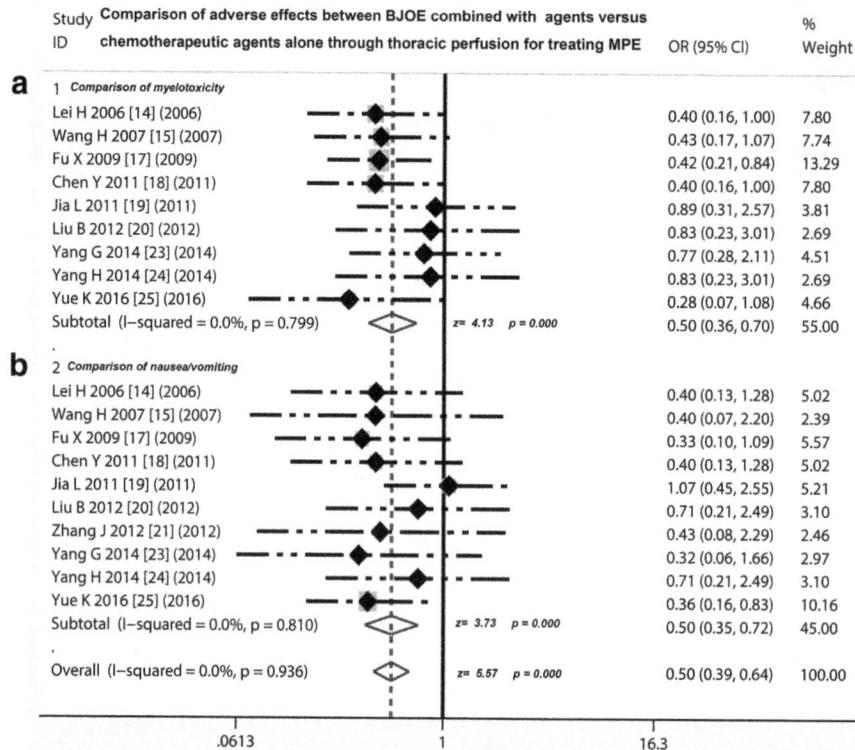

Fig. 3 Safety evaluation of BJOE combined with another agent versus another agent alone by thoracic perfusion for controlling MPE. **a** The BJOE combination therapy displayed a lower incidence rate of myelotoxicity than the project of other agents alone; **b** The BJOE combined with other agents had a lower incidence of digestive reactions than and other agents alone. BJOE, brucea javanica oil emulsion; MPE, malignant pleural effusion; OR, odds ratio

tumor cell apoptosis, which affects the process of cell cycle, disrupts the cellular energy metabolism, and depresses the expression of vascular endothelial growth factor [7]. So far, a great number of published studies have reported that BJOE can perform a synergetic effect for controlling MPE by improving tumor response and QOL and reducing the incidence of AEs [12–16, 19, 20, 26, 28–30].

We conducted a comprehensive literature search and screening, and finally 14 trials were selected as appropriate for this meta-analysis. By statistical verification and combining the clinical information of these studies, we found that these included RCTs had very good homogeneity and comparability, and further performed a meta-analysis. Our analysis showed that traditional chemotherapy drugs plus BJOE via intrapleural injection had a better ORR benefit compared with traditional chemotherapy drugs alone (odds ratio = 1.39) for controlling MPE, translating into a 22.95% absolute improvement. The results suggested that participation of BJOE exerted an important effect in treating MPE, indicating that BJOE can be used as an alternative drug for controlling the MPE in clinical practice. Previous studies show that the BJOE combination therapy could promote liver cancer cell apoptosis by regulating

the expression of soluble Fas/soluble Fas ligand [28] and BJOE also induces apoptosis in the colon cancer cells [28]. Another study finds that BJO-loaded liposomes inhibits the proliferation of hepatocellular cancer HepG2 cells, which appears be dose-dependent, possibly by inducing apoptosis of cancer cells [31]. However, in our study, the BJOE combination seemed to have the same DCR rate (odds ratio = 1.04, p = 0.663) compared with chemotherapeutic agents alone. High ORR indicates that the drug can control the disease progress of patients with MPE, meaning that the disease condition of patients was significantly alleviated. At this point, its significance is greater than the control rate because reversing the patient's disease condition is critical aim of treating malignant tumors [32]. Since the DCR of BJOE combination is comparable to the existing traditional chemotherapy drugs, and it has a high ORR, then the drug should have a certain application value.

Although the control of primary disease is very important, the improvement of QOL in patients is also very critical. Overall survival (OS) has always been considered the "gold standard" for tumor therapy in the study of the therapeutic effects of cancer patients. In today's clinical trials, the improvement in QOL in patients is increasingly

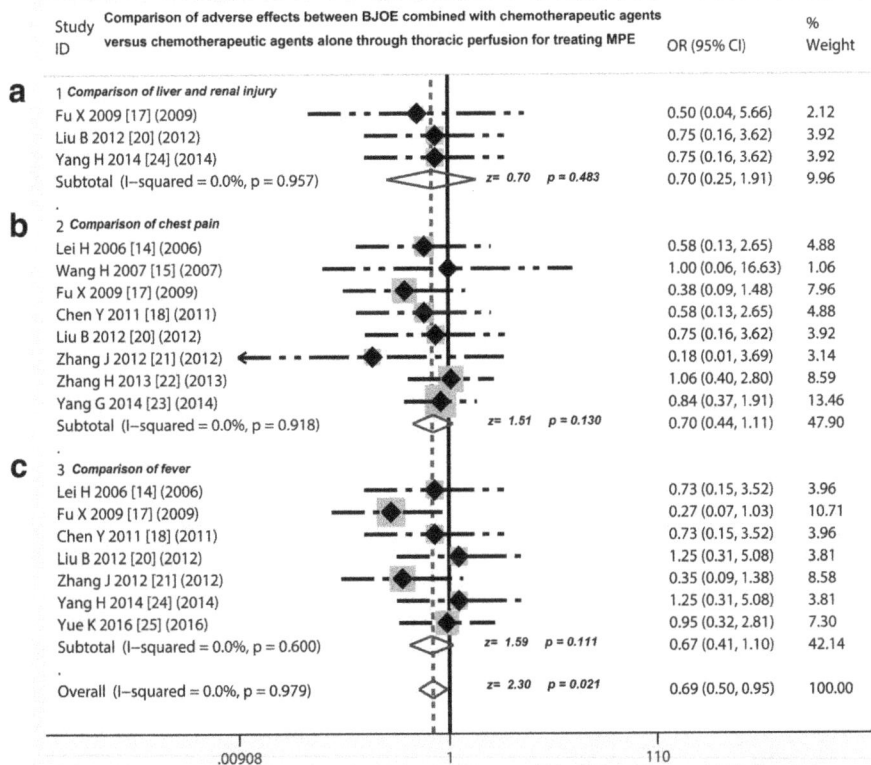

Fig. 4 Safety evaluation of BJOE combined with another agent versus another agent alone by thoracic perfusion for treating MPE. **a** No difference in incidence rate of liver and renal injury was testified between BJOE combined with other agents and other agents alone; **b** The incidence of chest pain caused by BJOE combination therapy had the same occurrence probability compared with the other agents alone; **c** The BJOE combined with other agents had the same incidence of fever with other agents alone. BJOE, brucea javanica oil emulsion; MPE, malignant pleural effusion; OR, odds ratio

being used to examine efficacy of therapy [32]. Our study showed that presence of BJOE remarkably elevated the QOL of patients with MPE (OR = 1.56, 95% CI 1.21 to 2.0), which responding an absolute 28.2% increase of the QOL, as compared with chemotherapeutic agents alone. That is to say that BJOE-containing therapy improves the ability of QOL of patients with MPE to be about 1.56 times compared with therapy of chemotherapy alone. Previous study points out that BJOE inhibits the proliferation of C6 glioma cells by suppressing the phosphoinositide 3-kinases (PI3K), protein Kinase B (AKT), and nuclear transcription factor-κB (NF-κB) protein expression, which also leads to inhibition of invasiveness of glioma cells, suggesting that the anti-tumor effect of BJOE relates to the inhibition of PI3K/AKT signal pathway [30]. The molecular mechanism that BJOE induces apoptosis of T24 bladder cancer cells may be the activation of caspase apoptotic pathway by upregulation of the expression of caspase-3 and caspase-9 proteins and inhibition of the expression of NF-κB and cyclo-oxygenase-2 (COX-2) proteins [29]. A meta-analysis has showed that intravenous therapy of BJOE plus chemoradiotherapy

may have positive effects on lung cancer patients in response rate, improvement of QOL, and reducing incidences of some AEs compared with chemoradiotherapy alone. However, the results need to be viewed with caution because of low quality of the included studies [33].

The antineoplastic agent cisplatin is widely used for treating lung cancer as it is highly effective. Unfortunately, the AEs are frequently encountered in platinum-based chemotherapy. With rising cancer survival rates, a greater proportion of patients with cancer are living with the AEs of their chemotherapy treatments. Consequently, the QOL of cancer survivors has now become a major concern for clinicians [34]. In our study, whether BJOE plus traditional chemotherapy drugs or traditional chemotherapy drugs alone via thoracic perfusion, the most common AEs are hematopoietic dysfunction and gastrointestinal symptoms, but most of them are grade 1 and grade 2, and patients are better tolerated. However, we excitedly found that the incidence of myelotoxicity and digestive reactions in treatment of traditional chemotherapy drugs plus BJOE was significantly lower than that in traditional chemotherapy drugs

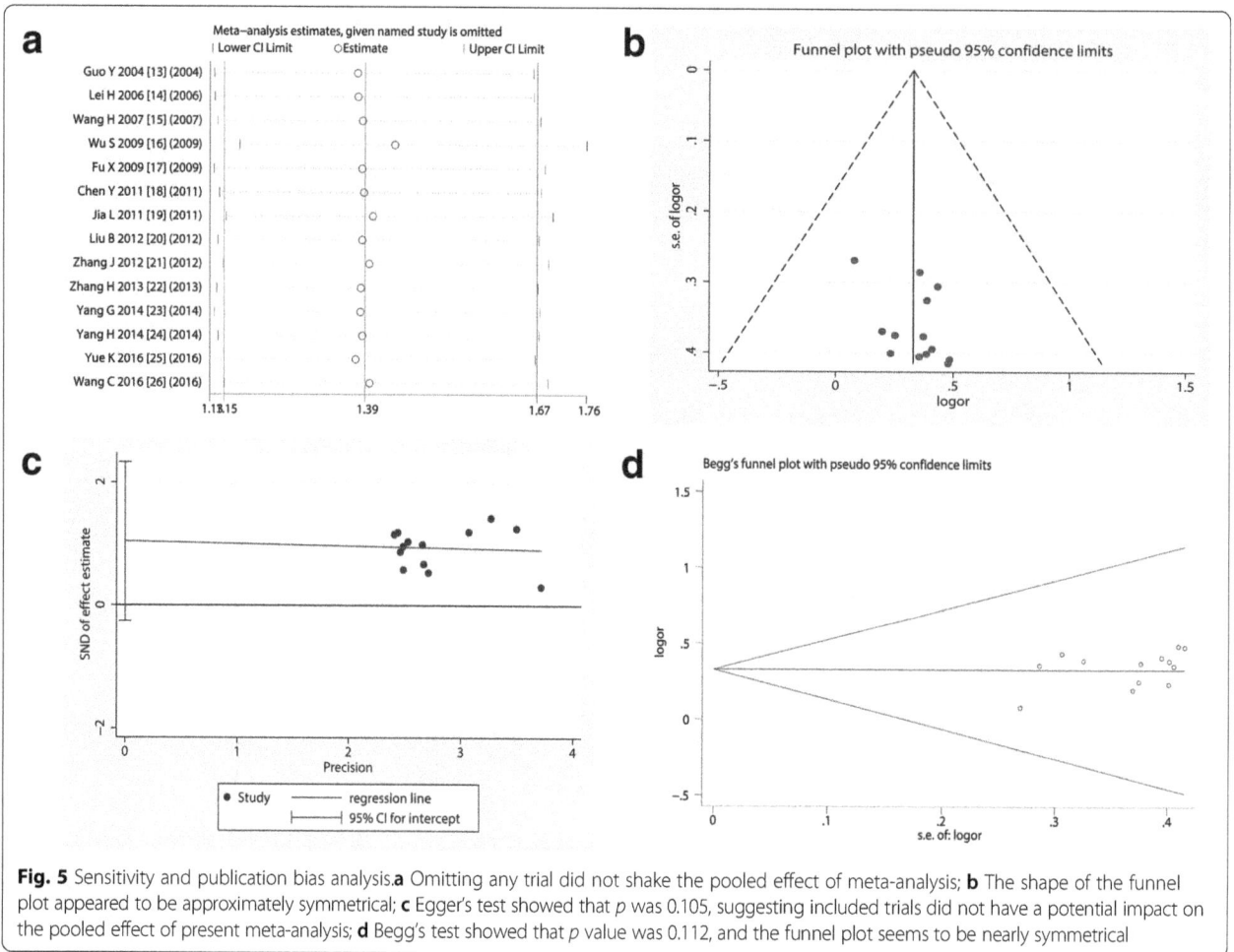

Fig. 5 Sensitivity and publication bias analysis. **a** Omitting any trial did not shake the pooled effect of meta-analysis; **b** The shape of the funnel plot appeared to be approximately symmetrical; **c** Egger's test showed that p was 0.105, suggesting included trials did not have a potential impact on the pooled effect of present meta-analysis; **d** Begg's test showed that p value was 0.112, and the funnel plot seems to be nearly symmetrical

alone, indicating that the BJOE not only exert a impact for treating MPE but also decrease the incidence of myelotoxicity and digestive reactions. Unlike traditional antineoplastic agents, previous studies show that BJOE can not only directly kill cancer cells, but also has enhanced immune function and bone marrow hematopoietic function [7, 11]. Our further analysis found that the incidence rate of liver and renal injury, chest pain and fever of BJOE combination therapy had the same occurrence compared with chemotherapeutic agents alone ($P > 0.05$), suggesting that BJOE participation did not increase the incidence of these AEs. So far, more data have exhibited that the BJOE therapy could be well tolerated and had a better safety for clinical application.

For meta-analysis, heterogeneity testing is important because the heterogeneity of the study will affect the overall statistical effect. In order to insure the comparability, it is necessary to do method comparison and bias evaluation. In the funnel plot analysis of publication biases (the contrast of homozygous genotype plotted against the precision) [35], the shape of the funnel plot appeared to be approximately symmetrical, and the magnitude of the main ORs

was in dispersion on the right side of 1. The Egger's test is based on a linear regression of the standard normal deviate against its precision [35]. In our study, the Egger's tests and the Begg's test all suggested that publication biases may not have a significant influence on the results. Sensitivity analysis can estimate the impact of a single study on overall statistical performance. Our study suggested that the included studies had excellent homogeneity and were comparable.

However, we also found some of the defects that existed in the meta-analysis study. First, the vast majority of the samples included in the study were small, thus reducing the test efficiency. Second, included studies in this meta-analysis rarely describes whether implements the allocation hiding, inadequate implementation may exaggerate efficacy. Third, most of patients were from China (because BJOE was approved by the China State Food and Drug Administration), which may lead to geographical and ethnic differences. In spite of this, our results still propose a significant suggestion that the BJOE is effective and safe, and it is an alternative for controlling MPE.

Conclusion

Intrapleural injection of traditional chemotherapy drugs plus BJOE has a better benefit of ORR for treating MPE and improves the QOL of MPE patients, compared with traditional chemotherapy drugs alone. In addition, the participation of BJOE can reduce the toxicity caused by chemotherapy drugs. However, rigorously RCTs should be needed before it is recommended widely.

Abbreviations

AEs: Adverse effects; AKT: Protein Kinase B; BJO: Brucea javanica oil; BJOE: Brucea javanica oil emulsion; CI: Confidence intervals; CNKI: China National Knowledge Infrastructure; COX-2: Cyclooxygenase-2; CR: Complete response; DCR: Disease control rate; EMBASE: Excerpt Medica Database; HRQOL: Health-related quality of life; KPS: Karnofsky score; MPE: Malignant pleural effusion; NF-Kb: Nuclear transcription factor-κB; NSCLC: Non-mall cell lung cancer; OR: Odds ratio; ORR: Overall response rate; OS: Overall survival; PD: Progressive disease; PI3K: Phosphoinositide 3-kinase; PR: Partial response; QOL: Quality of life; RCTs: Randomised controlled trials; RECIST: Response evaluation criteria in solid tumors; SD: Stable disease; sFas/sFasL: Soluble Fas/soluble Fas ligand; SFDA: China State Food and Drug Administration; TCMs: Traditional Chinese Medicines; WHO: World Health Organization; Yadanzi: The another name of BJOE in Chinese

Acknowledgements

We appreciate the great help of Mr. Rong BX, and Miss Li M as interviewers.

Funding

This work was supported by Natural Science Foundation of Gansu Provincial, China (No. 1606RJZA154). The funders of this project had no role in the design of the study and collection, analysis and in writing the manuscript.

Authors' contributions

D FH and G X conception, design and selection of data, L HY, W JY, G XM and C WX data collation, statistical analysis and composition of manuscript. All authors have read and approved the manuscript.

Competing interests

The authors declare that they have no competing interests.

Author details

[1]Department of Interventional Medicine, Gansu Provincial Hospital, 204 Dong gang West Road, Lanzhou 730000, China. [2]First Clinical Medical College, Institute of Hematology, Lanzhou University, Lanzhou, China.

References

1. Dixit R, Agarwal KC, Gokhroo A, Patil CB, Meena M, Shah NS, et al. Diagnosis and management options in malignant pleural effusions. Lung India. 2017;34(2):160–6.
2. Biaoxue R, Xiguang C, Hua L, Wenlong G, Shuanying Y. Thoracic perfusion of recombinant human endostatin (Endostar) combined with chemotherapeutic agents versus chemotherapeutic agents alone for treating malignant pleural effusions: a systematic evaluation and meta-analysis. BMC Cancer. 2016;16(1):888.
3. Biaoxue R, Hui P, Wenlong G, Shuanying Y. Evaluation of efficacy and safety for recombinant human adenovirus-p53 in the control of the malignant pleural effusions via thoracic perfusion. Sci Rep. 2016;6:39355.
4. Psallidas I, Kalomenidis I, Porcel JM, Robinson BW, Stathopoulos GT. Malignant pleural effusion: from bench to bedside. Eur Respir Rev. 2016; 25(140):189–98.
5. Azzopardi M, Porcel JM, Koegelenberg CF, Lee YC, Fysh ET. Current controversies in the management of malignant pleural effusions. Semin Respir Crit Care Med. 2014;35(6):723–31.
6. Biaoxue R, Shuxia M, Wenlong G, Shuanying Y. Thoracic perfusion of matrine as an adjuvant treatment improves the control of the malignant pleural effusions. World J Surg Oncol. 2015;13:329.
7. Xu W, Jiang X, Xu Z, Ye T, Shi Q. The efficacy of Brucea javanica oil emulsion injection as adjunctive therapy for advanced non-small-cell lung Cancer: a meta-analysis. Evid Based Complement Alternat Med. 2016;2016:5928562.
8. Ma S, Chen F, Ye X, Dong Y, Xue Y, Xu H, et al. Intravenous microemulsion of docetaxel containing an anti-tumor synergistic ingredient (Brucea javanica oil): formulation and pharmacokinetics. Int J Nanomedicine. 2013;8:4045–52.
9. Liu TT, Mu LQ, Dai W, Wang CB, Liu XY, Xiang DX. Preparation, characterization, and evaluation of antitumor effect of Brucea javanica oil cationic nanoemulsions. Int J Nanomedicine. 2016;11:2515–29.
10. Yan Z, Zhang B, Huang Y, Qiu H, Chen P, Guo GF. Involvement of autophagy inhibition in Brucea javanica oil emulsion-induced colon cancer cell death. Oncol Lett. 2015;9(3):1425–31.
11. Wang Q, Wang M, He X, Gao T, Cao H, Dou W, et al. Meta-analysis on treatment of non-small cell lung cancer with brucea javanica oil emulsion in combination with platinum-contained first-line chemotherapy. Zhongguo Zhong Yao Za Zhi. 2012;37(13):2022–9.
12. Liu J, Huang XE, Tian GY, Cao J, Lu YY, Wu XY, et al. Phase II study on safety and efficacy of Yadanzi(R) (Javanica oil emulsion injection) combined with chemotherapy for patients with gastric cancer. Asian Pac J Cancer Prev. 2013;14(3):2009–12.
13. Guo Y, Wu J, Yang H, Cao C. Treatment of malignant pleural effusion with Brucea javanica oil emulsion combined with cisplatin intravesical injection (in Chinese). J Oncol. 2004;10(2):129–30.
14. Lei H, Zhao Y, Su L. Treatment of 111 cases of malignant pleural effusion by brucea javanica oil emulsion combined with chemotherapy (in Chinese). Ningxia Med J. 2006;28(5):372–3.
15. Wang H, Liao G, Liu P, Qu Y, Xie G, Liu S. Brucea javanica oil emulsion combined with cisplatin treatment for 70 patients with malignant pleural effusion of lung cancer (in Chinese). Chinese cancer. 2007;16(12):1035–6.
16. Wu S, Rui L, Hong Y. Clinical observation on 68 cases of cancerous pleural effusion treated by brucea javanica oil emulsion combined with cisplatin (in Chinese). Hai Nan Med J. 2009;20(9):14–5.
17. Fu X, Fu S, Yang G, Xue Y, Chen L, Yu S. Observation on the curative effect of continuous drainage combined with brucea javanica oil and cisplatin in the treatment of malignant pleural effusion (in Chinese). Clin J Med Offic. 2009;37(5):818–20.
18. Chen Y. Therapeutic effect of brucea javanica oil emulsion combined with cisplatin in the treatment of malignant pleural effusion (in Chinese). Zhejiang J I T C W M. 2011;21(10):713–4.
19. Jia L, Wang Y, Geng L. Treatment of 35 cases of malignant pleural effusion using brucea javanica oil emulsion combined with oxaliplatin (in Chinese). J Tradit Chin Med. 2011;52(22):1956–7.
20. Liu B, Zhang L. Clinical observation of brucea javanica oil emulsion and cisplatinum on treating lung cancer malignant pleural effussion (in Chinese). China Modern Med. 2012;19(7):47–8
21. Zhang J, Liu X. The results of 28 patients with pleural effusion of lung cancer treated with brucea javanice oil emulsion combined with bleomycin hydrochloride for injection (in Chinese). Pract J Cancer. 2012;27(5):500–2.
22. Zhang H, Jing D, Zhao Y. Treatment of 34 cases of malignant pleural effusion with brucea javanica oil and cisplatin (in Chinese). Modern Distance Education of Chinese Med. 2013;11(5):41–2.
23. Yang G, Song C. Clinical observation of Brucea javanica oil emulsion combined with cisplatin in the treatment of malignant pleural effusion (in Chinese). China Foreign Med Treatment. 2014;13:142–5.
24. Yang H, Wu M. Clinical observation of cisplatin and interleukin-II combined with brucea javanica oil emulsion in the treatment of malignant pleural effusion caused by lung cancer (in Chinese). J Clin Pulmonary Med. 2014; 19(10):1857 62.
25. Yue K. Efficacy of Brucea javanica oil emulsion combined with cisplatin in the treatment of pleural effusion of lung cancer (in Chinese). J Med Theor Prac. 2016;29(9):1164–5.
26. Wang C, Sun C. Thirty cases of lung cancer pleural effusion treated with brucea javanica oil emulsion in combination with cisplatin (in Chinese). Henan Traditional Chinese Med. 2016;36(4):665–6.

27. Biaoxue R, Hua L, Wenlong G, Shuanying Y. Increased serum amyloid a as potential diagnostic marker for lung cancer: a meta-analysis based on nine studies. BMC Cancer. 2016;16(1):836.

28. Jin W, Han H, Zhou S, Wang Y, Dong T, Zhao C. Therapeutic efficacy of brucea javanica oil emulsion (BJOE) combined with transcatheter hepatic arterial chemoembolization (TACE) in patients with primary liver cancer. Int J Clin Exp Med. 2015;8(10):18954–62.

29. Lou GG, Yao HP, Xie LP. Brucea javanica oil induces apoptosis in T24 bladder cancer cells via upregulation of caspase-3, caspase-9, and inhibition of NF-kappaB and COX-2 expressions. Am J Chin Med. 2010;38(3):613–24.

30. Qin LJ, Jia YS, Zhao XQ, Zhang T, Zhang W, Sun N. Effect of Brucea Javanica oil emulsion on the invasiveness of glioma cells and its possible mechanism. Sichuan Da Xue Xue Bao Yi Xue Ban. 2016;47(3):347–50.

31. Yue Y, Yang Y, Shi L, Wang Z. Suppression of human hepatocellular cancer cell proliferation by Brucea javanica oil-loaded liposomes via induction of apoptosis. Arch Med Sci. 2015;11(4):856–62.

32. Anota A, Hamidou Z, Paget-Bailly S, Chibaudel B, Bascoul-Mollevi C, Auquier P, et al. Time to health-related quality of life score deterioration as a modality of longitudinal analysis for health-related quality of life studies in oncology: do we need RECIST for quality of life to achieve standardization? Qual Life Res. 2015;24(1):5–18.

33. Nie YL, Liu KX, Mao XY, Li YL, Li J, Zhang MM. Effect of injection of brucea javanica oil emulsion plus chemoradiotherapy for lung cancer: a review of clinical evidence. J Evid Based Med. 2012;5(4):216–25.

34. Waissbluth S, Peleva E, Daniel SJ. Platinum-induced ototoxicity: a review of prevailing ototoxicity criteria. Eur Arch Otorhinolaryngol. 2017;274(3):1187–96.

35. Biaoxue R, Shuanying Y, Xiguang C, Wei Z, Wei L. Differential diagnostic CYFRA 21-1 level for benign and malignant pleural effusions: a meta-analysis in the Chinese population. Arch Med Sci. 2012;8(5):756–66.

6

Erlotinib treatment after platinum-based therapy in elderly patients with non-small-cell lung cancer in routine clinical practice – results from the ElderTac study

Wolfgang M. Brueckl[1*], H. Jost Achenbach[2], Joachim H. Ficker[1] and Wolfgang Schuette[3]

Abstract

Background: In this prospective non-interventional study, the effectiveness and tolerability of erlotinib in elderly patients with non-small-cell lung cancer (NSCLC) after ≥1 platinum-based chemotherapy were assessed.

Methods: A total of 385 patients ≥65 years of age with advanced NSCLC receiving erlotinib were observed over 12 months. The primary endpoint was the 1-year overall survival (OS) rate.

Results: Patients were predominantly Caucasian (99.2%), a mean of 73 years old; 24.7% had an Eastern Cooperative Oncology Group performance status (ECOG PS) ≥2. Most common tumor histologies were adenocarcinoma (64.9%) and squamous cell carcinoma (22.3%). Of 119 patients tested, 15.1% had an activating epidermal growth factor receptor gene (EGFR) mutation. The 1-year OS rate was 31% (95% CI 25–36) with a median OS of 7.1 months (95% CI 6.0–7.9). OS was significantly better in females than males ($p = 0.0258$) and in patients with an EGFR mutation compared to EGFR wild-type patients ($p = 0.0004$). OS was not affected by age ($p = 0.3436$) and ECOG PS ($p = 0.5364$). Patients with squamous NSCLC tended to live longer than patients with non-squamous EGFR wild-type tumors (median OS: 8.6 vs 5.5 months). Cough and dyspnea improved during the observation period. The erlotinib safety profile was comparable to that in previous studies with rash (45.2%) and diarrhea (22.6%) being the most frequently reported adverse events.

Conclusions: Erlotinib represents a suitable palliative treatment option in further therapy lines for elderly patients with advanced NSCLC. The results obtained under real-life conditions add to our understanding of the benefits and risks of erlotinib in routine clinical practice.

Keywords: Aged, Epidermal growth factor receptor, Non-small-cell lung carcinoma, Second line, Tyrosine kinase inhibitor

Background

Lung cancer is the leading cause of cancer deaths worldwide [1]; about 85% of cases are diagnosed as non-small-cell lung cancer (NSCLC) [2]. The median age of NSCLC patients is 70 years and the disease is usually diagnosed in advanced stages, when curative surgery is no longer feasible [3]. In metastasized disease, first-line chemotherapy is often not successful and the 5-year survival rate is only 4.2% [3]. NSCLC is histologically classified into the major subtypes adenocarcinoma (~ 40%) [4, 5], squamous cell carcinoma (~ 30–40%) [6–9] and large cell carcinoma (~ 5–10%) [9]. Survival has improved for all subtypes in recent years, but the extent of improvement has been higher for adenocarcinoma than squamous tumors [10]. Recurring mutations have been reported in genes coding for epidermal growth factor receptors (EGFR) in 10–40% of adenocarcinomas [11–13], but these mutations are rare in squamous tumors [14]. EGFR mutations can lead to constitutive activation of anti-apoptotic

* Correspondence: Wolfgang.Brueckl@klinikum-nuernberg.de
[1]Department of Respiratory Medicine, Allergology and Sleep Medicine, Paracelsus Medical University Nuernberg, General Hospital Nuernberg, Prof.-Ernst-Nathan-Str. 1, Nuremberg, Germany
Full list of author information is available at the end of the article

and proliferation signaling pathways, which promote cancer progression [15].

EGFR tyrosine kinase inhibitors (TKI) are the preferred first-line treatment for advanced NSCLC with *EGFR* mutations [16, 17], and the EGFR-TKI erlotinib (Roche Pharma, Tarceva®, Basel, Switzerland) is also approved in Europe for treatment of patients with *EGFR* wild-type tumors after failure of at least one prior chemotherapy regimen [18].

Treating NSCLC is challenging because of the advanced age of patients. As EGFR-TKI avoid the systemic side effects of traditional chemotherapy they might be more suitable for treating elderly patients [19]. A large phase-3 trial with erlotinib including 586 younger and 163 elderly patients demonstrated a similar survival and quality of life (QoL) in both age groups, although a somewhat higher toxicity in the elderly was observed [20]. Clinical studies examining the elderly population are limited and often firm conclusions cannot be drawn [21, 22]. In this study (ElderTac: erlotinib in routine clinical practice in elderly patients with NSCLC), we examined the effectiveness and tolerability of erlotinib in elderly NSCLC patients with progressive disease on ≥1 platinum-based chemotherapy in Germany.

Methods
Study design
ElderTac was a multicenter, non-comparative, non-interventional, single-arm surveillance study documenting erlotinib treatment during routine clinical practice in Germany between April 2011 and August 2014. The observation period was 12 months. Information was gathered during examinations by the physician at baseline and after 3, 6, 9, and 12 months.

This study was conducted in accordance with the German Medicines Act (AMG chapter 67, section 6). It was registered with the German Federal Institute for Drugs and Medical Devices (BfArM) and at ClinicalTrials.gov (NCT01535729). Regular monitoring of study documentation in every center was performed by AMS Advanced Medical Services GmbH, Mannheim, Germany.

Patients and treatment
Elderly patients (≥65 years) with advanced or metastatic UICC stage IV NSCLC, confirmed by histological analysis, were recruited. Histological and immunohistochemical analysis was used to distinguish different types of NSCLC. Patients were eligible if they had progressive disease on ≥1 platinum-based chemotherapy treatment. Erlotinib was prescribed to patients in accordance with the terms of the marketing authorization. Specific treatment and diagnostic procedures were at the discretion of the treating physician.

Outcome measurements
The main outcome parameter was the 1-year overall survival (OS) rate. In addition, OS, 1-year progression-free survival (PFS) rate, PFS, objective response rate (ORR), disease control rate (DCR), symptom control, and adverse events (AE) were assessed. The ORR was defined as the proportion of patients with at least a partial response. The DCR was defined as the complete response + partial response + stable disease. Response to treatment was assessed by the investigator using RECIST criteria (version 1.1). AEs were coded by the Medical Dictionary for Regulatory Activities (MedDRA) (version 15.1).

EGFR mutation status
As erlotinib is approved in Europe for second–/third-line therapy of metastatic NSCLC irrespective of *EGFR* mutation status [18], *EGFR* mutation testing was performed at the discretion of the participating centers. *EGFR* testing using sequencing strategies was done by certified molecular pathology departments collaborating with the individual study centers. Results were documented as: not tested, not available, *EGFR* activating mutation or wild-type.

Statistics
To accurately estimate the 1-year OS, 400 patients were considered necessary, assuming a survival rate of 33 ± 4.6%, and using a symmetric 95% confidence interval (CI, calculated using Greenwood's standard error estimate). The survival rate was estimated to be 33% based on publications of four big international studies [23–26]. Other data were analyzed descriptively.

The effectiveness and safety for all patients who received ≥1 dose of erlotinib were analyzed. Continuous and categorical data were described as median (minimum, maximum) and frequencies/percentages, respectively.

Survival was analyzed by Kaplan Meier methodology and survival curves were compared using an unstratified log-rank test. Survival and response data were analyzed overall and in the following subgroups: age (65–69, 70–74, 75–79, ≥80 years or < 75 and ≥ 75 years), *EGFR* mutation (positive or wild type), Eastern Cooperative Oncology Group performance status (ECOG PS) (0, 1, ≥2) and gender. The influence of age, gender and *EGFR* mutation status on the OS was additionally investigated using Cox regression models (considering single and multiple factors). Post-hoc analysis was performed to compare younger with older patients (< 75 or ≥ 75 years) and non-squamous *EGFR* wild-type carcinoma with squamous carcinoma.

No correction for missing data was performed.

Results
Patients
In 102 centers, 465 patients were screened for eligibility. Eighty patients were excluded for the following reasons:

no previous failed platinum-based chemotherapy (33), NSCLC UICC stage IV histology not confirmed (20), < 65 years old (11), erlotinib not administered (9), patient records unavailable (5), lack of informed consent (1) and screening failure (1). In total, 385 patients were included in the analysis. At 3 months, data were available for 380 patients (98.7%). This decreased to 159 patients (41.3%) at 6 months, 80 (20.8%) at 9 months, and 54 (14.0%) at 12 months. The main reason for discontinuation was disease progression (60% patients).

The patients' baseline data are presented in Table 1. The median age was 72 years (range: 62–90 years). The most common tumor histology was adenocarcinoma (64.9%), followed by squamous cell carcinoma (22.3%), and large cell carcinoma (4.2%). EGFR mutation screening was performed in 31% of patients and 15.1% had a positive EGFR mutation status. Although EGFR mutation testing was mainly performed in patients with adenocarcinoma, other histological tumor types cannot be excluded. Thus, we refer to non-squamous EGFR wild-type carcinoma hereafter.

At baseline, 16.6% and 54.5% of patients had an ECOG PS of 0 or 1, respectively, while 24.7% had an ECOG PS ≥2. This did change slightly at the 3-month visit, where 9.1% and 35.6% had an ECOG PS of 0 or 1, respectively. The percentage of patients with an ECOG PS ≥3 was < 3% for the rest of the observation period. The majority of patients had concomitant diseases (86.2%). The main comorbid conditions were chronic obstructive pulmonary disease (33.0%), diabetes mellitus (21.6%), heart failure (8.1%), coronary heart disease/angina pectoris (14.0%), peripheral arterial occlusion disease (10.4%), and stroke (6.8%).

All patients had previously received chemotherapy, mainly based on carboplatin (72.5%) and/or cisplatin (32.2%) (Table 1). Six or more cycles of chemotherapy were completed in 43.3% of patients, and only one cycle was completed in 4.5% of patients. Radiotherapy had been previously administered to 35.8% of patients. Additionally, 24.9% of patients had received previous surgical treatment; 43.8% of these with curative intent.

Treatment
At baseline, 91.7% of patients received the recommended daily dose of 150 mg erlotinib. Erlotinib dose was modified during the study course as follows: 3/6 months: increased in 4/3 patients (1.1/1.9%), reduced in 32/11 patients (8.7/7.1%), interrupted in 20/10 patients (5.4/6.5%), and discontinued in 192/64 patients (35/41.6%) out of 368/154 remaining patients. The main reason for dose reduction was intolerance (3/6 months: 27/6 patients [7.3/3.9%]). The main reason for discontinuation was disease progression (3/6 months: 132/49 patients [35.8/31.8%]).

Table 1 Patient baseline characteristics (N = 385)

Patient characteristics		Patients, n (%)
Age, years	65–69	110 (28.6)
	70–74	140 (36.4)
	75–79	94 (24.4)
	≥ 80	37 (9.6)
	NR	4 (1.0)
Gender	Male	258 (67)
	Female	127 (33)
Ethnicity	Caucasian	382 (99.2)
	Asian	2 (0.5)
	Afro-American	0 (0)
	Other	1 (0.3)
ECOG PS	0	64 (16.6)
	1	210 (54.5)
	2	92 (23.9)
	3	3 (0.8)
	NR	16 (4.2)
Smoking status	Never smoked	91 (23.7)
	Former smoker	198 (51.4)
	Current smoker	77 (20.0)
	NR	19 (4.9)
Tumor histology	Adenocarcinoma	250 (64.9)
	Squamous cell carcinoma	86 (22.3)
	Large cell carcinoma	16 (4.2)
	Bronchoalveolar carcinoma	11 (2.9)
	Adenoid squamous cell carcinoma	10 (2.6)
	Other	12 (3.1)
EGFR mutation status	Tested	119 (30.9)
	Positive	18 (15.1)
	Wild-type	98 (82.4)
	Indefinite	3 (2.5)
Previous chemotherapy	Carboplatin	279 (72.5)
	Cisplatin	124 (32.2)
	Docetaxel	54 (14.0)
	Gemcitabine	96 (24.9)
	Paclitaxel	56 (14.5)
	Vinorelbine	92 (23.9)
	Other	182 (47.3)

EGFR epidermal growth factor receptor gene, ECOG PS Eastern Cooperative Oncology Group performance status, NR not recorded

Effectiveness of erlotinib treatment in elderly patients
Treatment response
Six months after treatment onset in the overall population, 2 of the 127 patients evaluated (1.6%) had a complete

response, 12 (9.4%) had a partial response and 55 (43.3%) had stable disease. In *EGFR* wild-type patients, 1 of the 22 evaluated (3.6%) had a complete response, 1 (3.6%) had a partial response and 9 (40.9%) had stable disease after six months. ORR and DCR at the 3-month and the 6-month visit and treatment responses stratified according to tumor histology are displayed in Table 2.

Survival
Overall, the 1-year OS rate was 31% (95% CI 25–36) with a median OS of 7.1 months (95% CI 6.0–7.9) (Table 2, Fig. 1a). The 1-year PFS rate and the median PFS were 19% (95% CI 15–23) and 3.5 months (95% CI 3.2–4.0), respectively.

The OS curve was significantly affected by gender ($p = 0.0258$), demonstrating 1-year OS rates of 41.8% and 25.4% for females and males, respectively. The log-rank test additionally revealed a significant difference in the OS curves for the subgroup *EGFR* status ($p = 0.0004$, Fig. 1b). In contrast, OS curves were not significantly different between the four age groups ($p = 0.3436$) and the three ECOG PS groups ($p = 0.5364$) (Table 2). Cox regression models with adjustment for single factors showed a significant influence of gender ($p = 0.027$) and *EGFR* status ($p = 0.001$) on OS. Accordingly, females had an almost 30% reduced risk of death compared to males (hazard ratio [HR] 0.717, 95% CI 0.535–0.962). Patients with an *EGFR* mutation had an almost 80% reduced risk of death compared to wild-type patients (HR 0.211, 95% CI 0.083–0.539). In the Cox regression with adjustment for several parameters simultaneously, the association with reduced risk was maintained for positive *EGFR* mutation status ($p = 0.002$, HR 0.177, 95% CI 0.060–0.522). Age did not significantly influence the OS in either analysis (reference 65–74 years, $p > 0.05$).

Patients with squamous NSCLC tended to live longer (median OS: 8.6 months) than patients with documented non-squamous *EGFR* wild-type disease (median OS: 5.5 months) (Table 2; Fig. 1b, c). In addition, patients ≥75 years with non-squamous *EGFR* wild-type carcinoma had a tendency to live longer than their younger counterparts (median OS: 7.93 vs 5.16 months; $p = 0.2895$) (Fig. 1c).

Symptom control
Symptoms were effectively managed during the observation period. At baseline, 41.6% of patients had cough and 44.4% dyspnea of predominantly mild to moderate intensity. Both symptoms improved at follow-up (Fig. 2). Based on the remaining patients under observation at each visit, only ≤2% of the patients had severe cough at each follow-up visit and severe dyspnea was observed in ≤6.45% of the patients during follow-up (Fig. 2). Post-hoc analysis of *EGFR* wild-type patients showed a similar

symptom control compared to the overall population (data not shown).

Safety and tolerability of erlotinib treatment in elderly patients
During the study, 982 AEs were observed in 296 patients (76.9%) (Table 3). According to the common toxicity criteria for adverse events (CTC), 27.3% of patients had AEs of grade ≥ 3. Serious AEs were reported in 29.1% of patients that led to death in 13.0% of patients. The most commonly reported AEs were rash (45.2%) and diarrhea (22.6%), followed by dyspnea, fatigue, and cough. AEs led to permanent treatment discontinuation in 107 patients (27.8%): Main reasons were rash (26 patients, 6.8%), dyspnea (20 patients, 5.2%), and malignant neoplasm progression (17 patients, 4.4%). The frequency of AEs was not significantly affected by age or *EGFR* mutation status (data not shown). All AEs reported were consistent with those described in the summary of product characteristics [18].

Discussion
Few data regarding targeted cancer therapy in pretreated elderly NSCLC patients exist. Available study results in elderly patients with advanced NSCLC treated with erlotinib are summarized in Table 4.

In most studies, patients received erlotinib as first-line treatment [27–29] or the treatment line was not defined [30, 31]. Four studies included exclusively Asian patients [27, 31–33], who are known to have a better outcome with EGFR-TKI treatment compared to Caucasian patients [34]. In the phase-3 trial BR.21, involving 731 patients after progression on ≥1 platinum-based chemotherapy, erlotinib demonstrated prolonged survival [26] and improved QoL compared to placebo [35]. A retrospective subgroup analysis revealed that older (≥70 years) and younger patients had the same survival and QoL benefit, with a somewhat greater toxicity in the elderly [20]. However, the elderly population receiving erlotinib in that study ($n = 112$) [20] was small and a retrospective design involves a greater risk for bias compared with a prospective design.

The ElderTac study was designed to examine the effectiveness and tolerability of erlotinib as a second –/third-line treatment for advanced NSCLC in elderly patients in real life. In accordance with previous findings, females treated with erlotinib lived longer than males [36, 37]. The effectiveness of erlotinib in ElderTac was comparable with that in the BR.21 trial in which median OS/PFS durations of 7.6/3.0 months were observed in elderly patients receiving second- or third-line treatment with erlotinib [20]. Likewise, symptom control – as a surrogate for QoL – was improved in our population, confirming the results of the BR.21 trial [20, 26]. Maintenance of QoL is particularly important in patients

Table 2 Clinical endpoints stratified by patient baseline characteristics for the overall population, in patients with squamous NSCLC, and in patients with non-squamous *EGFR* wild-type tumors

	ORR 3/6 months (%)	DCR 3/6 months (%)	Median PFS (months)	Median OS (months)	1-year OS (%)
		All patients (*N* = 385)			
Overall	5.7/3.6	30.9/17.9	3.5	7.1	30.6
Age (years)					
65–69	4.5/1.8	25.5/12.7	3.3	7.0	26.6
70–74	4.3/2.9	27.1/18.6	3.4	6.6	29.8
75–79	7.4/6.4	42.6/23.4	5.0	7.9	37.2
≥ 80	10.8/5.4	32.4/16.2	2.9	6.0	25.6
< 75[a] (*n* = 250)	4.4/2.4	26.4/16.0	3.3	6.8	28.3
≥ 75[a] (*n* = 131)	8.4/6.1	39.7/21.4	4.0	7.8	34
ECOG PS					
0	6.3/3.1	28.1/17.2	3.3	8.4	37.6
1	6.2/3.3	31.4/16.7	3.5	6.3	29.9
≥ 2	4.2/5.3	33.7/23.2	3.7	7.3	29.1
Gender					
Male	5.8/2.7	31.8/16.7	3.4	6.3	25.4
Female	5.5/5.5	29.1/20.5	4.1	8.1	41.8
Post-hoc analysis: Squamous cell histology (*n* = 86)					
Overall	8.1/1.2	34.9/18.6	3.5	8.6	32.4
Age (years)					
< 75 (*n* = 55)	5.5/1.8	29.1/18.2	3.5	9.5	33.1
≥ 75 (*n* = 30)	13.3/0	43.3/16.7	3.6	7.8	29.1
ECOG PS					
0 (*n* = 12)	8.3/0	50.0/16.7	4.6	8.7	31.4
1 (*n* = 44)	11.4/0	34.1/20.5	3.7	11.2	43.3
≥ 2 (*n* = 27)	3.7/3.7	33.3/18.5	3.5	7.3	19.2
Gender					
Male (*n* = 66)	6.1/1.5	33.3/16.7	3.5	8.6	28.7
Female (*n* = 20)	15.0/0	40.0/25.0	4.4	9.5	44.5
Post-hoc analysis: Non-squamous *EGFR* wild-type (*n* = 91)					
Overall	3.3/2.2	20.9/11.0	3.1	5.5	28.8
Age (years)					
< 75 (*n* = 60)	1.7/0	20.0/8.3	3.1	5.2	22.3
≥ 75 (n = 30)	6.7/6.7	23.3/16.7	3.2	7.9	41.7
ECOG PS					
0 (*n* = 18)	5.6/0	22.5/5.6	2.2	7.0	30.9
1 (*n* = 50)	2.0/2.0	20.0/10.0	2.6	5.5	23.7
≥ 2 (n = 18)	0/5.6	22.2/22.2	4.2	6.8	39.2
Gender					
Male (*n* = 54)	1.9/0	18.5/5.6	2.1	4.7	16.2
Female (*n* = 37)	5.4/5.4	24.3/18.9	5.0	9.3	47.9

[a]post-hoc analysis

EGFR epidermal growth factor receptor gene, *NSCLC* non-small-cell lung cancer, *OS* overall survival, *PFS* progression-free survival, *ORR* objective response rate, *DCR* disease control rate, *ECOG PS* Eastern Cooperative Oncology Group performance status

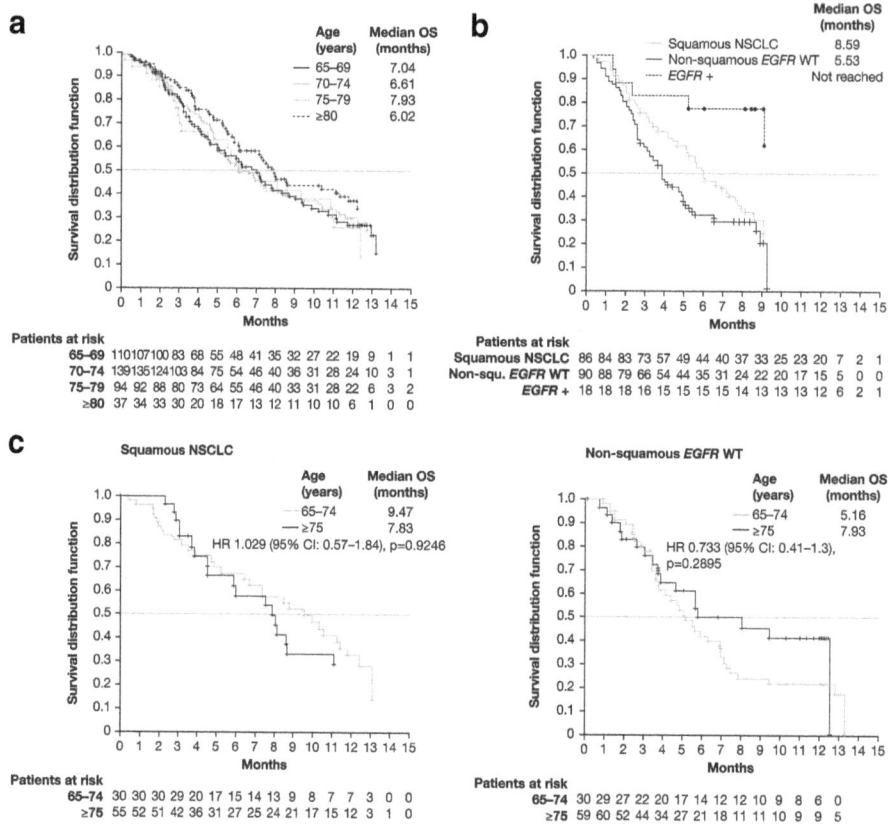

Fig. 1 Kaplan-Meier curves on 1-year overall survival in erlotinib-treated patients. **a)** Overall survival in the whole study population according to prespecified age group. **b)** Overall survival in patients with squamous carcinoma, patients with non-squamous *EGFR* wild-type carcinoma and patients with *EGFR* activating mutations. **c)** Overall survival according to age group (< 75 vs ≥75 years) in patients with squamous carcinoma and in patients with non-squamous *EGFR* wild-type carcinoma. CI, confidence interval; *EGFR*, epidermal growth factor receptor gene; HR, hazard ratio; NSCLC, non-small-cell lung cancer; OS, overall survival; WT, wild-type.

with advanced disease receiving second- or third-line treatment. A recent clinical trial demonstrated a similar efficacy for erlotinib and chemotherapy as a second-line treatment for advanced NSCLC in unselected patients and the authors suggested that second-line treatment should be given on patient preference and individual toxicity-risk profiles [24]. However, this recommendation was based on a patient population with a median age of 59 years [24]. In our study, the median age was 72 years and a quarter of patients had an ECOG PS ≥2. Therefore, we have demonstrated that patients with a low performance status, who are not eligible for further

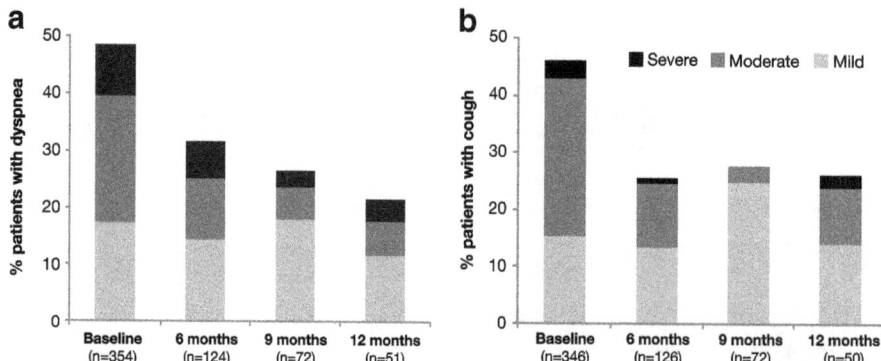

Fig. 2 Occurrence of symptoms during the study period. Percentage of patients with mild, moderate and severe dyspnea (**a**) and cough (**b**) at baseline and 6, 9 and 12 months. Percentages were based on patients remaining in the study at the respective timepoints

Table 3 Overall adverse events (N = 385)

	Patients, n (%)
Patients with ≥1 AE	296 (76.9)
Patients with ≥1 AE CTC grade ≥ 3	105 (27.3)
Patients with ≥1 SAE	112 (29.1)
Treatment discontinuations due to AE	107 (27.8)
Most common AEs (frequency ≥ 5%)	
Rash	174 (45.2)
Diarrhea	87 (22.6)
Dyspnea	66 (17.1)
Fatigue	65 (16.9)
Cough	44 (11.4)
Malignant neoplasm progression	31 (8.1)
Decreased appetite	28 (7.3)
Nausea	24 (6.2)
General physical health deterioration	21 (5.5)
Affected system organ class	
Skin	194 (50.4)
Respiratory system	107 (27.8)
Gastrointestinal system	105 (27.3)
General disorders	99 (25.7)
Infections and infestations	44 (11.4)
Neoplasms	40 (10.4)
Metabolic system	35 (9.1)

AE adverse event, CTC common toxicity criteria, SAE serious adverse event

chemotherapy, can still benefit from erlotinib. The tolerability of erlotinib in our study was consistent with previous clinical findings in elderly and non-elderly populations, with a tolerable toxicity profile and rash and diarrhea being the most frequently reported AEs [20, 26–28, 30, 38]. No new safety signals were observed. Erlotinib therefore represents a potential palliative treatment for elderly patients with advanced NSCLC.

Based on the mode of action, erlotinib is a more effective treatment for *EGFR*-mutated tumors. As expected, patients with an activating *EGFR* mutation had the greatest benefit from erlotinib treatment, in agreement with previous findings [28, 39]. Nonetheless, consistent with the results of two phase-3 trials [40], our response rates show that *EGFR* wild-type patients can also benefit from erlotinib treatment. A systematic review of the literature and metaanalysis revealed a significant improvement in OS with erlotinib versus other management options in patients with *EGFR* wild-type tumors [41]. In contrast, in the TAILOR and DELTA studies, chemotherapy with docetaxel was more effective than erlotinib for second- or third-line treatment of *EGFR* wild-type patients [42, 43]. However, the populations in TAILOR and DELTA are hardly comparable to the ElderTac population: Patients in

TAILOR and DELTA were about six or five years younger and 92.7% or 96.0% of patients had an ECOG PS ≤1, respectively, compared to only 71.2% in ElderTac [42, 43]. Additionally, clinical parameters between the study cohorts in TAILOR were not balanced, as its original concept was not a comparison between erlotinib and docetaxel [42]. In the DELTA study, the subgroup analysis in the unselected population revealed no PFS benefit for docetaxel over erlotinib in patients ≥70 years of age [43], demonstrating that age is an important factor for the treatment decision.

Interestingly, erlotinib-treated patients with squamous tumors tended to live longer than patients with non-squamous *EGFR* wild-type carcinoma, which contradicts previous findings that the prognosis of adenocarcinoma patients is generally better than that of patients with squamous tumors [10]. The finding is unexpected considering the very low *EGFR* mutation rate in squamous tumors but may be explained by *EGFR* gene amplifications frequently found in these tumors [44, 45]. In a phase-4 trial in 1093 patients with metastatic squamous NSCLC, 95% of patients had tumors expressing detectable EGFR and 38% of tumors had a high EGFR expression as confirmed by immunohistochemistry [46]. The LUX-Lung 8 study revealed that the ErbB family blocker afatinib was superior to erlotinib in the treatment of squamous NSCLC [47]. However, the study exclusively included fit patients with an ECOG PS ≤1, and a statistically significant OS benefit for afatinib over erlotinib was only apparent in the subgroup of patients < 65 years of age (HR 0.68, 95% CI 0.55–0.85) but not in patients ≥65 years (HR 0.95, 95% CI 0.76–1.19) [47]. In contrast, our results demonstrate a benefit of erlotinib treatment in older patients (≥65 years) with squamous carcinoma, including unfit patients with an ECOG > 1. A recent case report of a 65-year-old man with *EGFR*-wildtype squamous lung cancer who had an unexpected prolonged response to third-line erlotinib confirms our results [48]. Because genomic alterations have not been comprehensively characterized in squamous tumors, no molecular-targeted therapies have been developed for this NSCLC type so far [45]. Meanwhile, immune checkpoint inhibitors are established first- and/or second-line treatments for NSCLC including squamous tumors [49–52], so that EGFR-TKI will likely move to further therapy lines in patients with squamous *EGFR* wild-type tumors.

A further unexpected result was that older patients with non-squamous *EGFR* wild-type carcinoma (≥75 years) tended to live longer than their younger counterparts. This finding is confirmed by results from a Japanese study with gefitinib in which an age < 75 years was an independent negative factor affecting PFS after EGFR-TKI therapy in patients with advanced NSCLC [53].

Most limitations of our study relate to the nature of a non-interventional trial, especially the lack of a control

Table 4 Overview of studies with erlotinib in elderly patients (≥70 years) with advanced NSCLC

Study	Treatment line	Design	Comparator	Participants	Activating EGFR mutation	Outcomes
Jackman et al. (2007) [28]	First line	Open-label, phase 2	None	N = 80; 95% Caucasian	9/43 patients tested	• Median OS: 10.9 months (95% CI 7.8–14.6) • 1-year survival rate 46% • Well tolerated: most common AEs were rash (79%) and diarrhea (69%)
Chen et al. (2012) [27]	First line	Open-label, randomized, phase 2	Vinorelbine (V)	N = 113; 57 (E) vs. 56 (V); 100% Taiwanese	24/60 patients tested	• Median OS: 17.3 months (E) vs. 22.6 months (V) • Mild toxicities: most frequent treatment-related AEs were rash (64.91%), diarrhea (29.82%), and mouth ulceration (14.04%)
TRUST elderly subgroup [29]	First line	Open-label, phase 4 (subgroup analysis)	None	N = 485; 82% Caucasian; 16% Asian	2/18 patients tested	• Median OS: 7.29 months (95% CI 6.27–8.67), non-Asian population: 7.19 months • 1-year survival rate: 36.6% • Disease control rate 79% (compared with 69% for the overall population; p < 0.0001) • Good tolerability: only 4% had grade ≥ 3 treatment-related AEs, 7% had treatment-related SAEs (compared with 4% of the overall population)
Stinchcombe et al. (2011) [30]	Any	Open-label, randomized, phase 2	Gem, E +Gem	N = 146; 51 (E) vs. 51 E/gem; US study (included ethnicities not reported)	Unknown	• Median OS with E: 5.8 months (95% CI 3.0–8.3) • Acneiform rash with E: 45% • No significant difference in 6-month PFS, OS and toxicity rates among the groups
POLARSTAR [31]	Any	Open-label,phase 4	None	N = 9907a; Age-stratified: 7848 (<75 years), 1911 (75–84 years), 148 (≥85 years); 100% Japanese	Unknown	• Efficacy and incidence of non-hematologic and hematologic toxicities were comparable between age groups
BR.21 Study elderly subgroup [20]	≥Second line	Double-blind, randomized, phase 3 (retrospective subgroup analysis)	Placebo	Erlotinib: 112 (elderly) vs. 376 (young); 9.2% Asian, 90.8% other	15/115 patients tested	• Median OS (elderly vs. young): 7.6 months (elderly) vs. 6.4 months (young): HR 1.02 (95% CI 0.81–1.30) • More overall and severe (grade 3–4) toxicity with erlotinib in elderly vs. younger patients (35% vs 18%; p < 0.001)
Keio Lung Oncology Group Study 001 [33]	≥Second line	Phase 2	None	N = 38; 100% Japanese	13/35 tested	• Median OS: 17.3 months (95% CI 13.3–21.3) • Main AE was skin rash (76%)
Lung Oncology Group in Kyushu (LOGiK-0802) [32]	≥Second line	Phase 2	None	N = 40b; 100% Japanese	10/29 tested	• Median OS: 12.2 months (95% CI 6.1–24.7) • Major toxicities: skin disorders, fatigue, anorexia • 32.5% required dose reduction
ElderTac (present study)	≥Second line	Prospective, non-interventional	None	N = 465c; 99.2% Caucasian	18/119 patients tested	• Median OS: 7.1 months • 1-year survival rate: 30.6% • No new safety signals; most frequently reported AEs were rash (45.2%) and diarrhea (22.6%)

AE adverse event, CI confidence interval, E erlotinib, EGFR epidermal growth factor receptor gene, Gem gemcitabine, NSCLC non-small-cell lung cancer, OS overall survival, PFS progression-free survival, SAE serious adverse event

aSafety analysis population

bAge ≥ 75 years

cAge ≥ 65 years

group and the open-label design. The low rate of *EGFR* mutation testing hampered the comparison of erlotinib effectiveness in a larger group of patients with or without *EGFR* mutations. It, however, reflects the clinical routine in Germany at the time the study was performed, with *EGFR* mutation analysis being done in less than 50% of NSCLC patients [54]. The high rate of treatment discontinuations due to the severely ill patient population might have had an influence on data analysis and interpretation. Furthermore, the results of post-hoc analyses have to be interpreted with caution. Nevertheless, our observational study generated invaluable results for real-life treatment decisions.

Conclusion

We have demonstrated that erlotinib is a suitable palliative treatment option in further therapy lines for elderly patients with recurrent/advanced NSCLC, especially in patients with an activating *EGFR* mutation and squamous histology. Our results were obtained under real-life conditions and therefore demonstrate effectiveness and tolerability of erlotinib in routine clinical practice.

Abbreviations
AE: Adverse event; CI: Confidence interval; DCR: Disease control rate; ECOG PS: Eastern Cooperative Oncology Group performance status; EGFR: Epidermal growth factor receptor; *EGFR*: Epidermal growth factor receptor gene; ElderTac: Erlotinib in routine clinical practice in elderly patients with NSCLC; HR: Hazard ratio; NSCLC: Non-small-cell lung cancer; ORR: Objective response rate; OS: Overall survival; PFS: Progression-free survival; PS: Performance state; QoL: Quality of life; TKI: Tyrosine kinase inhibitor

Acknowledgements
The authors thank all patients and physicians who contributed to the study, which was sponsored by Roche Pharma AG, Grenzach-Wyhlen, Germany. Medical writing assistance was provided by Jutta Walstab, Physicians World Europe GmbH, Mannheim, Germany.

Funding
The study was funded by Roche Pharma AG, Grenzach-Wyhlen, Germany, who provided funding for data analysis and medical writing support.

Authors' contributions
WMB, HJA, JHF and WS made substantial contributions to data acquisition, data interpretation and manuscript revision. WMB, HJA, JHF and WS gave final approval of the version to be published. The authors had complete access to the data that support this publication. WMB, HJA, JHF and WS agreed to be accountable for all content and editorial decisions.

Competing interests
WMB received lecture and consultancy fees from Astra Zeneca, Boehringer Ingelheim, BMS, Lilly, MSD and Roche Pharma. JHF received lecture and consultancy fees from AstraZeneca, Boehringer Ingelheim, Lilly, Novartis, Pfizer, and Roche Pharma. WS declares receiving payments for lectures and consultancy from Roche Pharma. HJA received lecture and consultancy fees, as well as travel support from Bristol-Myers-Squibb, Boehringer Ingelheim, Grifols, Insmed, Lilly, Novartis, PneumRx, and Roche Pharma.

Author details
[1]Department of Respiratory Medicine, Allergology and Sleep Medicine, Paracelsus Medical University Nuernberg, General Hospital Nuernberg, Prof.-Ernst-Nathan-Str. 1, Nuremberg, Germany. [2]Lung Clinic Lostau, Department of Thoracic Oncology, Lindenstr. 2, Lostau, Nuremberg, Germany. [3]Hospital Martha-Maria Halle-Doelau, Klinik für Innere Medizin II, Röntgenstr. 1, Halle, Germany.

References
1. Torre LA, Bray F, Siegel RL, Ferlay J, Lortet-Tieulent J, Jemal A. Global cancer statistics, 2012. CA Cancer J Clin. 2015;65(2):87–108.
2. American Cancer Society: https://www.cancer.org/cancer/non-small-cell-lung-cancer/about/what-is-non-small-cell-lung-cancer.html. Accessed 19 Mar 2018.
3. SEER Cancer Statistics: http://seer.cancer.gov/statfacts/html/lungb.html. Accessed 2 Dec 2015.
4. Travis WD. Pathology of lung cancer. Clin Chest Med. 2011;32(4):669–92.
5. Chang JS, Chen LT, Shan YS, Lin SF, Hsiao SY, Tsai CR, Yu SJ, Tsai HJ. Comprehensive analysis of the incidence and survival patterns of lung Cancer by Histologies, including rare subtypes, in the era of molecular medicine and targeted therapy: a nation-wide Cancer registry-based study from Taiwan. Medicine (Baltimore). 2015;94(24):e969.
6. Jimenez Massa AE, Alonso Sardon M, Gomez Gomez FP. Lung cancer: how does it appear in our hospital? Rev Clin Esp. 2009;209(3):110–7.
7. Kukulj S, Popovic F, Budimir B, Drpa G, Serdarevic M, Polic-Vizintin M. Smoking behaviors and lung cancer epidemiology: a cohort study. Psychiatr Danub. 2014;26(Suppl 3):485–9.
8. Missaoui N, Hmissa S, Landolsi H, Korbi S, Joma W, Anjorin A, Ben Abdelkrim S, Beizig N, Mokni M. Lung cancer in Central Tunisia: epidemiology and clinicopathological features. Asian Pac J Cancer Prev. 2011;12(9):2305–9.
9. Novaes FT, Cataneo DC, Ruiz Junior RL, Defaveri J, Michelin OC, Cataneo AJ. Lung cancer: histology, staging, treatment and survival. J Bras Pneumol. 2008;34(8):595–600.
10. Olszewski AJ, Ali S, Witherby SM. Disparate survival trends in histologic subtypes of metastatic non-small cell lung cancer: a population-based analysis. Am J Cancer Res. 2015;5(7):2229–40.
11. Marchetti A, Martella C, Felicioni L, Barassi F, Salvatore S, Chella A, Camplese PP, Larussi T, Mucilli F, Mezzetti A, et al. EGFR mutations in non-small-cell lung cancer: analysis of a large series of cases and development of a rapid and sensitive method for diagnostic screening with potential implications on pharmacologic treatment. J Clin Oncol. 2005;23(4):857–65.
12. Sugio K, Uramoto H, Ono K, Oyama T, Hanagiri T, Sugaya M, Ichiki Y, So T, Nakata S, Morita M, et al. Mutations within the tyrosine kinase domain of EGFR gene specifically occur in lung adenocarcinoma patients with a low exposure of tobacco smoking. Br J Cancer. 2006;94(6):896–903.
13. Varghese AM, Sima CS, Chaft JE, Johnson ML, Riely GJ, Ladanyi M, Kris MG. Lungs don't forget: comparison of the KRAS and EGFR mutation profile and survival of collegiate smokers and never smokers with advanced lung cancers. J Thorac Oncol. 2013;8(1):123–5.
14. Lopes GL, Vattimo EF, Castro Junior G. Identifying activating mutations in the EGFR gene: prognostic and therapeutic implications in non-small cell lung cancer. J Bras Pneumol. 2015;41(4):365–75.
15. Yarden Y, Sliwkowski MX. Untangling the ErbB signalling network. Nat Rev Mol Cell Biol. 2001;2(2):127–37.
16. Novello S, Barlesi F, Califano R, Cufer T, Ekman S, Levra MG, Kerr K, Popat S, Reck M, Senan S, et al. Metastatic non-small-cell lung cancer: ESMO clinical practice guidelines for diagnosis, treatment and follow-up. Ann Oncol. 2016; 27(suppl 5):v1–v27.
17. Brueckl WM. Treatment choice in EGFR-mutant non-small-cell lung cancer. Lancet Oncol. 2017; https://doi.org/10.1016/S1470-2045(17)30684-8. [Epub ahead of print]
18. Tarceva®. Summary of product characteristics. In: Last updated 12; 2017.
19. Gridelli C, Maione P, Rossi A, Ferrara ML, Castaldo V, Palazzolo G, Mazzeo N. Treatment of advanced non-small-cell lung cancer in the elderly. Lung Cancer. 2009;66(3):282–6.
20. Wheatley-Price P, Ding K, Seymour L, Clark GM, Shepherd FA. Erlotinib for advanced non-small-cell lung cancer in the elderly: an analysis of the National Cancer Institute of Canada clinical trials group study BR.21. J Clin Oncol. 2008;26(14):2350–7.

21. Lewis JH, Kilgore ML, Goldman DP, Trimble EL, Kaplan R, Montello MJ, Housman MG, Escarce JJ. Participation of patients 65 years of age or older in cancer clinical trials. J Clin Oncol. 2003;21(7):1383–9.

22. Vora N, Reckamp KL. Non-small cell lung cancer in the elderly: defining treatment options. Semin Oncol. 2008;35(6):590–6.

23. Karampeazis A, Voutsina A, Souglakos J, Kentepozidis N, Giassas S, Christofillakis C, Kotsakis A, Papakotoulas P, Rapti A, Agelidou M, et al. Pemetrexed versus erlotinib in pretreated patients with advanced non-small cell lung cancer: a Hellenic oncology research group (HORG) randomized phase 3 study. Cancer. 2013;119(15):2754–64.

24. Ciuleanu T, Stelmakh L, Cicenas S, Miliauskas S, Grigorescu AC, Hillenbach C, Johannsdottir HK, Klughammer B, Gonzalez EE. Efficacy and safety of erlotinib versus chemotherapy in second-line treatment of patients with advanced, non-small-cell lung cancer with poor prognosis (TITAN): a randomised multicentre, open-label, phase 3 study. Lancet Oncol. 2012; 13(3):300–8.

25. Reck M, van Zandwijk N, Gridelli C, Baliko Z, Rischin D, Allan S, Krzakowski M, Heigener D. Erlotinib in advanced non-small cell lung cancer: efficacy and safety findings of the global phase IV Tarceva lung Cancer survival treatment study. J Thorac Oncol. 2010;5(10):1616–22.

26. Shepherd FA, Rodrigues Pereira J, Ciuleanu T, Tan EH, Hirsh V, Thongprasert S, Campos D, Maoleekoonpiroj S, Smylie M, Martins R, et al. Erlotinib in previously treated non-small-cell lung cancer. N Engl J Med. 2005;353(2):123–32.

27. Chen YM, Tsai CM, Fan WC, Shih JF, Liu SH, Wu CH, Chou TY, Lee YC, Perng RP, Whang-Peng J. Phase II randomized trial of erlotinib or vinorelbine in chemonaive, advanced, non-small cell lung cancer patients aged 70 years or older. J Thorac Oncol. 2012;7(2):412–8.

28. Jackman DM, Yeap BY, Lindeman NI, Fidias P, Rabin MS, Temel J, Skarin AT, Meyerson M, Holmes AJ, Borras AM et al: Phase II clinical trial of chemotherapy-naive patients > or = 70 years of age treated with erlotinib for advanced non-small-cell lung cancer. J Clin Oncol 2007, 25(7):760–766.

29. Merimsky O, Cheng CK, Au JS, von Pawel J, Reck M. Efficacy and safety of first-line erlotinib in elderly patients with advanced non small cell lung cancer. Oncol Rep. 2012;28(2):721–7.

30. Stinchcombe TE, Peterman AH, Lee CB, Moore DT, Beaumont JL, Bradford DS, Bakri K, Taylor M, Crane JM, Schwartz G et al.: A randomized phase II trial of first-line treatment with gemcitabine, erlotinib, or gemcitabine and erlotinib in elderly patients (age >/=70 years) with stage IIIB/IV non-small cell lung cancer. J Thorac Oncol 2011, 6(9):1569–1577.

31. Yoshioka H, Komuta K, Imamura F, Kudoh S, Seki A, Fukuoka M. Efficacy and safety of erlotinib in elderly patients in the phase IV POLARSTAR surveillance study of Japanese patients with non-small-cell lung cancer. Lung Cancer. 2014;86(2):201–6.

32. Yamada K, Azuma K, Takeshita M, Uchino J, Nishida C, Suetsugu T, Kondo A, Harada T, Eida H, Kishimoto J, et al. Phase II trial of Erlotinib in elderly patients with previously treated non small cell lung Cancer: results of the lung oncology Group in Kyushu (LOGiK-0802). Anticancer Res. 2016;36(6):2881–7.

33. Miyawaki M, Naoki K, Yoda S, Nakayama S, Satomi R, Sato T, Ikemura S, Ohgino K, Ishioka K, Arai D, et al. Erlotinib as second- or third-line treatment in elderly patients with advanced non-small cell lung cancer: Keio lung oncology group study 001 (KLOG001). Mol Clin Oncol. 2017;6(3):409–14.

34. Soo RA, Kawaguchi T, Loh M, Ou SH, Shieh MP, Cho BC, Mok TS, Soong R. Differences in outcome and toxicity between Asian and caucasian patients with lung cancer treated with systemic therapy. Future Oncol. 2012;8(4):451–62.

35. Bezjak A, Tu D, Seymour L, Clark G, Trajkovic A, Zukin M, Ayoub J, Lago S, de Albuquerque Ribeiro R, Gerogianni A, et al. Symptom improvement in lung cancer patients treated with erlotinib: quality of life analysis of the National Cancer Institute of Canada clinical trials group study BR.21. J Clin Oncol. 2006;24(24):3831–7.

36. Cioffi P, Marotta V, Fanizza C, Giglioni A, Natoli C, Petrelli F, Grappasonni I. Effectiveness and response predictive factors of erlotinib in a non-small cell lung cancer unselected European population previously treated: a retrospective, observational, multicentric study. J Oncol Pharm Pract. 2013;19(3):246–53.

37. Van Meerbeeck J, Galdermans D, Bustin F, De Vos L, Lechat I, Abraham I. Survival outcomes in patients with advanced non-small cell lung cancer treated with erlotinib: expanded access programme data from Belgium (the TRUST study). Eur J Cancer Care (Engl). 2014;23(3):370–9.

38. Rosell R, Carcereny E, Gervais R, Vergnenegre A, Massuti B, Felip E, Palmero R, Garcia-Gomez R, Pallares C, Sanchez JM, et al. Erlotinib versus standard chemotherapy as first-line treatment for European patients with advanced EGFR mutation-positive non-small-cell lung cancer (EURTAC): a multicentre, open-label, randomised phase 3 trial. Lancet Oncol. 2012;13(3):239–46.

39. Vale CL, Burdett S, Fisher DJ, Navani N, Parmar MK, Copas AJ, Tierney JF. Should Tyrosine Kinase Inhibitors Be Considered for Advanced Non-Small-Cell Lung Cancer Patients With Wild Type EGFR? Two Systematic Reviews and Meta-Analyses of Randomized Trials. Clin Lung Cancer. 2015;16(3):173–182.e174.

40. Osarogiagbon RU, Cappuzzo F, Ciuleanu T, Leon L, Klughammer B. Erlotinib therapy after initial platinum doublet therapy in patients with EGFR wild type non-small cell lung cancer: results of a combined patient-level analysis of the NCIC CTG BR.21 and SATURN trials. Transl Lung Cancer Res. 2015;4(4):465–74.

41. Jazieh AR, Al Sudairy R, Abu-Shraie N, Al Suwairi W, Ferwana M, Murad MH. Erlotinib in wild type epidermal growth factor receptor non-small cell lung cancer: a systematic review. Ann Thorac Med. 2013;8(4):204–8.

42. Garassino MC, Martelli O, Broggini M, Farina G, Veronese S, Rulli E, Bianchi F, Bettini A, Longo F, Moscetti L, et al. Erlotinib versus docetaxel as second-line treatment of patients with advanced non-small-cell lung cancer and wild-type EGFR tumours (TAILOR): a randomised controlled trial. Lancet Oncol. 2013;14(10):981–8.

43. Kawaguchi T, Ando M, Asami K, Okano Y, Fukuda M, Nakagawa H, Ibata H, Kozuki T, Endo T, Tamura A, et al. Randomized phase III trial of erlotinib versus docetaxel as second- or third-line therapy in patients with advanced non-small-cell lung cancer: docetaxel and Erlotinib lung Cancer trial (DELTA). J Clin Oncol. 2014;32(18):1902–8.

44. Hirsch FR, Varella-Garcia M, Bunn PA Jr, Di Maria MV, Veve R, Bremmes RM, Baron AE, Zeng C, Franklin WA. Epidermal growth factor receptor in non-small-cell lung carcinomas: correlation between gene copy number and protein expression and impact on prognosis. J Clin Oncol. 2003;21(20):3798–807.

45. The Cancer Genome Atlas Research Network. Comprehensive genomic characterization of squamous cell lung cancers. Nature. 2012;489(7417):519–25.

46. Thatcher N, Hirsch FR, Luft AV, Szczesna A, Ciuleanu TE, Dediu M, Ramlau R, Galiulin RK, Balint B, Losonczy G, et al. Necitumumab plus gemcitabine and cisplatin versus gemcitabine and cisplatin alone as first-line therapy in patients with stage IV squamous non-small-cell lung cancer (SQUIRE): an open-label, randomised, controlled phase 3 trial. Lancet Oncol. 2015;16(7): 763–74.

47. Soria JC, Felip E, Cobo M, Lu S, Syrigos K, Lee KH, Goker E, Georgoulias V, Li W, Isla D, et al. Afatinib versus erlotinib as second-line treatment of patients with advanced squamous cell carcinoma of the lung (LUX-lung 8): an open-label randomised controlled phase 3 trial. Lancet Oncol. 2015;16(8):897–907.

48. Gambale E, Carella C, Amerio P, Buttitta F, Patea RL, Natoli C, De Tursi M. Extraordinary and prolonged erlotinib-induced clinical response in a patient with EGFR wild-type squamous lung cancer in third-line therapy: a case report. Int Med Case Rep J. 2017;10:173–5.

49. Rittmeyer A, Barlesi F, Waterkamp D, Park K, Ciardiello F, von Pawel J, Gadgeel SM, Hida T, Kowalski DM, Dols MC, et al. Atezolizumab versus docetaxel in patients with previously treated non-small-cell lung cancer (OAK): a phase 3, open-label, multicentre randomised controlled trial. Lancet. 2017;389(10066):255–65.

50. Reck M, Rodriguez-Abreu D, Robinson AG, Hui R, Csoszi T, Fulop A, Gottfried M, Peled N, Tafreshi A, Cuffe S, et al. Pembrolizumab versus chemotherapy for PD-L1-positive non-small-cell lung Cancer. N Engl J Med. 2016;375(19): 1823–33.

51. Herbst RS, Baas P, Kim DW, Felip E, Perez-Gracia JL, Han JY, Molina J, Kim JH, Arvis CD, Ahn MJ, et al. Pembrolizumab versus docetaxel for previously treated, PD-L1-positive, advanced non-small-cell lung cancer (KEYNOTE-010): a randomised controlled trial. Lancet. 2016;387(10027):1540–50.

52. Brahmer J, Reckamp KL, Baas P, Crino L, Eberhardt WE, Poddubskaya E, Antonia S, Pluzanski A, Vokes EE, Holgado E, et al. Nivolumab versus docetaxel in advanced squamous-cell non-small-cell lung Cancer. N Engl J Med. 2015;373(2):123⁻35.

53. Masago K, Fujita S, Togashi Y, Kim YH, Hatachi Y, Fukuhara A, Nagai H, Sakamori Y, Mio T, Mishima M. Clinicopathologic factors affecting the progression-free survival of patients with advanced non-small-cell lung cancer after gefitinib therapy. Clin Lung Cancer. 2011;12(1):56–61.
54. Bertram M, Petersen V, Heßling J, Tessen HW, Münz M, Jänicke M, Spring L. N M: EGFR mutation testing and treatment with tyrosin-kinase inhibitors in patients with metastatic non-small cell lung cancer treated by office based medical oncologists in Germany - data from the clinical registry on lung cancer (TLK). Oncol Res Treat. 2015;38(suppl 5):V886.

7

Dietary patterns, *BCMO1* polymorphisms, and primary lung cancer risk in a Han Chinese population

Fei He[1,2†], Ren-dong Xiao[3†], Tao Lin[1,2], Wei-min Xiong[1,2], Qiu-ping Xu[1,2], Xu Li[3], Zhi-qiang Liu[1,2], Bao-chang He[1,2], Zhi-jian Hu[1,2] and Lin Cai[1,2*]

Abstract

Background: We investigated whether *BCMO1* variants and dietary patterns are associated with lung cancer risk.

Methods: Case-control study including 1166 lung cancer cases and 1179 frequency matched controls was conducted for three *BCMO1* variants (rs6564851, rs12934922, and rs7501331) and four dietary patterns were investigated. Logistic regression was used to estimate odds ratios (ORs) and 95% confidence intervals (95% CIs).

Results: The rs6564851, rs12934922, and rs7501331 were not found to be associated with lung cancer risk ($P > 0.05$). In multivariable-adjusted models, compared to the lowest quartile of the score on the "fruits and vegetables" pattern, the highest quintile was associated with a 78.4% decreased risk (OR $_{Q4\ vs.\ Q1}$ = 0.216; 95% CI, 0.164–0.284; P for trend < 0.001). Other patterns were not found the association. The "fruits and vegetables" pattern was associated with a reduced risk of lung cancer with all 3 SNPs irrespective of genotypes (all P for trend< 0.001). The association for the "Frugal" pattern was associated with increased risk of lung cancer among smokers (P for interaction = 0.005). The protective effects of the "cereals/wheat and meat" pattern was more evident for squamous cell carcinoma and other histological type.

Conclusions: We did not observe associations of *BCMO1* variants and lung cancer. Diets rich in fruits and vegetables may be protective against lung cancer.

Keywords: Dietary patterns, *BCMO1* polymorphisms, Primary lung cancer, Chinese, Case-control study

Background

The International Agency for Research on Cancer reported a lung cancer incidence rate of 23.1/100,000 and a lung cancer mortality rate of 19.7/100,000 for 2012 [1]. Although China does not yet have a well-established cancer registry system, the data available for 2015 indicate that lung cancer is the most common and most deadly cancer in China [2]. Because of the poor prognosis and often aggressive nature of lung cancer, the 5-year overall survival rate for lung cancer is only 10–15%, putting a heavy burden on patients, patient's families, and governments [3]. Although tobacco smoking is the most salient cause of lung cancer, several other risk factors may contribute to the disease [4, 5].

It has been reported that about a third of all tumors may related to dietary factors [6]. Currently, most studies that have examined the influence of dietary factors on lung cancer risk have focused on a single food or a limited combination of certain foods or nutrients, and their results have not been consistent [7–10]. However, generally, people do not consume single foods or nutrients. Moreover, different categories of foods and nutrients may have interactions with one another. Hence, exploring specific foods and nutrients in isolation is not representative of real-life diets.

* Correspondence: x117x@163.com
†Equal contributors
[1]Department of Epidemiology, School of Public Health, Fujian Medical University, Fuzhou 350108, China
[2]Key Laboratory of Ministry of Education for Gastrointestinal Cancer, Fujian Medical University, Fuzhou 350108, China
Full list of author information is available at the end of the article

Consequently, researchers have become interested in examining the influence of dietary patterns and holistic dietary status on lung cancer risk [11–18]. Although the findings are uncertain, they argue that a diet with high vegetable is related with a reduced risk of lung cancer [19], while a high fat and red meat diet is related with increased risk. However, most of these studies were conducted outside of China, where eating habit vary greatly across different regions. Examination of the possible influence of Chinese dietary patterns on lung cancer is lacking.

Importantly, any observed correlation between dietary patterns and lung cancer could be related to other factors, such as smoking, social-economic status, and physical activity [19]. Although intake of vegetables and fruits has been suggested to reduce the risk of lung cancer [10], β-carotene (BC)—a retinal (form of vitamin A) precursor found in many edible plants—has been suggested to increase the risk of lung cancer in smokers [7], perhaps due to a complex gene-diet interaction. In this regard, Tu and colleagues suggested recently that the association between dietary patterns and lung cancer risk may be modified by genetic background [17].

Dietary BC is cleaved into two retinal molecules by β-carotene-15,15′-monooxygenase (BCMO1) [20]. Single nucleotide morphisms (SNPs) of the human *BCMO1* gene, which is located on chromosome 16, have been reported to influence blood concentrations of BC, suggesting that *BCMO1* SNPs may affect the efficiency of BC transformation into vitamin A in vivo [21]. If so, then it is possible that *BCMO1* SNPs may also influence the effects of dietary patterns on lung cancer risk. To test this hypothesis, we conducted a case-control study to explore the potential influence of three *BCMO1* SNPs, namely rs6564851, rs12934922, and rs7501331, on the association between dietary patterns and lung cancer risk in a case-control study of ethnic Han Chinese participants.

Methods

Study subjects

We recruited 1166 patients with newly diagnosed (the time of cancer diagnosis and the time of enrolling into the study was the same) primary lung cancer (cases) from three area hospitals (The First Clinical Medical College of Fujian Medical University, The Affiliated Union Hospital of Fujian Medical University and Fuzhou General Hospital) between July 2006 and February 2013 and the participate rate for patients was 96.20%. The non-responders included 32 male and 14 female, average age was 58.93 ± 15.44 years, so there were no differences between the responders and non-responders. One thousand one hundred seventy-nine gender- and age-matched healthy controls (±2 years) randomly selected from the community between July 2006 and February 2013. Individuals who were direct relatives to the cases or had a previous history of

cancer were excluded. The rate for control subjects was 90.01%. The non-responders included 92 male and 39 female, average age was 59.66 ± 12.17 years, so there were no differences between the responders and non-responders. All cases and controls were Fujian Province residents. This study was approved by the Institutional Review Board of Fujian Medical University (Fuzhou, China) and all participants signed informed consent forms ([2014] Fu Yi Ethics Review (No. 98)).

Data collection

All epidemiological data were obtained by in-person interviews with a standardized questionnaire, which collected information on demographic characteristics, disease and family cancer history, food, tobacco use, tea and wine consumption, environmental tobacco exposure. Using the inquiry method for surveying dietary habits, respondents recalled their average frequency of consumption of foods (grams per day) in last year (the year prior to study enrolment for all objects) for a variety food items including cereals/wheat, potatoes, meat (pork, beef, mutton, poultry), eggs, seafood (fish, shellfish, snails, salted fish), kelp and seaweed, beans (soy products, dried beans), milk, fruits, vegetables, salted vegetables. The questionnaire has been shown to be a valid and reliable food frequency survey tool across various populations [22–24].

Smokers were defined as individuals who had smoked at least 100 cigarettes during their lifetime. Environmental tobacco smoke (ETS) was defined as exposure to ETS at home and/or at work for more than 15 min per day. Drinking alcohol was defined as drinking at least once a week for more than half a year. Drinking tea was defined as drinking at least 1 cup a week for more than half a year. A 5-ml non-fasting blood sample was collected from each participant for genotyping.

Selection of SNPs

We selected three common (minor allele frequency > 5%) SNPs for analysis, namely rs6564851, rs12934922, and rs7501331. Two of these (rs12934922 and rs7501331) are non-synonymous mutations, identified as yielding a 57% reduction in the catalytic activity of BCMO1 ($P < 0.001$) [25]. The third SNP, rs6564851, was identified by a genome-wide association study, wherein it was associated with elevated plasma β-carotene and low plasma lutein [26].

Genotyping

Genomic DNA was extracted from the blood samples with a protease K digestion and phenol-chloroform extraction and purification system according to standard procedures. The genomic DNA was stored at − 20 °C until being subjected to SNP genotyping with the Sequenom platform according to the manufacturer's iPLEX

Application Guide (Sequenom, Inc., San Diego, CA). The samples were scanned through a matrix assisted laser desorption ionization-time of flight mass spectrometry system and genotyped with a MassArrayTyper 3.4 (Sequenom Inc. San Diego, CA). Approximately 10% of the samples (randomly selected) were re-run for quality control purposes. Genotyping call rates were > 90% and the concordance rate reached 99.5%.

Statistical methods

Descriptive statistics were performed to characterize the study subjects. In the preliminary stage of statistical analysis, the chi-square test was employed to examine differences in demographic variables between cases and controls.

We identified dietary patterns using principal components factor analysis based on responses to the baseline questionnaire. We designated 11 food items. Using the food frequency survey, we collected information about the types and quantities of dietary intake from all subjects for the past year (i.e., the 12 months before the survey was administered). We standardized the quantity values to a mean of 0 and a standard deviation (SD) of 1.0. Each of the standardized quantity variables were entered in the factor analysis; based on inspection of scree plots, eight factors were retained. The factors were rotated using the quartimax procedure to facilitate interpretability of the factors. Factor scores were categorized into quartiles based on the sex-specific distribution in the control group.

The associations between each factor and the risk of lung cancer were estimated by calculating the crude and adjusted odds ratio (OR) for confounders and a 95% confidence interval (CI) with unconditional logistic regressions for factor scores on each of the four factors, the multivariate models adjusted for potential confounders based on a priori knowledge. And we also investigated the associations between dietary patterns and lung cancer risk striated by smoking status and SNP of interest. To detect trends, we entered the factor scores into the model as continuous terms. A two-tailed p-value less than 0.05 was considered to be statistically significant. All statistical analyses were performed in the R software package (v. 3.3.1).

Results

Characteristics of study subjects

The demographic characteristics and risk factors for cases ($N = 1166$) and controls ($N = 1179$) are summarized in Table 1. A lower BMI ($P < 0.001$), lower income ($P = 0.031$), tobacco smoking (OR = 2.451; 95% CI, 2.075–2.894), and ETS exposure (OR = 2.859; 95% CI, 2.412–3.388), together with family cancer history (OR = 1.373, 95% CI, 1.105–1.706) and lung disease history (OR = 1.697; 95% CI, 1.301–2.214) were associated with lung cancer. In contrast, a high educational background

emerged as a protective factor against lung cancer ($P < 0.001$). Additionally, different occupations had different associated risks for lung cancer ($P < 0.001$).

SNP effects on lung cancer risk

The genotype frequencies for all three SNPs examined conformed to the Hardy-Weinberg equilibrium (HWE) in the control group ($P_{controls} = 0.09$–0.88). The genotype frequency data for these SNPs in the case and control groups are reported in Table 2 with the corresponding ORs for lung cancer. Neither the rs6564851, rs12934922, nor rs7501331 variant genotypes of *BCMO1* were found to be associated with lung cancer risk, with or without controlling for the effects of potentially confounding factors.

Dietary patterns analysis

Before rotation, the four primary dietary pattern factors identified by our principal components factor analysis explained 49.53% of the variance in cases and controls. The foods and factor weightings for each factor are shown in Additional file 1: Table S1. For the first factor, the highest factor weight was concentrated in high quality protein, such as seafood, kelp and seaweed, egg and beans. The second factor was milk, fruits and vegetables. The most heavily weighted foods in the third factor were traditional pattern, including cereals/wheat and meat. Sweet potato and salty vegetables were the highest weighted contributors to the fourth factor. The four dietary patterns were named "high quality protein", "fruits and vegetables", "cereals/wheat and meat" and "frugal pattern". All patterns complied with the dietary characteristic and traditions of the Fujian people in China, indicating that the factors captured distinct sources of local dietary variation.

Baseline characteristics of all subjects by quartile (Q) of factor score

The characteristics of the individuals associated with each of the four dietary patterns are summarized in Additional file 2: Table S2. Relative to the other participants, people with a sea food-dominant diet (high quality protein pattern) were younger, were more likely to be college graduates, exposure to less ETS and consumed more tea. Meanwhile, those with the fruits and vegetables pattern were associated with higher education background, and to have more frequent exposure to smoking, increased tea intake, and decreased ETS. High scores for cereals/wheat and meat pattern were younger, with adenocarcinoma, more common in female than male and were associated with family history of lung cancer, decreased tobacco and tea use, and increased ETS. The frugal pattern was associated with a lower education level and income, and greater ETS exposure.

Table 1 Distribution of selected variables among cases and controls

Variables	Case (%) (n = 1166)	Control (%) (n = 1179)	P value	OR (95% CI)
Age (yrs.) mean ± SD	58.28 ± 11.28	59.19 ± 10.78	0.149	
< 50	223(19.1)	264(22.4)		1
51–69	739(63.4)	716(60.7)		1.222 (0.995–1.501)
≥ 70	204(17.5)	199(16.9)		1.214 (0.932–1.581)
Income(yuan/month)				
≤ 3500	797(67.6)	836(71.7)	0.031	1
> 3500	382 (32.4)	330 (28.3)		0.824 (0.690–0.982)
Gender			0.542	
Male	842 (72.2)	838 (71.1)		1
Female	324 (27.8)	341 (28.9)		0.946 (0.790–1.132)
Education			< 0.001	
Illiteracy	185(15.9)	133(11.3)		1
Middle school and below	686(58.8)	647(54.9)		0.762 (0.595–0.976)
High school and above	295(25.3)	399(33.8)		0.532 (0.406–0.696)
Marital status			0.15	
Married	1099(94.3)	1094(92.8)		1
Single	67(5.7)	85(7.2)		0.785(0.564–1.092)
Occupation			< 0.001	
Worker	266(22.8)	297(25.2)		1
Farmer	333(28.6)	245(20.8)		1.518 (1.201–1.917)
Enterprises and employees	321(27.5)	433(36.7)		0.828 (0.665–1.031)
Cook	18(1.5)	9(0.8)		2.233 (0.986–5.055)
Others	228(19.6)	195(16.5)		1.305 (1.014–1.681)
Family history of lung cancer			0.004	
No	942(80.8)	1005(85.2)		1
Yes	224(19.2)	174(14.6)		1.373(1.105–1.706)
History of lung diseases			< 0.001	
No	1009(86.5)	1080(91.6)		1
Yes	157(13.5)	99(8.4)		1.697(1.301–2.214)
BMI (kg/m^2)			< 0.001	
18.5–23.9	720(61.9)	638(54.5)		1
< 18.5	133(11.4)	51(4.4)		2.311(1.645–3.246)
≥ 24	311(26.7)	481(41.1)		0.573(0.479–0.685)
Tea			0.729	
No	578(49.6)	576(48.9)		1
Yes	588(50.4)	603(51.1)		0.972(0.826–1.143)
Alcohol			0.353	
No	884(75.8)	913(77.4)		1
Yes	282(24.2)	266(22.6)		1.095(0.904–1.326)
Smoking			< 0.001	
No	427(36.6)	691(58.6)		1
Yes	739(63.4)	488(41.4)		2.451(2.075–2.894)

Table 1 Distribution of selected variables among cases and controls *(Continued)*

Variables	Case (%) (n = 1166)	Control (%) (n = 1179)	P value	OR (95% CI)
ETS			< 0.001	
No	348(29.8)	647(54.9)		1
Yes	818(70.2)	532(45.1)		2.859(2.412–3.388)
Histology				
Adenocarcinoma	551(47.3)			
Squamous cell carcinoma	324(27.8)			
Others	290(24.9)			

Associations of dietary pattern and lung cancer risk

Multivariable-adjusted associations of dietary patterns with lung cancer risk are presented in Table 3. In multivariable-adjusted models, compared to the lowest quartile of the score on the "fruits and vegetables" pattern, the highest quintile was associated with a 78.4% decreased risk and dose-response relationship (OR $_{Q4}$ vs. $_{Q1}$ = 0.216; 95% CI, 0.164–0.284; P for trend < 0.001). Other patterns were not found the association. The stratified associations by histological type of lung cancer is also summarized in Table 3. The "fruits and vegetables" pattern was associated with risks of all histological types. The protective effects of the "cereals/wheat and meat" pattern was more evident for squamous cell carcinoma and other histological type.

Stratified associations by smoking status

The negative association of the "fruits and vegetables" pattern with lung cancer risk was present among never or smokers, and the P for interaction was 0.002. The "Cereals/wheat and meat" pattern was associated with an increased risk of lung cancer among never smokers and a decreased risk of lung cancer among smokers, with the P for interaction (< 0.001) was statistically significant. The association for the "Frugal" pattern was associated with increased risk of lung cancer among smokers (P for interaction = 0.005). The association for the "High quality protein" pattern did not differ by smoking status (P for interaction = 0.570) (Table 4).

Stratified associations by BCMO1 loci

The stratified associations of dietary patterns with lung cancer risk by *BCMO1* genotype at 3 SNPs are summarized in Table 5. The "fruits and vegetables" pattern was associated with a reduced risk of lung cancer with all 3 SNPs irrespective of genotypes and a dose-response relationship (all P for trend< 0.001). In contrast, the "High quality protein" pattern was associated with an increased

Table 2 Distribution of *BCMO1* single nucleotide polymorphisms and their associations with lung cancer

Locus	Case (n = 1166)	Control (n = 1179)	Unadjusted OR 95% CI	Adjusted OR* 95% CI	P_{trend} value
rs6564851(P_{HWE} = 0.57)	1097	1102			0.729
GG	743 (67.7%)	724 (65.7%)	1	1	
GT	310 (28.3%)	342 (31.0%)	0.883 (0.734–1.062)	0.922 (0.754–1.128)	
TT	44 (4.0%)	36 (3.3%)	1.191 (0.758–1.872)	1.311 (0.805–2.134)	
GT + TT	354 (32.3%)	378 (34.3%)	0.913 (0.764–1.090)	0.959 (0.791–1.163)	
rs12934922(P_{HWE} = 0.88)	1121	1146			0.672
AA	839 (74.8%)	861 (75.1%)	1	1	
AT	261 (23.3%)	264 (23.0%)	1.015 (0.834–1.234)	0.955 (0.772–1.182)	
TT	21 (1.9%)	21 (1.8%)	1.026 (0.556–1.893)	0.813 (0.424–1.561)	
AT+TT	282 (25.2%)	285 (24.8%)	1.015 (0.840–1.228)	0.944 (0.768–1.160)	
rs7501331(P_{HWE} = 0.09)	1060	1084			0.117
CC	707 (66.7%)	696 (64.2%)	1	1	
CT	308 (29.1%)	334 (30.8%)	0.908 (0.753–1.094)	0.862 (0.704–1.056)	
TT	45 (4.2%)	54 (5.0%)	0.820 (0.545–1.235)	0.829 (0.531–1.294)	
CT + TT	353 (33.3%)	388 (35.8%)	0.896 (0.749–1.070)	0.858 (0.707–1.041)	

*adjusted by incomes, occupation, education, family history of lung cancer, history of lung diseases, environmental tobacco smoke, smoking status, BMI

Table 3 Associations between dietary patterns by quartile (Q) and lung cancer risk by histological types

Dietary pattern	Controls	Adenocarcinoma		Squamous cell carcinoma		Others		All	
		N	adjusted OR*(95% CI)	N	adjusted OR*(95% CI)	N	adjusted OR*(95% CI)	N	adjusted OR*(95% CI)
High quality protein									
Q1(low)	294	126	1	74	1	77	1	277	1
Q2	296	130	1.119 (0.824–1.520)	85	1.250 (0.856–1.824)	75	1.068 (0.735–1.552)	290	1.141 (0.891–1.460)
Q3	295	142	1.196 (0.883–1.618)	88	1.341 (0.920–1.954)	62	0.906 (0.615–1.336)	292	1.134 (0.885–1.452)
Q4(high)	294	153	1.400 (0.999–1.890)	77	1.254 (0.853–1.845)	76	1.192 (0.820–1.734)	306	1.283 (0.999–1.643)
P for trend			0.170		0.406		0.785		0.063
Fruits and vegetables									
Q1(low)	294	283	1	160	1	160	1	603	1
Q2	295	121	0.439 (0.332–0.581)	79	0.513 (0.365–0.720)	61	0.398 (0.280–0.565)	261	0.447 (0.354–0.566)
Q3	296	85	0.282 (0.208–0.384)	51	0.330 (0.225–0.484)	40	0.247 (0.166–0.369)	176	0.285 (0.221–0.368)
Q4(high)	294	62	0.213 (0.152–0.298)	34	0.235 (0.152–0.363)	29	0.188 (0.120–0.295)	125	0.216 (0.164–0.284)
P for trend			< 0.001		< 0.001		< 0.001		< 0.001
Cereals/wheat and meat									
Q1(low)	294	117	1	92	1	84	1	293	1
Q2	295	146	1.149 (0.847–1.561)	93	0.848 (0.592–1.215)	78	0.820 (0.569–1.182)	317	0.973 (0.759–1.246)
Q3	296	127	0.920 (0.673–1.257)	83	0.816 (0.565–1.179)	70	0.744 (0.512–1.081)	280	0.846 (0.658–1.086)
Q4(high)	294	164	1.179 (0.871–1.597)	56	0.534 (0.358–0.796)	58	0.588 (0.397–0.872)	278	0.831 (0.645–1.070)
P for trend			0.342		0.012		0.021		0.230
Frugal pattern									
Q1(low)	294	126	1	75	1	63	1	264	1
Q2	296	117	0.857 (0.627–1.171)	72	0.841 (0.569–1.243)	66	0.951 (0.638–1.417)	255	0.873 (0.675–1.129)
Q3	295	118	0.827 (0.605–1.131)	81	0.894 (0.610–1.311)	73	1.022 (0.690–1.514)	272	0.897 (0.695–1.159)
Q4(high)	294	190	1.337 (0.998–1.790)	96	1.029 (0.710–1.491)	88	1.216 (0.831–1.779)	374	1.235(0.966–1.581)
P for trend			0.050		0.791		0.267		0.073

*adjusted by incomes, occupation, education, family history of lung cancer, history of lung diseases, environmental tobacco smoke, smoking status, BMI

risk of lung cancer only among those with one copy of the minor allele of rs6564851 (OR $_{Q4\ vs.\ Q1}$ = 1.870; 95% CI,1.206–2.900; P for trend = 0.001; P for interaction = 0. 019). The "Frugal" pattern was associated with an increased risk of lung cancer among those with the wild genotype at rs6564851 and rs7501331 (P for trend < 0. 05). No statistically significant were found between "Cereals/wheat and meat" patterns and all 3 SNPs (Table 5).

Discussion

In this study, we did not observe any associations of SNPs in *BCMO1* with lung cancer or dietary pattern related to lung cancer in a case-control study of 2345 unrelated Fujian Han Chinese participants. Because of the lack of linkage disequilibrium, we could not construct a haplotype of the three examined SNPs. Our factor analysis yielded four dietary patterns based on traditional Fujian dietary habits. The results of our analysis of baseline characteristics and lung cancer risk suggest that a diet rich in fruits and vegetables may be protective against lung cancer and the "cereals/wheat and meat"

pattern was associated with a reduced risk and the protective effects were more evident for squamous cell carcinoma and other histological types and among smokers. In contrast, the "Frugal pattern" pattern was associated with an increased risk and the harmful effects were more pronounced for smokers. Finally, for the first time, we found that the effects of the "high quality protein" pattern was further modified by rs6564851.

Because BC, which is ubiquitous in edible plants, and BC metabolites have important biological functions, BC is generally considered to be a health promoting compound. However, lung exposure to BC in Bcmo1$^{-/-}$ mice has been reported to alter gene expression in a manner that augments the Gene Ontology terms "oncogenes", "cell proliferation", and "cell cycle". BC has also been reported to have adverse effects on lung tissues in human subjects, including increasing the risk of lung cancer [21, 27, 28]. BC absorption and conversion into retinal is extremely variable across individuals, with as many 45% of the people being classified as low responders to dietary BC [29]. Two *BCMO1* coding-

Table 4 Associations between dietary patterns by quartile (Q) and lung cancer risk by smoking status

Dietary pattern	Never smokers		Smokers	
	Cases/controls	Adjusted OR*(95% CI)	Cases/controls	Adjusted OR*(95% CI)
High quality protein				
Q1(low)	104/172	1	173/122	1
Q2	102/177	1.085 (0.753–1.563)	189/119	1.226 (0.865–1.737)
Q3	108/169	1.244 (0.864–1.790)	184/126	1.151 (0.813–1.631)
Q4(high)	113/173	1.397 (0.972–2.008)	193/121	1.310 (0.924–1.857)
P for trend		0.053		0.187
Fruits and vegetables				
Q1(low)	239/154	1	364/140	1
Q2	88/165	0.365 (0.258–0.517)	173/130	0.529 (0.383–0.730)
Q3	53/184	0.180 (0.121–0.266)	123/112	0.410 (0.289–0.580)
Q4(high)	47/188	0.159 (0.106–0.239)	79/106	0.270 (0.184–0.395)
P for trend		< 0.001		< 0.001
Cereals/wheat and meat				
Q1(low)	85/189	1	208/105	1
Q2	82/167	1.136 (0.774–1.666)	229/128	0.827 (0.588–1.164)
Q3	120/168	1.351 (0.935–1.951)	161/128	0.556 (0.392–0.794)
Q4(high)	137/167	1.517 (1.053–2.184)	141/127	0.463 (0.322–0.666)
P for trend		0.016		< 0.001
Frugal pattern				
Q1(low)	117/163	1	147/131	1
Q2	94/176	0.661 (0.458–0.956)	161/120	1.142 (0.799–1.633)
Q3	90/177	0.620(0.428–0.898)	182/118	1.278 (0.895–1.824)
Q4(high)	126/175	0.865 (0.607–1.232)	249/119	1.713 (1.215–2.416)
P for trend		0.436		0.002

*adjusted by incomes, occupation, education, family history of lung cancer, history of lung diseases, ETS and BMI

region SNPs examined in this study (rs12934922 and rs7501331) were shown previously to result in reduced BCMO1 catalytic activity, confirming that these variants at least contribute to a low-responder phenotype. In vitro biochemical characterization of a double mutant BCMO1 protein encoded by recombinant gene carrying bot the rs12934922 and rs7501331 SNPs indicated that the double mutation reduced catalytic activity of BCMO1 by 57% ($P < 0.001$) [25]. Meanwhile, the homozygous rs6564851 genotype of BCMO1 has been reported to result in a 48% reduction in the catalytic activity of BCMO1 as reflected by in vivo plasma level data in adult female human volunteers [29].

We speculated that efficiency-reducing BCMO1 SNPs would allow accumulation of BC in vivo, which may support uncontrolled proliferation of lung cells. Our hypothesis that the low BC→retinal efficiency BCMO1 variant genotypes would thus be associated with lung cancer risk was not supported by the present results. Although the sample size of the current study is not small, the association of BCOM1 polymorphisms can be

examined with a larger study with a more comprehensive genotyping on BCOM1 gene. This study was the first, to our knowledge, to examine the relationship between these variants and lung cancer directly. A prior Italian genome-wide association study did reveal an association between rs6564851 and higher than average BC levels, but the authors expected it would nonetheless be associated with a lower risk of cancer [26]. In our study, we observed that the effects of the "high quality protein" pattern was further modified by rs6564851. It showed there may have been some genetic mechanisms need to explore.

Notably, this study had the strength of employing dietary pattern analysis, which can better reveal dietary habit interactions and health benefits than studies of isolated nutrients. The results of a recent meta-analysis suggest that a healthful dietary pattern (a.k.a. a prudent pattern)—characterized by a high intake of vegetables, fruits, white meat, fish, and whole-grain breads and a low intake of red meat, fatty foods, and refined grains—is associated with a reduced lung cancer risk, and thus

Table 5 Associations between dietary patterns and lung cancer risk by genotype at 3 SNPs

Dietary patterns	Cases/controls rs6564851:GG	Adjusted OR (95% CI)	Cases/controls rs6564851:GT + TT	Adjusted OR (95% CI)	P for interaction
High quality protein		$P_{trend} = 0.655$		$P_{trend} = 0.001$	0.019
Q1(low)	186/169	1.00(ref)	80/111	1.00(ref)	
Q2	195/180	1.112 (0.807–1.531)	76/99	1.186 (0.758–1.855)	
Q3	176/184	0.999 (0.722–1.381)	97/82	1.869 (1.200–2.910)	
Q4(high)	186/191	1.120 (0.811–1.547)	98/86	1.870 (1.206–2.900)	
Fruits and vegetables		$P_{trend} < 0.001$		$P_{trend} < 0.001$	0.792
Q1(low)	386/186	1.00(ref)	181/91	1.00(ref)	
Q2	162/182	0.413 (0.304–0.559)	82/94	0.511 (0.339–0.770)	
Q3	114/176	0.300 (0.216–0.416)	53/99	0.280 (0.179–0.437)	
Q4(high)	81/180	0.217 (0.153–0.309)	38/94	0.227 (0.140–0.367)	
Cereals and meat		$P_{trend} = 0.036$		$P_{trend} = 0.541$	0.1
Q1(low)	188/165	1.00(ref)	89/119	1.00(ref)	
Q2	203/191	0.857 (0.622–1.181)	91/85	1.230 (0.797–1.899)	
Q3	170/185	0.726 (0.523–1.008)	92/89	1.163 (0.757–1.787)	
Q4(high)	182/183	0.729 (0.525–1.012)	82/85	1.163 (0.748–1.809)	
Frugal pattern		$P_{trend} = 0.028$		$P_{trend} = 0.445$	0.371
Q1(low)	165/192	1.00(ref)	83/86	1.00(ref)	
Q2	173/183	1.016 (0.734–1.408)	59/95	0.569 (0.354–0.915)	
Q3	174/176	1.053 (0.759–1.461)	85/93	0.785 (0.499–1.234)	
Q4(high)	231/173	1.423 (1.036–1.956)	127/104	1.034 (0.672–1.592)	
	rs12934922:AA		rs12934922:AT+TT		
High quality protein		$P_{trend} = 0.065$		$P_{trend} = 0.119$	0.69
Q1(low)	203/213	1.00(ref)	65/79	1.00(ref)	
Q2	209/221	1.132 (0.844–1.519)	72/64	1.400 (0.838–2.339)	
Q3	203/214	1.180 (0.877–1.588)	78/67	1.610 (0.965–2.686)	
Q4(high)	224/213	1.321 (0.984–1.773)	67/75	1.470 (0.878–2.463)	
Fruits and vegetables		$P_{trend} < 0.001$		$P_{trend} < 0.001$	0.447
Q1(low)	426/214	1.00(ref)	156/73	1.00(ref)	
Q2	185/227	0.430 (0.326–0.567)	59/65	0.432 (0.266–0.701)	
Q3	135/210	0.309 (0.229–0.416)	38/74	0.263 (0.156–0.443)	
Q4(high)	93/210	0.224 (0.162–0.309)	29/73	0.216 (0.124–0.376)	
Cereals and meat		$P_{trend} = 0.701$		$P_{trend} = 0.035$	0.129
Q1(low)	206/216	1.00(ref)	77/74	1.00(ref)	
Q2	217/226	0.903 (0.674–1.210)	82/59	1.275 (0.767–2.118)	
Q3	200/212	0.864 (0.641–1.164)	68/77	0.836 (0.510–1.370)	
Q4(high)	216/20/	0.953 (0.707–1.283)	55/75	0.624 (0.369–1.053)	
Frugal pattern		$P_{trend} = 0.079$		$P_{trend} = 0.725$	0.619
Q1(low)	179/217	1.00(ref)	72/66	1.00(ref)	
Q2	191/223	0.933 (0.689–1.263)	55/69	0.701 (0.412–1.193)	
Q3	1194/207	0.938 (0.691–1.273)	71/77	0.821 (0.492–1.368)	
Q4(high)	275/214	1.287 (0.960–1.727)	84/73	1.031 (0.627–1.695)	
	rs7501331:CC		rs7501331:CT + TT		

Table 5 Associations between dietary patterns and lung cancer risk by genotype at 3 SNPs *(Continued)*

Dietary patterns	Cases/controls rs6564851:GG	Adjusted OR (95% CI)	Cases/controls rs6564851:GT + TT	Adjusted OR (95% CI)	P for interaction
High quality protein		$P_{trend} = 0.097$		$P_{trend} = 0.134$	0.902
Q1(low)	180/181	1.00(ref)	77/89	1.00(ref)	
Q2	172/177	1.139 (0.826–1.571)	92/101	1.189 (0.751–1.883)	
Q3	182/168	1.323 (0.957–1.827)	81/95	1.089 (0.678–1.748)	
Q4(high)	173/170	1.269 (0.917–1.756)	103/103	1.483 (0.934–2.354)	
Fruits and vegetables		$P_{trend} < 0.001$		$P_{trend} < 0.001$	0.487
Q1(low)	359/173	1.00(ref)	191/101	1.00(ref)	
Q2	160/175	0.464 (0.341–0.630)	65/99	0.372 (0.241–0.574)	
Q3	115/182	0.291 (0.210–0.402)	51/86	0.332 (0.209–0.528)	
Q4(high)	73/166	0.212 (0.147–0.305)	46/102	0.274 (0.172–0.435)	
Cereals and meat		$P_{trend} = 0.110$		$P_{trend} = 0.948$	0.44
Q1(low)	169/177	1.00(ref)	100/102	1.00(ref)	
Q2	202/179	1.083 (0.786–1.494)	77/89	0.778 (0.493–1.229)	
Q3	176/166	1.005 (0.725–1.395)	84/104	0.694 (0.443–1.088)	
Q4(high)	160/174	0.769 (0.550–1.074)	92/93	1.032 (0.662–1.610)	
Frugal pattern		$P_{trend} = 0.014$		$P_{trend} = 0.727$	0.253
Q1(low)	150/180	1.00(ref)	88/92	1.00(ref)	
Q2	153/175	0.979 (0.700–1.370)	76/100	0.709 (0.446–1.127)	
Q3	180/170	1.172 (0.842–1.630)	71/95	0.651 (0.405–1.048)	
Q4(high)	224/171	1.433 (1.036–1.982)	118/101	1.055 (0.682–1.632)	

provide evidence for favoring diet pattern shifts in the general population [19].

The patterns identified in this analysis were reflective of real-world consumption in the Fujian Han population rather than an ideal dietary pattern. A potential criticism of this approach is that the dietary pattern factors are dependent on the study population for their validity. Thus, a different set of patterns may emerge with a different study population, which limits the interpretive value of these dietary patterns. However, it is important to note that our high quality protein (seafood in majority), fruits and vegetables patterns are analogous to patterns that have emerged repeatedly in many studies that used factor analysis to study dietary patterns [30, 31].

Our association findings for four patterns are consistent with findings from previous studies on dietary pattern and lung cancer. Previous factor-analysis studies [15–17] have related healthful eating to a decreased risk of lung cancer, similar to findings obtained with index-based dietary patterns, supporting the current dietary guidance of increasing consumption of fruits, vegetables, whole grains, lean meats or meat alternatives, and low-fat dairy [11]. In addition, the Mediterranean dietary pattern was thought to be negatively related with risk of lung cancer, whereas a "Western" dietary pattern was found to be associated with lung cancer risk [13].

On the other hand, our study showed a positive relationship between frugal pattern and lung cancer risk, which has not, to our knowledge, been reported previously. The participants in our study with high scores on the frugal pattern showed with a lower income. In Fujian, poor people usually take dried sweet potato and salted vegetables as staple food. This pattern showed increased incidence of lung cancer that suggests that there may have been relationship between economics and lung cancer. However, the potential mechanisms linking strong adherence to frugal pattern with an increased risk of lung cancer are unknown.

Our study had several strengths and limitations. The strengths include our large sample size, which tends to reduce type II errors. Additionally, extensive information on lifestyle factors were collected to enable adjustment for confounding factors. Several potential limitations of the present study should also be considered. Firstly, there was a recruitment bias related to the retrospective case-control study design; however, the results did not appear to be seriously affected by this bias given the HWEs in the control group. Secondly, our study was subject to potential dietary intake recall bias and we do not use 3-day measuring method or other methods to validate for each of the dietary patterns. It exits potential bias on the findings. Nevertheless, the directions and magnitudes of the associations for our patterns were consistent with other prospective studies. Finally, we did not employ a food-frequency questionnaire (FFQ) and thus may have missed the opportunity to capture data on more types of foods. Further studies in large population-based cohorts by using a FFQ are warranted to identify the role of dietary habits in lung cancer in Fujian, China.

Conclusions

In summary, our study adds to the growing evidence indicating that diet plays an important role in lung carcinogenesis, which is often assumed to be caused solely by smoking. In particular, our study suggests that a diet rich in fruits and vegetables may reduce lung cancer risk.

Abbreviations

BC: β-carotene; BMI: Body mass index; CI: Confidence interval; ETS: Environmental tobacco smoking; HWE: Weinberg equilibrium; SNPs: Single nucleotide morphisms

Acknowledgements

We thank all the staffs from Department of Thoracic Surgery, The first affiliated hospital of Fujian Medical University. And we also would like to express our appreciation to the patients participated in our study.

Funding

This study was supported by grants from the National Natural Science Foundation of China (Nos 81402738), Fujian Provincial Natural Science Foundation Project (Nos 2016 J01355) and the projects of environmental science and technology of Fujian Province (Nos 2015R012). All funding supported the design of the study and collection, analysis, and interpretation of data and in writing the manuscript.

Authors' contributions

HF and XRD carried out the molecular genetic studies, participated in the drafted the manuscript. XWM, XQP, LZQ, LT and HBC carried out experiments and collected samples. HF and LC participated in the design of the study and performed the statistical analysis. LX and HZJ conceived of the study, and participated in its design and coordination and helped to draft the manuscript. All authors read and approved the final manuscript.

Competing interests

The authors declare that they have no competing interests.

Author details

[1]Department of Epidemiology, School of Public Health, Fujian Medical University, Fuzhou 350108, China. [2]Key Laboratory of Ministry of Education for Gastrointestinal Cancer, Fujian Medical University, Fuzhou 350108, China. [3]Department of Thoracic Surgery, The first affiliated hospital of Fujian Medical University, Fuzhou 350005, China.

References

1. Torre LA, Bray F, Siegel RL, Ferlay J, Lortet-Tieulent J, Jemal A. Global cancer statistics, 2012. CA Cancer J Clin. 2015;65(2):87–108. https://doi.org/10.3322/caac.21262.
2. Chen W, Zheng R, Baade PD, Zhang S, Zeng H, Bray F, Jemal A, Yu XQ, He J. Cancer statistics in China, 2015. CA Cancer J Clin. 2016;66(2):115–32. https://doi.org/10.3322/caac.21338.
3. Zhao H, Fan Y, Ma S, Song X, Han B, Cheng Y, Huang C, Yang S, Liu X, Liu Y, Lu S, Wang J, Zhang S, Zhou C, Wang M, Zhang L, investigators I. Final overall survival results from a phase III, randomized, placebo-controlled, parallel-group study of gefitinib versus placebo as maintenance therapy in patients with locally advanced or metastatic non-small-cell lung cancer (INFORM; C-TONG 0804). J Thorac Oncol. 2015;10(4):655–64. https://doi.org/10.1097/JTO.0000000000000445.
4. Filaire E, Dupuis C, Galvaing G, Aubreton S, Laurent H, Richard R, Filaire M. Lung cancer: what are the links with oxidative stress, physical activity and nutrition. Lung Cancer. 2013;82(3):383–9. https://doi.org/10.1016/j.lungcan.2013.09.009.
5. Proctor RN. Tobacco and the global lung cancer epidemic. Nat Rev Cancer. 2001;1(1):82–6. https://doi.org/10.1038/35094091.
6. Baena Ruiz R, Salinas HP. Diet and cancer: risk factors and epidemiological evidence. Maturitas. 2014;77(3):202–8. https://doi.org/10.1016/j.maturitas.2013.11.010.
7. Bolland MJ, Grey A, Reid IR. Vitamin and mineral supplements in the primary prevention of cardiovascular disease and cancer. Ann Intern Med. 2014;160(9):655–6. https://doi.org/10.7326/L14-5009-4.
8. Cho E, Hunter DJ, Spiegelman D, Albanes D, Beeson WL, van den Brandt PA, Colditz GA, Feskanich D, Folsom AR, Fraser GE, Freudenheim JL, Giovannucci E, Goldbohm RA, Graham S, Miller AB, Rohan TE, Sellers TA, Virtamo J, Willett WC, Smith-Warner SA. Intakes of vitamins A, C and E and folate and multivitamins and lung cancer: a pooled analysis of 8 prospective studies. Int J Cancer. 2006;118(4):970–8. https://doi.org/10.1002/ijc.21441.
9. Song J, Su H, Wang BL, Zhou YY, Guo LL. Fish consumption and lung cancer risk: systematic review and meta-analysis. Nutr Cancer. 2014;66(4):539–49. https://doi.org/10.1080/01635581.2014.894102.
10. Wang Y, Li F, Wang Z, Qiu T, Shen Y, Wang M. Fruit and vegetable consumption and risk of lung cancer: a dose-response meta-analysis of prospective cohort studies. Lung Cancer. 2015;88(2):124–30. https://doi.org/10.1016/j.lungcan.2015.02.015.
11. Anic GM, Park Y, Subar AF, Schap TE, Reedy J. Index-based dietary patterns and risk of lung cancer in the NIH-AARP diet and health study. Eur J Clin Nutr. 2016;70(1):123–9. https://doi.org/10.1038/ejcn.2015.122.
12. Balder HF, Goldbohm RA, van den Brandt PA. Dietary patterns associated with male lung cancer risk in the Netherlands cohort study. Cancer Epidemiol Biomark Prev. 2005;14(2):483–90. https://doi.org/10.1158/1055-9965.EPI-04-0353.
13. Couto E, Boffetta P, Lagiou P, Ferrari P, Buckland G, Overvad K, Dahm CC, Tjonneland A, Olsen A, Clavel-Chapelon F, Boutron-Ruault MC, Cottet V, Trichopoulos D, Naska A, Benetou V, Kaaks R, Rohrmann S, Boeing H, von Ruesten A, Panico S, Pala V, Vineis P, Palli D, Tumino R, May A, Peeters PH, Bueno-de-Mesquita HB, Buchner FL, Lund E, Skeie G, Engeset D, Gonzalez CA, Navarro C, Rodriguez L, Sanchez MJ, Amiano P, Barricarte A, Hallmans G, Johansson I, Manjer J, Wirfart E, Allen NE, Crowe F, Khaw KT, Wareham N, Moskal A, Slimani N, Jenab M, Romaguera D, Mouw T, Norat T, Riboli E, Trichopoulou A. Mediterranean dietary pattern and cancer risk in the EPIC cohort. Br J Cancer. 2011;104(9):1493–9. https://doi.org/10.1038/bjc.2011.106.
14. De Stefani E, Boffetta P, Ronco AL, Deneo-Pellegrini H, Acosta G, Gutierrez LP, Mendilaharsu M. Nutrient patterns and risk of lung cancer: a factor analysis in Uruguayan men. Lung Cancer. 2008;61(3):283–91. https://doi.org/10.1016/j.lungcan.2008.01.004.
15. Gorlova OY, Weng SF, Hernandez L, Spitz MR, Forman MR. Dietary patterns affect lung cancer risk in never smokers. Nutr Cancer. 2011;63(6):842–9. https://doi.org/10.1080/01635581.2011.589958.
16. Gnagnarella P, Maisonneuve P, Bellomi M, Rampinelli C, Bertolotti R, Spaggiari L, Palli D, Veronesi G. Nutrient intake and nutrient patterns and risk of lung cancer among heavy smokers: results from the COSMOS screening study with annual low-dose CT. Eur J Epidemiol. 2013;28(6):503–11. https://doi.org/10.1007/s10654-013-9803-1.
17. Tu H, Heymach JV, Wen CP, Ye Y, Pierzynski JA, Roth JA, Wu X. Different dietary patterns and reduction of lung cancer risk: a large case-control study in the U.S. Sci Rep. 2016;6:26760. https://doi.org/10.1038/srep26760.
18. De Stefani E, Ronco AL, Boffetta P, Deneo-Pellegrini H, Correa P, Acosta G. Nutritional patterns and lung cancer risk in Uruguayan men. Cancer Ther. 2006;4:153–62.
19. Sun Y, Li Z, Li J, Li Z, Han J. A healthy dietary pattern reduces lung Cancer risk: a systematic review and meta-analysis. Nutrients. 2016;8(3):134. https://doi.org/10.3390/nu8030134.
20. van Helden YG, Heil SG, van Schooten FJ, Kramer E, Hessel S, Amengual J, Ribot J, Teerds K, Wyss A, Lietz G, Bonet ML, von Lintig J, Godschalk RW,

Keijer J. Knockout of the Bcmo1 gene results in an inflammatory response in female lung, which is suppressed by dietary beta-carotene. Cell Mol Life Sci. 2010;67(12):2039–56. https://doi.org/10.1007/s00018-010-0341-7.

21. Gong X, Marisiddaiah R, Rubin LP. Beta-carotene regulates expression of beta-carotene 15,15′-monoxygenase in human alveolar epithelial cells. Arch Biochem Biophys. 2013;539(2):230–8. https://doi.org/10.1016/j.abb.2013.09.013.

22. Cui Y, Morgenstern H, Greenland S, Tashkin DP, Mao JT, Cai L, Cozen W, Mack TM, Lu QY, Zhang ZF. Dietary flavonoid intake and lung cancer–a population-based case-control study. Cancer. 2008;112(10): 2241–8. https://doi.org/10.1002/cncr.23398.

23. Jin YR, Lee MS, Lee JH, Hsu HK, Lu JY, Chao SS, Chen KT, Liou SH, Ger LP. Intake of vitamin A-rich foods and lung cancer risk in Taiwan: with special reference to garland chrysanthemum and sweet potato leaf consumption. Asia Pac J Clin Nutr. 2007;16(3):477–88.

24. Lin Y, Cai L. Environmental and dietary factors and lung cancer risk among Chinese women: a case-control study in Southeast China. Nutr Cancer. 2012;64(4):508–14. https://doi.org/10.1080/01635581.2012.668743.

25. Leung WC, Hessel S, Meplan C, Flint J, Oberhauser V, Tourniaire F, Hesketh JE, von Lintig J, Lietz G. Two common single nucleotide polymorphisms in the gene encoding beta-carotene 15,15′-monoxygenase alter beta-carotene metabolism in female volunteers. FASEB J. 2009;23(4):1041–53. https://doi. org/10.1096/fj.08-121962.

26. Ferrucci L, Perry JR, Matteini A, Perola M, Tanaka T, Silander K, Rice N, Melzer D, Murray A, Cluett C, Fried LP, Albanes D, Corsi AM, Cherubini A, Guralnik J, Bandinelli S, Singleton A, Virtamo J, Walston J, Semba RD, Frayling TM. Common variation in the beta-carotene 15,15′-monooxygenase 1 gene affects circulating levels of carotenoids: a genome-wide association study. Am J Hum Genet. 2009;84(2):123–33. https://doi.org/10.1016/j.ajhg.2008.12.019.

27. Piga R, van Dartel D, Bunschoten A, van der Stelt I, Keijer J. Role of Frizzled6 in the molecular mechanism of beta-carotene action in the lung. Toxicology. 2014;320:67–73. https://doi.org/10.1016/j.tox.2014.03.002.

28. van Helden YG, Godschalk RW, Swarts HJ, Hollman PC, van Schooten FJ, Keijer J. Beta-carotene affects gene expression in lungs of male and female Bcmo1 (–/–) mice in opposite directions. Cell Mol Life Sci. 2011;68(3):489–504. https://doi.org/10.1007/s00018-010-0461-0.

29. Lietz G, Oxley A, Leung W, Hesketh J. Single nucleotide polymorphisms upstream from the beta-carotene 15,15′-monoxygenase gene influence provitamin a conversion efficiency in female volunteers. J Nutr. 2012;142(1): 161S–5S. https://doi.org/10.3945/jn.111.140756.

30. Bradshaw PT, Siega-Riz AM, Campbell M, Weissler MC, Funkhouser WK, Olshan AF. Associations between dietary patterns and head and neck cancer: the Carolina head and neck cancer epidemiology study. Am J Epidemiol. 2012;175(12):1225–33. https://doi.org/10.1093/aje/kwr468.

31. Nanri A, Yoshida D, Yamaji T, Mizoue T, Takayanagi R, Kono S. Dietary patterns and C-reactive protein in Japanese men and women. Am J Clin Nutr. 2008;87(5):1488–96.

8

CTHRC1 induces non-small cell lung cancer (NSCLC) invasion through upregulating MMP-7/MMP-9

Weiling He[1,2†], Hui Zhang[1†], Yuefeng Wang[1†], Yanbin Zhou[3], Yifeng Luo[3], Yongmei Cui[1], Neng Jiang[1], Wenting Jiang[1], Han Wang[1], Di Xu[4], Shuhua Li[1], Zhuo Wang[1], Yangshan Chen[1], Yu Sun[1], Yang Zhang[5], Hsian-Rong Tseng[6], Xuenong Zou[7], Liantang Wang[1] and Zunfu Ke[1*]

Abstract

Background: The strong invasive and metastatic nature of non-small cell lung cancer (NSCLC) leads to poor prognosis. Collagen triple helix repeat containing 1 (CTHRC1) is involved in cell migration, motility and invasion. The object of this study is to investigate the involvement of CTHRC1 in NSCLC invasion and metastasis.

Methods: A proteomic analysis was performed to identify the different expression proteins between NSCLC and normal tissues. Cell lines stably express CTHRC1, MMP7, MMP9 were established. Invasion and migration were determined by scratch and transwell assays respectively. Clinical correlations of CTHRC1 in a cohort of 230 NSCLC patients were analysed.

Results: CTHRC1 is overexpressed in NSCLC as measured by proteomic analysis. Additionally, CTHRC1 increases tumour cell migration and invasion in vitro. Furthermore, CTHRC1 expression is significantly correlated with matrix metalloproteinase (MMP)7 and MMP9 expression in sera and tumour tissues from NSCLC. The invasion ability mediated by CTHRC1 were mainly MMP7- and MMP9-dependent. MMP7 or MMP9 depletion significantly eradicated the pro-invasive effects mediated by CTHRC1 on NSCLC cells. Clinically, patients with high CTHRC1 expression had poor survival.

Conclusions: CTHRC1 serves as a pro-metastatic gene that contributes to NSCLC invasion and metastasis, which are mediated by upregulated MMP7 and MMP9 expression. Targeting CTHRC1 may be beneficial for inhibiting NSCLC metastasis.

Keywords: Lung cancer, CTHRC1, MMP7, MMP9, Invasion/metastasis

Background

Lung cancer is one of the most common malignant tumours and remains the leading cause of cancer-related death in China and around the world [1]. Among all the lung cancers, non-small cell lung cancer (NSCLC) is the most common and aggressive type, accounting for ~ 85% of cases [2, 3]. Surgical resection remains the preferred clinical treatment for NSCLC patients in the early stages of disease. Despite advances in radio- and chemotherapy and the development of new targeted therapies in the past few years, 5-year survival rate remains poor in NSCLC patients due to unresectable advanced or metastatic disease at diagnosis. The high mortality and low cure rates for NSCLC are largely attributed to the strong ability of lung cancer cells to invade surrounding tissue or metastasize to other remote sites [4–6]. Hence, understanding the molecular mechanisms underlying NSCLC invasion and metastasis is essential.

Tumor metastasis is a complex process involving cell adhesion and proteolytic degradation of the extracellular matrix (ECM) [7, 8]. Matrix metalloproteinases (MMPs) are characterized by their ability to degrade extracellular matrix (ECM) proteins and expose cryptic sites within

* Correspondence: kezunfu@mail.sysu.edu.cn
†Equal contributors
[1]Department of Pathology, The First Affiliated Hospital, Sun Yat-sen University, No. 58, ZhongShan Second Road, Guangdong 510080, China
Full list of author information is available at the end of the article

the matrix molecules to facilitate tumour invasion and metastasis [9–12]. A previous study has shown MMP7 in promoting ovarian cancer cell invasion [13]. Additionally, mice deficient in MMP9 are resistant to tumour metastasis [14]. MMP9 is highly involved in strengthening the invasion capability of NSCLC [15]. Clinically, MMP7 and MMP9 expression correlates with poor prognosis of NSCLC [16–18]. To further understand MMP modulation mechanisms in NSCLC to search for new therapeutic targets is thus imperative.

Collagen triple helix repeat containing 1 (CTHRC1) was originally identified in balloon-injured rat arteries, and its overexpression in fibroblasts is associated with increased cell migration, motility and invasion [19]. CTHRC1 is widely upregulated in several solid tumours, including melanoma and cancers of the gastrointestinal tract, breast, thyroid, liver and pancreas [20]. Furthermore, recombinant CTHRC1 protein augments the migration and invasion capacities of primary gastrointestinal stromal tumours [21]. According to Chen et al. [22], CTHRC1 promotes tumour invasion and predicts poor prognosis in hepatocellular carcinoma. In our previous study, CTHRC1 overexpression in NSCLC cells was associated with tumour aggressiveness [23]; however, how CTHRC1 is involved in tumour cell migration and metastasis has yet to be fully elucidated. In a recent study by Park et al. [24], CTHRC1 regulated pancreatic cancer migration and adhesion by inducing Src, MEK and Rac1 activation. We previously showed the ability of CTHRC1 to increase the invasive capability of epithelial ovarian cancer cells by provoking constitutive activation of Wnt/β-catenin signalling [25]. However, whether CTHRC1 is involved in cancer cell invasion and metastasis has not been completely clarified. Additionally, the mechanisms employed by CTHRC1 to regulate MMPs remain uncharacterized by previous investigations.

In our present study, we detected CTHRC1 overexpression in NSCLC tissues by performing a proteomic analysis and further confirmed the results through western blotting and in IHC assays at the tissue and cell levels. Furthermore, IHC analysis revealed a close relationship between CTHRC1 overexpression and lymph node metastasis, clinical stage and overall survival. Moreover, we demonstrated that CTHRC1 promoted tumour invasion by regulating MMP7 and MMP9 expression, which is mediated by the AP-1/c-Jun and NF-κB pathways, respectively. Additionally, serum concentration of CTHRC1 correlates with metastasis, clinical stage and circulating tumour cell (CTC) number and functions as an important prognostic factor for NSCLC patients. In summary, our findings represent an important step forward in understanding the role of CTHRC1 in NSCLC metastasis.

Methods
Patient and tissue information
Sera and primary tumour tissues were collected from a total of 230 cases of clinically and immunohistologically verified NSCLC (obtained from 2006 to 2011) identified in the pathology archives of the Affiliated First Hospital, Sun Yat-sen University, and the Central Hospital of Wuhan. NSCLC was verified by performing haematoxylin and eosin (HE) staining and immunohistochemistry as shown in Additional file 1: Figure S1A. Patients' clinical characteristics are listed in Additional file 1: Table S1.

Proteomic analysis
Proteomic analysis was performed. NSCLC tissues ($n = 20$) and adjacent non-tumour tissues ($n = 20$) were used to extract proteins for analysis. Tumour tissues were homogenized in lysis buffer via sonication on ice. A 2-D CleanQ2-Up Kit (Amersham Biosciences, UK) and a 2-D Quant Kit (GE Healthcare, London, UK) were used for protein purification and concentration qualification, respectively, according to the manufacturers' instructions. Two-dimensional gel electrophoresis was performed using an immobilized pH gradient (IPG) strip (24 cm, pH 3–10 NL; GE Healthcare), in which proteins were separated according to their isoelectric point (pI) and molecular weight. Visualized stained proteins were selected using an Ettan Spot Handling Workstation (GE Healthcare), and spots of interest were digested with trypsin. Peptide mass mapping was performed via matrix-assisted laser desorption time-of-flight mass spectrometry (MALDI-TOF MS) using an ABI Voyager DE-STR mass spectrometer. The MASCOT Database (http://www.matrixscience.com/search_form_select.html) was employed to identify the original proteins. The search criteria were as follows: Homo sapiens, trypsin cleavage, and no constraints on either the molecular weight or the isoelectric point of the protein.

Western blot
After electrophoresis, Membranes were incubated with primary antibodies in 5% milk/TBST at 4 °C overnight. The membranes were then washed with TBST and subsequently incubated with HRP-conjugated anti-rabbit IgG at room temperature for 60 min. Membranes were washed with TBST, and signals were detected via enhanced chemiluminescence (ECL). Cell nucleoprotein was extracted using EpiQuik Nuclear Extraction Kit (Epigentek, Farmingdale, NY) according to the manufacturer's instructions.

Reverse dot hybridization
All assays were performed as previously described [26] and in strict accordance with the instructions provided with the kit (Roche, USA). Specific probes targeting

MMP genes were designed and listed in Additional file 1: Table S2. siRNA sequences and RT-PCR primers are listed in Additional file 1: Tables S3 and S4 respectively.

Luciferase reporter gene assay

NCI-H1975 cells were seeded in 24-well plates in triplicate and allowed to adhere for 24 h. Luciferase reporter plasmids (200 ng) containing different fragments of the MMP7 or MM9 promoters were transfected into cells using Lipofectamine 2000 with 1 ng of pRL-SV40 Renilla luciferase as an internal control. Cell extracts were prepared 24 h after transfection, and luciferase signals were measured using the Dual-Luciferase Reporter Assay System (Promega, USA) according to the manufacturer's instructions.

Chromatin immunoprecipitation (ChIP)

ChIP was performed using a Chromatin Immunoprecipitation Kit (Upstate) according to the manufacturer's instructions. Briefly, NCI-H1975 cells were treated with 1% formaldehyde to cross-link proteins to DNA in a 100-mm culture dish. Sonication was applied to the cell debris to shear DNA into 300–1000-bp fragments. Equal amounts of chromatin supernatants, containing an antibody against CTHRC1 (1 µg) or an equal amount of control IgG, were incubated overnight at 4 °C with shaking. PCR was performed after the reverse cross-linking of protein/DNA complexes to release DNA.

Immunohistochemistry

Paraffin-embedded tissues were sectioned (4 µm) and incubated with anti-CTHRC-1 (Abcam, Cambridge, UK), anti-MMP7 (Abcam, Cambridge, UK) and anti-MMP9 (Abcam, Cambridge, UK) primary antibodies at 4 °C overnight. After washing with PBS, sections were then incubated with an HRP-conjugated goat anti-rabbit secondary antibody for 1 h at room temperature. Peroxidase was visualized with 3,3′-diaminobenzidine, and haematoxylin was used as a counterstain.

CTC enrichment using the NanoVelcro system

CTC were detected by NanoVelcro system as we previously described [27]. Blood specimens were collected in EDTA tubes. Blood samples were processed within 24 h. NH_4Cl was added to whole blood at a ratio of 10:1 v/v and incubated for 20 min at room temperature to lyse the red blood cells. Samples were centrifuged at 200 g for 5 min, and the supernatants were removed. Cell pellets were re-suspended. Immunocytochemistry was applied to visualize cells captured on the SiNW substrate. The microchannels were loaded with 100 µl of fluorophore-labelled antibody solution (20 µl/1 ml of the initial concentration) and incubated at 4 °C overnight.

CTCs were identified based on positive staining for cytokeratin (PE) and negative staining for CD45 (FITC). An experienced pathologist characterized the phenotypes and morphologies of tumour cells.

Enzyme-linked immunosorbent assay (ELISA)

Sera were collected from NSCLC patients or healthy controls. The concentrations of CTHRC1 in the sera were measured by ELISA as previous described [28].

Statistical analysis

All above experiments were performed at least three times. Statistical analysis was carried out using SPSS software (version 16.0; SPSS, Chicago, IL, USA). The $\chi 2$ test was applied to analyse the relationships between CTHRC1, MMP7, and MMP9 expression and clinicopathologic parameters. An unpaired, two-tailed Student's t-test was used to determine the between- group significance. Bivariate correlation analysis was calculated as Spearman's rank correlation coefficient. Survival curves were plotted using the Kaplan-Meier method and compared with the log-rank test. ROC curve analysis was carried out to determine the CTHRC1 cut-off points for metastasis and recurrence status. P values < 0.05 were considered significant.

Results

CTHRC1 overexpression in NSCLC tissues correlates with clinical metastasis status in NSCLC

Comparative proteomic analysis simultaneously revealed 34 differential spots in NSCLC tissues compared with corresponding adjacent non-tumour tissues (ANTs). All protein spots of interest on silver-stain gels (Fig. 1a) were identified by MALDI-TOF/MS and further confirmed via a comparative sequence search in the MASCOT database. The identified proteins are summarized in Additional file 1: Table S5. In general, CTHRC1 was upregulated in all 20 NSCLC individuals. Representative peptide mass fingerprinting (PMF) of CTHRC1 is shown in Fig. 1b. We also confirmed that CTHRC1 is overexpressed in all the NSCLC cell lines (Additional file 1: Figure S1B).

CTHRC1 overexpression is reportedly associated with tumour invasion and metastasis [20, 29]. To investigate whether NSCLC also exhibits strong CTHRC1 expression compared to ANTs, we first measured CTHRC1 expression in twenty paired NSCLC and ANT samples by performing western blotting. Compared to individual corresponding ANTs, CTHRC1 expression was significantly higher in NSCLC tissues (Fig. 1c), which was further confirmed at the RNA level by RT-PCR (Additional file 1: Figure S1C). Consistent with the western blot and RT-PCR results, IHC data further verified the upregulation of CTHRC1 in primary NSCLC tissues

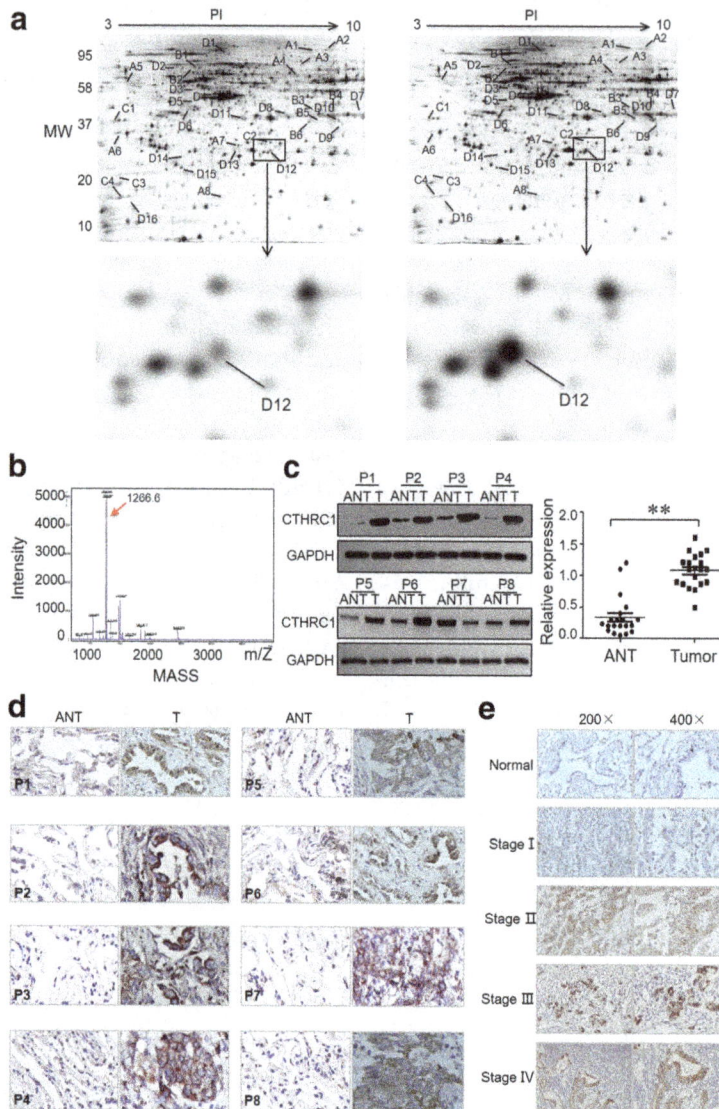

Fig. 1 Differential protein expression in NSCLC and corresponding adjacent nontumor tissues (ANTs) samples and the correlation with tumor metastasis. Thirty-four differential protein spots were identified from NSCLC (**a**, right) and ANT (**a**, left) samples in the representative silver-stained 2D gel image, and the outlined areas show CTHRC1 upregulation in NSCLC tissues ($n = 20$). **b** MS identification analysis of CTHRC1. The red arrow marks the specific peak corresponding to the CTHRC1 protein. **c, d** Comparative CTHRC1 protein quantification in paired primary NSCLC tissues (T) and their corresponding ANTs in the left panel ($n = 20$) as measured by western blotting and IHC (******$p < 0.01$). **e** CTHRC1 levels increase as tumour grade (I–IV) progresses, as determined by IHC staining ($n = 230$). Representative western blot bands and IHC images are presented. Three independent experiments were performed

(Fig. 1d). Next, we investigated the correlation between CTHRC1 expression and NSCLC metastasis. Pathologically verified NSCLC tumour tissues and ANTs were collected. According to the IHC results, CTHRC1 was expressed at very low levels in normal lung tissue. In contrast, CTHRC1 expression was very high in 55.2% of primary NSCLC tissues, and furthermore, CTHRC1 expression in NSCLC tissues was associated with tumour metastasis (Additional file 1: Table S1). Additionally, compared to early stages, advanced stages characterized

by localized invasion or distant metastasis had significantly higher levels of CTHRC1 (Fig. 1e).

CTHRC1 promotes NSCLC cell migration and invasion

Based on the above data, CTHRC1 was overexpressed and associated with disease invasion and metastasis in NSCLC. To provide direct evidence supporting the contribution of CTHRC1 to NSCLC invasion and migration, we first selected NCI-H1975 and NCI-H2122 to establish cell lines in which CTHRC1 was stably overexpressed or knocked down. Overexpression or depletion efficiencies were confirmed by performing western blot as shown in Additional file 1: Figure S2. An adhesion assay demonstrated decreased tumour cell adhesion accompanying the ectopic overexpression of CTHRC1, while depletion of CTHRC1 increased tumour cell adhesion (Fig. 2a, d). Additionally, CTHRC1 overexpression increased the ability of tumour cells to invade through a Transwell gel, and CTHRC1 depletion suppressed tumour cell invasion (Fig. 2b, c, e, f). Furthermore, tumour cell migration speed increased with CTHRC1 overexpression but was inhibited with CTHRC1 depletion (Fig. 2g-j).

CTHRC1 regulates MMP7 and MMP9 expression in vitro and in vivo

Based on our data, CTHRC1 regulated the invasion and metastasis of NSCLC in vitro and in vivo. To further understand the underlying mechanisms through which CTHRC1 promotes tumour invasion and metastasis, we performed ELISAs to detect CTHRC1 in 92 clinical NSCLC serum samples. Several MMPs correlated with CTHRC1 expression. Among them, MMP7 and MMP9, were the two MMPs that were highly correlated with CTHRC1 (Fig. 3a, c, Additional file 1: Figure S3A). To further study the

correlation between CTHRC1 and MMP7 as well as MMP9 in fresh primary tumour tissues, we measured the expression of CTHRC1 and MMPs by performing reverse dot blot hybridization. Consistent with the ELISA data, CTHRC1 expression was significantly correlated with MMP7 and MMP9 expression in primary tumour tissues (Fig. 3b, d, Additional file 1: Figure S3B). The correlation between CTHRC1 and MMP7 and MMP9 expression was further confirmed by IHC results obtained from 230 clinical NSCLC tumour samples. Among 127 cases with CTHRC1 high expression, 114 and 115 cases exhibited high MMP7 and MMP9 expression, respectively. Simultaneously, 92 and 85 cases exhibited low MMP7 and MMP9 expression, respectively, out of a total of 103 cases with low CTHRC1 expression (Additional file 1: Figure S3C, 3D).

We next examined the CTHRC1-mediated regulation of MMP7 and MMP9 in in vitro experiments. Both MMP7 and MMP9 were upregulated when CTHRC1 was overexpressed in NSCLC cells. In contrast, CTHRC1 knockdown in NCI-H1975 and NCI-H2122 cells downregulated MMP7 and MMP9 expression at the protein level, as measured by western blotting (Fig. 3e-h).

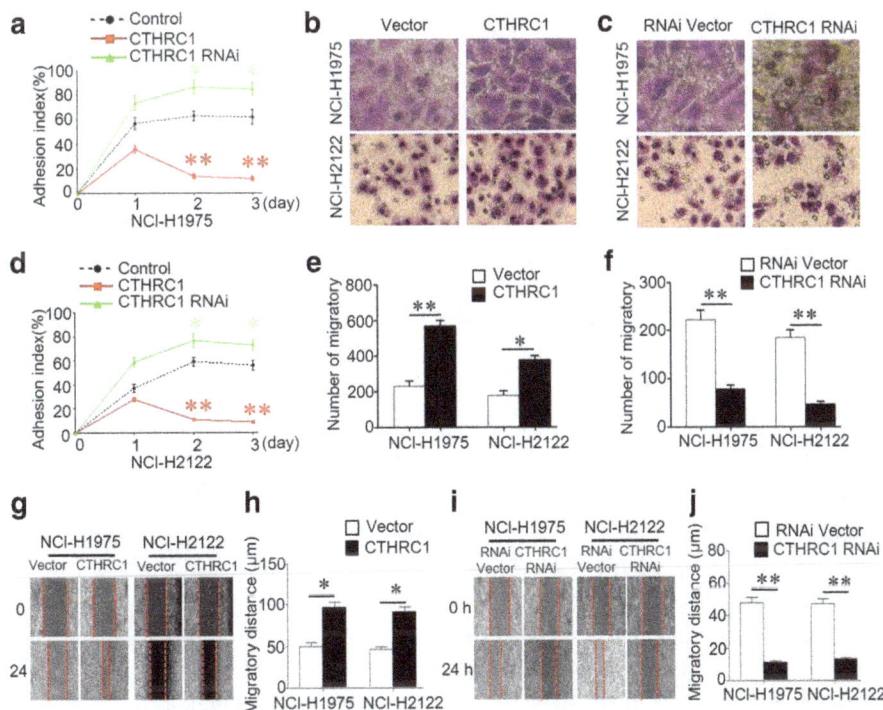

Fig. 2 CTHRC1 inhibits adhesion and promotes NSCLC cell migration and invasion of in vitro and metastasis in vivo. a, d CTHRC1 overexpression inhibited cell adhesion; CTHRC1 knockdown increased cell adhesion; (b-f) Transwell assay results indicated that ectopic overexpression of CTHRC1 promoted cell invasion; knockdown of endogenous CTHRC1 inhibited cell invasion. Migratory cells were stained with HE and qualitatively assessed, as summarized in the bar graphs. g-j A wound assay indicated CTHRC1 overexpression increased tumour cell migration; CTHRC1 knockdown inhibited tumour cell migration. Migration distances were measured and are summarized in the bar graphs; *p < 0.05 and **p < 0.01

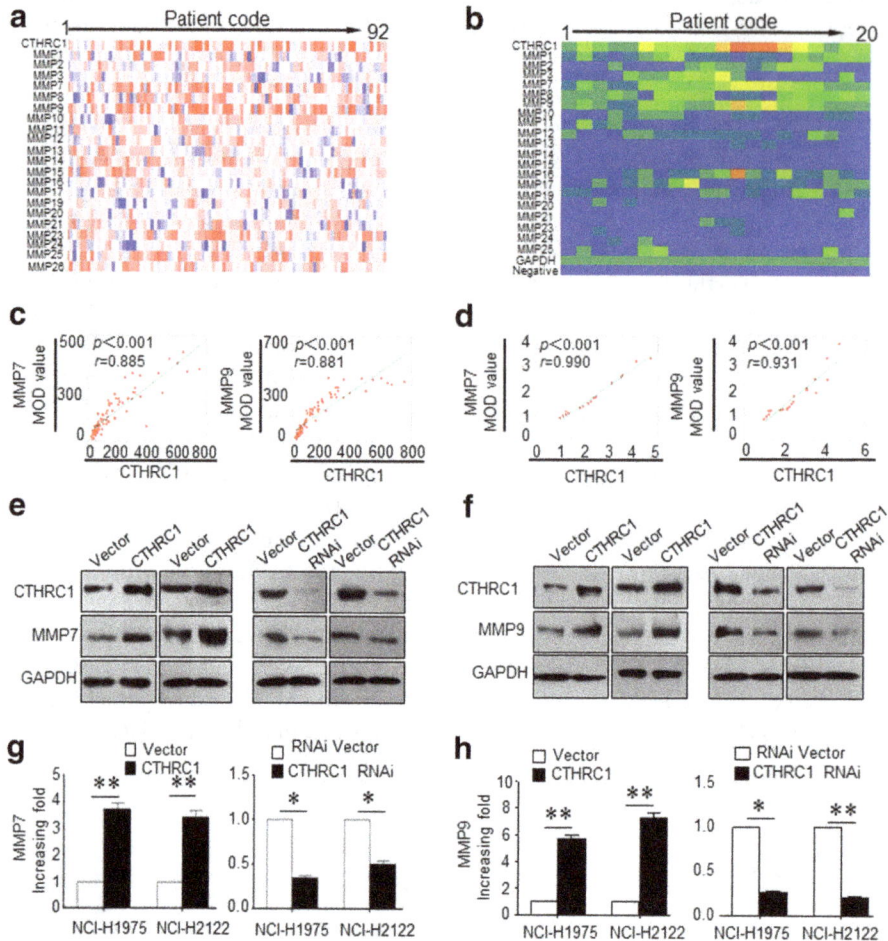

Fig. 3 CTHRC1 regulates MMP7 and MMP9 expression in vitro and in vivo. **a** The heat map shows the concentration distributions of CTHRC1 and diverse MMPs in the sera of NSCLC patients as measured by ELISA ($n = 92$). **b** mRNA levels of CTHRC1 and diverse MMPs in NSCLC tissues were further analysed by reverse dot blot hybridization ($n = 20$). **c, d** CTHRC1 expression was positively correlated with MMP7 and MMP9 in both sera and primary tumour tissues. **e, f** Western blot analysis demonstrated increased MMP7 and MMP9 production accompanying the ectopic overexpression of CTHRC1; CTHRC1 knockdown downregulated MMP7 and MMP9 expression. **g, h** The western blot results were semi-quantified and shown in bar graph form. Representative images were shown and all the experiments had been repeated 3 times. *$p < 0.05$ and **$p < 0.01$

NSCLC invasion and migration mediated by CTHRC1 are MMP7- and MMP9-dependent

Based on our data, MMP7 and MMP9 were modulated by CTHRC1 in NSCLC cells. We then sought to determine whether NSCLC invasion and metastasis mediated by CTHRC1 requires MMP7 or MMP9. siRNA was applied to NCI-H1975-CTHRC1 and NCI-H2122-CTHRC1 cells to achieve MMP7 or MMP9 downregulation. Knockdown efficiency was confirmed by RT-PCR, the results of which are shown as a bar graph (Additional file 1: Figure S4A, 4B). CTHRC1 overexpression decreased NSCLC cell adhesion ability, and the adhesion index was significantly increased by either MMP7 or MMP9 downregulation (Fig. 4a). According to our Transwell results, CTHRC1 overexpression increased

tumour invasion. However, when MMP7 or MMP9 was knocked down in CTHRC1-overexpressing cells, respectively, they exhibited significant difference in invasion ability compared to those CTHRC1-overexpressing cells without MMP7 or MMP9 knock-down (Fig. 4b, c). Additionally, significant difference was observed in a scratch assay between CTHRC1-overexpressing cells with and without MMP7 or MMP9 knocked-down, respectively (Fig. 4d-f). More significant difference was observed in a adhesion, Transwell and scratch assay in CTHRC1-overexpressing cells with both MMP7 and MMP9 knocked-down, compared with those with MMP7 or MMP9 knocked-down, respectively. Furthermore, we did not observe the changed expression of MMP7 or MMP9 when MMP9 or MMP7 was knocked down (Additional file 1: Figure S4C, 4D).

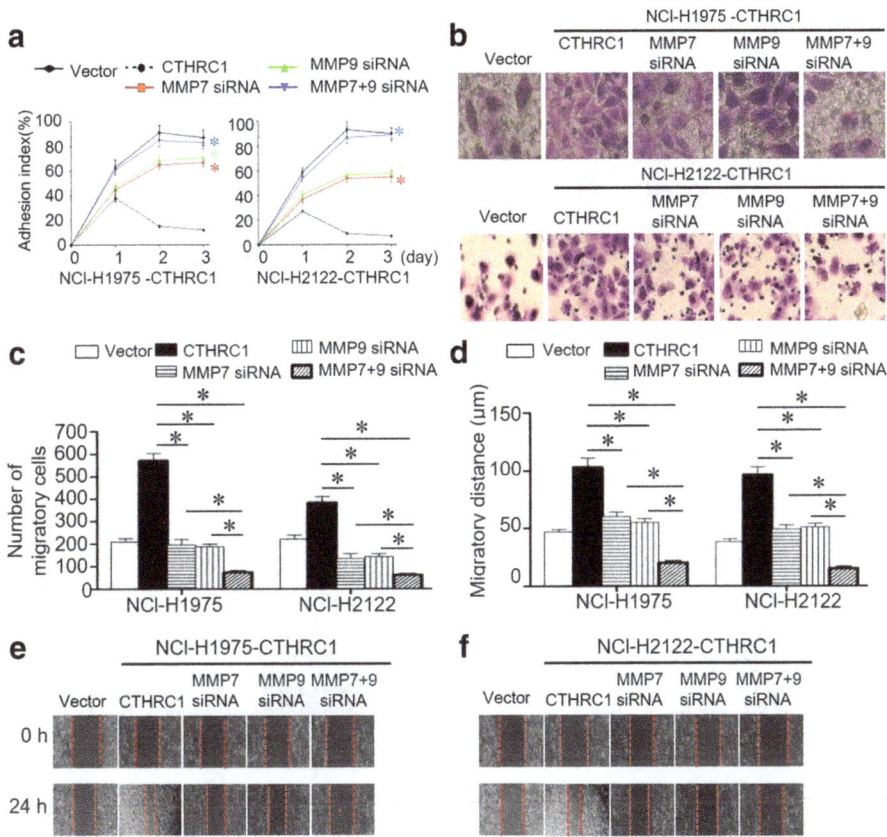

Fig. 4 The regulation of CTHRC1 on adhesion, migration, invasion and metastasis of tumor cells was mediated by MMP7 and MMP9. **a** Tumour cell adhesion ability decreased in CTHRC1-overexpressing cells. This decreased adhesion ability was elevated when either MMP7 or MMP9 was knocked down. **b, c** HE staining of cells invading through the Transwell gel demonstrated increased tumour cell invasion accompanying the ectopic overexpression of CTHRC1, which was inhibited by knocking down either MMP7 or MMP9. **d-f** A wound assay showing increased migration distance accompanying CTHRC1 overexpression. Knocking down either MMP7 or MMP9 inhibited the increased migration distance mediated by CTHRC1. $*p < 0.05$ and $**p < 0.01$

CTHRC1 enhances MMP7 promoter activity through AP-1/c-Jun pathway

To further characterize how CTHRC1 upregulates MMP7 expression, a luciferase reporter gene assay was carried out after the nuclear localization of CTHRC1 was confirmed by western blot in NCI-H1975 and NCI-H2122 cells (Additional file 1: Figure S5). NCI-H1975 and NCI-H2122 cells were co-transfected with the MMP7 promoter-luciferase construct pGL3 together with pcDNA3.1-CTHRC1 or a control vector, or CTHRC1 siRNA or scrambled RNA. As shown in Fig. 5a, MMP7 promoter-mediated luciferase activity was enhanced by the co-transfection of pcDNA3.1-CTHRC1 in a dose-dependent manner. In contrast, luciferase activity driven by the MMP7 promoter declined in both NCI-H1975 and NCI-H2122 cells transfected with CTHRC1-RNAi (Fig. 5b). Additionally, serial nucleotide sequences, specifically – 120 to + 50 (P1) and – 534 to + 50 (P2) in the MMP7 promoter region, were cloned into pGL3 (Fig. 5c). Compared to vector-

treated cells, the corresponding effects of these serial nucleotide sequences on luciferase activity were significantly increased by the ectopic overexpression of CTHRC1 or decreased by CTHRC1 knockdown. However, the MMP7 promoter fragment spanning – 534 to – 120 (P3) on the luciferase activity appeared to exert no differential effects when combined with either CTHRC1 overexpression or knockdown, compared to matched controls (Fig. 5d, Additional file 1: Figure S6A). Thus, CTHRC1 expression may be involved in the regulation of MMP7 promoter activity through the P1 and P2 regions (nucleotides – 120 to + 50 and – 534 to + 50).

According to the PCR results obtained from the ChIP assay, the physical interaction site between CTHRC1 and the MMP7 gene may be located in region 2 (nucleotides – 176 to + 50) of the MMP7 promoter (Fig. 5e, f). Because CTHRC1 itself does not contain DNA-binding sites, thus, there may be other transcription factors that cooperate with CTHRC1 to enhance promoter activity. Next, the MMP7 promoter region was screened for

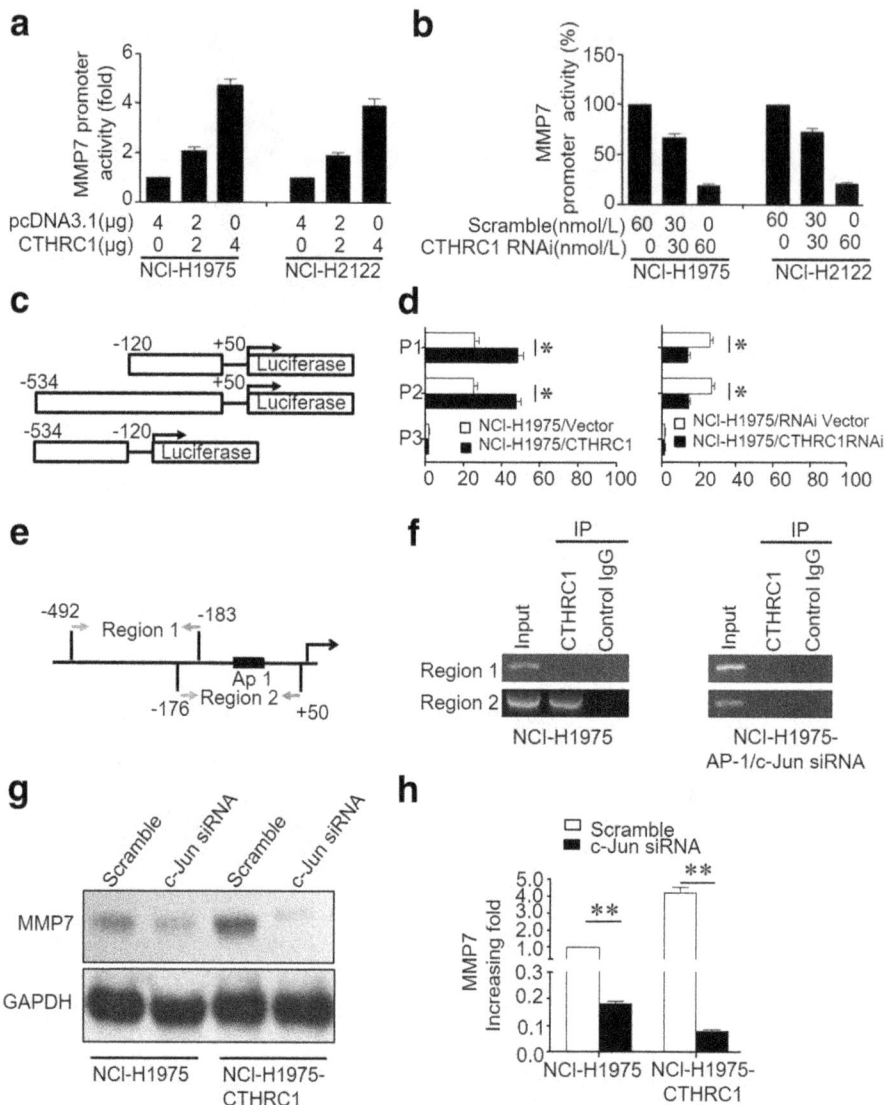

Fig. 5 CTHRC1 transcriptionally modulates MMP7 expression through c-JUN. **a** CTHRC1 overexpression increased MMP7 promoter activity. **b** MMP7 promoter activity was inhibited when CTHRC1 was downregulated. **c** The MMP7 promoter region was cloned as three fragments (P1 to P3). **d** Transactivating activity of CTHRC1 on serial MMP7 promoter fragments, as indicated in NCI-H1975 cells. CTHRC1 overexpression enhanced promoter activity in P1 and P2. CTHRC1 knockdown weakened promoter activity in P1 and P2. **e** Schematic illustration showing the PCR-amplified fragments of the MMP7 promoter. **f** Regions of the MMP7 promoter that were physically associated with CTHRC1 were analysed in a ChIP assay. IgG was used as a negative control. PCR amplification indicated the binding efficiency to region 2 was significantly decreased in NCI-H1975-AP-1/c-Jun siRNA cells. **g** CTHRC1 overexpression upregulated the expression of MMP7, and the upregulation of MMP7 was abolished when c-JUN was knocked down as measured by western blot. Representative bands are shown. **h** The western blot results were semi-quantified and are shown in bar graph form. Experiments had been repeated three times. *$p < 0.05$, **$p < 0.01$

transcriptional binding sites using prediction tools. A potential binding site in region 2, specifically nucleotides − 176 to + 50 within the MMP7 promoter, was identified as an activator protein (AP)-1–binding element (ABE), as indicated in Fig. 5e. Furthermore, silencing AP-1/c-Jun using siRNA significantly inhibited the binding efficiency of CTHRC1 to the MMP7 promoter (Fig. 5f), implying that AP-1 served as a "bridge protein" between CTHRC1 and MMP7 promoter. Moreover, according to our western blot and RT-PCR results, MMP7 expression

was significantly increased in NCI-H1975-CTHRC1 cells compared to NCI-H1975 cells. However, the increased expression of MMP7 in NCI-H1975-CTHRC1 cells was abolished when c-Jun siRNA was introduced (Fig. 5g, h), and MMP7 concentrations in the culture supernatants, as measured by ELISA, significantly decreased when c-Jun was depleted (Additional file 1: Figure S7A, C). Taken together, these findings confirm the involvement of the AP-1 pathway in the CTHRC1-mediated regulation of MMP7.

CTHRC1 enhances MMP9 promoter activity through the NF-κB and AP-1 pathways

Employing the same assay described above, we observed the dose-dependent effects of both CTHRC1 and CTHRC-RNAi on MMP9 promoter luciferase activity, similar to those observed for the MMP7 promoter (Fig. 6a, b). We also tested the luciferase activity driven by serial nucleotide fragments within the MMP9 promoter region, specifically -102 to $+31$ (P1), -312 to $+31$ (P2), -510 to $+31$ (P3), -810 to $+31$ (P4), -810 to -510 (P5), -510 to -312 (P6) and -312 to -102 (P7), as shown in Fig. 6c and d. CTHRC1 overexpression increased MMP9 promoter activity but

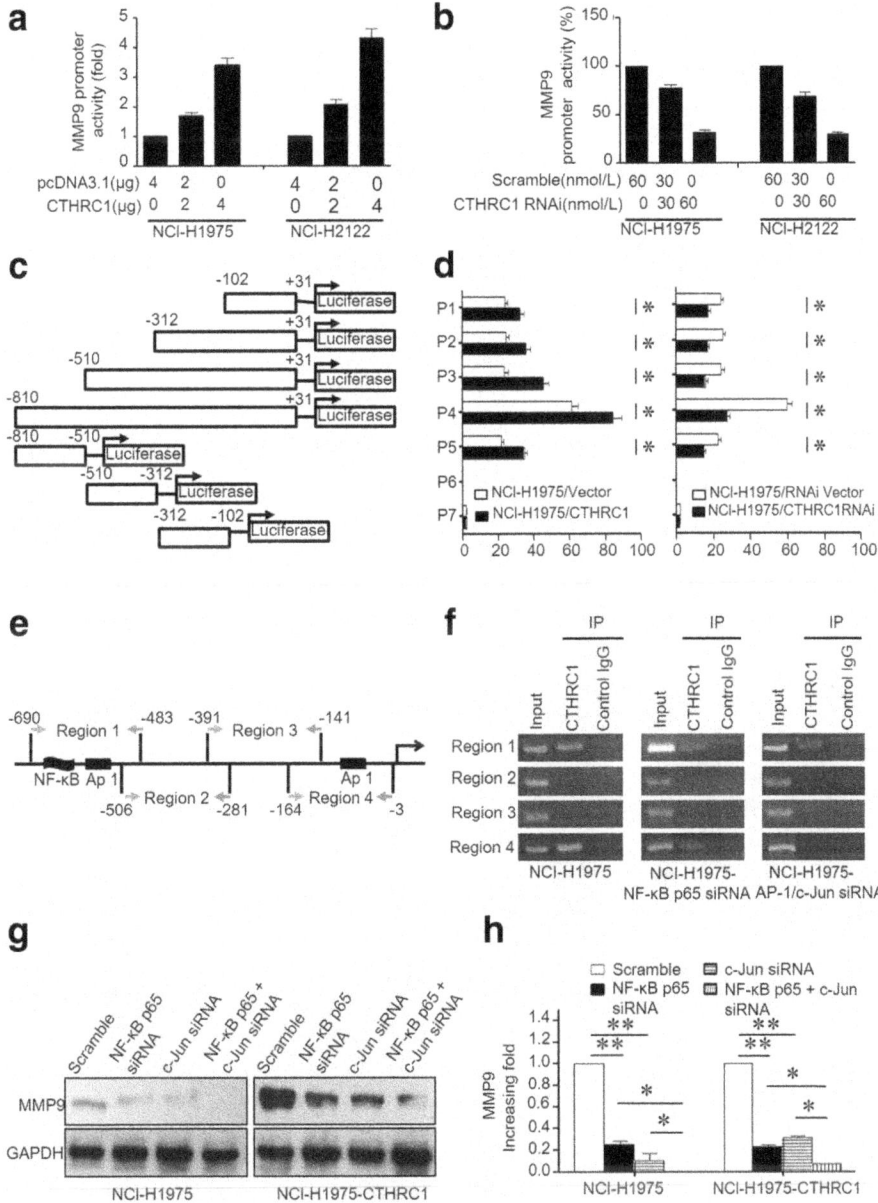

Fig. 6 CTHRC1 transcriptionally modulates MMP9 expression through c-JUN and NF-κB signals. **a** CTHRC1 overexpression increased MMP9 promoter activity. **b** MMP9 promoter activity was inhibited when CTHRC1 was downregulated. **c** The promoter region was cloned as seven fragments (P1 to P7). **d** Transactivating activity of CTHRC1 on serial MMP9 promoter fragments as indicated in NCI-H1975 cells. CTHRC1 overexpression enhanced the promoter activity in P1–5, while CTHRC1 knockdown weakened promoter activity in P1–5. **e** Schematic illustration showing the PCR-amplified fragments of the MMP9 promoter. **f** Regions of the MMP9 promoter that were physically associated with CTHRC1 were analysed in a ChIP assay. IgG was used as a negative control. PCR amplification indicated the binding efficiencies to region 1 and region 4 were decreased in NCI-H1975-AP-1/c-Jun siRNA cells, and binding efficiency to region 1 was significantly decreased in NCI-H1975-NF-κB siRNA cells. **g** Western blotting revealed upregulated MMP9 expression accompanying the ectopic overexpression of CTHRC1; this MMP9 upregulation was abolished when either NF-κB or c-JUN was knocked down. Knockdown of NF-κB and c-JUN together further decreased MMP9 expression. Representative bands are shown. **h** The western blot results were semi-quantified and are shown in bar graph form. Experiments had been repeated 3 times. *$p < 0.05$, **$p < 0.01$

decreased when CTHRC1 was knocked down (Fig. 6c, d and Additional file 1: Figure S6B). Potential binding sites within the MMP9 promoter region were identified in region 1 for NF-κB and Ap-1 (nucleotides – 690 to – 483) and within region 4 for Ap-1 (nucleotides – 164 to – 3) (Fig. 6e). Additionally, the binding efficiencies of CTHRC1 to MMP9 promoter regions 1 and 4 were reduced by the application of AP-1/c-Jun siRNA. NF-κB p65 siRNA significantly suppressed the binding capacity of CTHRC1 for region 1 within the MMP9 promoter (Fig. 6f). Moreover, western blot and ELISA results further verified the upregulation of MMP9 expression by CTHRC1 through NF-κB and AP-1 pathways at both the protein and mRNA levels (Fig. 6g, h, Additional file 1: Figure S7B, D).

Increased expression of CTHRC1 was correlated with CTC and predicts progression and poor prognosis of NSCLC

Further investigation is required to understand the relationship between CTHRC1 and clinical metastasis in NSCLC. Tumour cells are detectable in the circulating blood of cancer patients but not in that of healthy individuals or patients with non-malignant diseases. The increased numbers of CTCs indicate a higher chance for tumour metastasis. In the present study, we detected CTC numbers using a NanoVelcro system and measured serum CTHRC1 concentrations by ELISA ($n = 143$) in the same NSCLC patients. Compared to normal controls, serum levels of CTHRC1 were significantly higher in NSCLC patients ($n = 40$). CTHRC1 concentrations in NSCLC patients correlated with metastasis. Advanced disease stages characterized by local invasion or distant metastasis exhibited much higher serum CTHRC1 levels (Additional file 1: Figure S8A-C). Furthermore, CTHRC1 concentration significantly correlated with CTC counts (Fig. 7a, b). Additionally, the CTHRC1 cut-off had optimal sensitivity and specificity for metastasis with an area under the curve of 0.97 (95% CI: 0.941–1.000; $p < 0.001$). The CTHRC1 cut-off also had optimal sensitivity and specificity for recurrence with an area under the curve of 0.691 (95% CI: 0.604–0.788; $p < 0.001$) (Fig. 7c, d).

Given the role of CTHRC1 in the tumor invasion and metastasis, we made further efforts to identify the clinical significance of CTHRC1 for prognosis prediction in NSCLC patients. Patients with high CTHRC1 expression had significant lower 5-year survival rate (2.4%) than those with low CTHRC1 expression (51.5%) (Fig. 7e). Moreover, early stage (stages I and II) and late stage (stages III and IV) patients with high CTHRC1 expression had shorter survival durations than those with low CTHRC1 expression (Fig. 7f-h). In the early and advanced stages, 5-year survival rates for low CTHRC1 expression were 55.1% and 21.4%, respectively. All the advanced

stage patients with high CTHRC1 expression died within 5 years.

In a univariate analysis, CTHRC1 levels were correlated with overall survival (Additional file 1: Table S6). Further, a multivariate analysis performed using the COX proportional hazard regression model indicated CTHRC1 overexpression was an independent prognosis-related marker for NSCLC (Additional file 1: Table S7). We then evaluated how predictive prognostic power was related to the combined expression of CTHRC1, MMP7 and MMP9 in NSCLC patients. Compared to patients with a low expression pattern, patients with a high expression pattern for CTHRC1, MMP7 and MMP9 appeared to have poorer survival (Fig. 7i, j).

Discussion

Cancer invasion and metastasis are among the biological hallmarks acquired during the multistep development of human tumours. Underlying these hallmarks is genome instability, which leads to the genetic diversity that eventually expedites their acquisition [30, 31]. In this report, CTHRC1 upregulation was associated with lymphatic metastasis, distant metastasis, and MMP7 and MMP9 overexpression in NSCLC patients, indicating CTHRC1 plays a critical role in promoting cancer invasiveness. Consistent with the above findings, we identified MMP7 and MMP9 as substrates of CTHRC1 and revealed an unknown function of CTHRC1 in promoting strong cell invasion in an MMP7- and MMP9-dependent manner through the transcriptional upregulation of MMP7 and MMP9 via interactions with their corresponding promoters.

The most common causes of cancer-associated mortality are the occurrence of local invasion or distant metastasis, rather than the presence of the primary tumours themselves. Among clinically diagnosed NSCLC patients, almost half have confirmed distant metastases [32]. As a candidate tumour marker in this study, CTHRC1 was identified in NSCLC samples by performing quantitative assessments involving 2D-PAGE gels and mass spectrometry in comparison with adjacent non-tumour tissues. Furthermore, elevated preoperative serum CTHRC1 levels were associated with tumour metastasis. According to previous studies [20, 22, 29], and our own [23], CTHRC1 promotes cancer progression and activates relevant signalling molecules, which urged us to determine whether CTHRC1 plays a similar role in determining the aggressiveness of NSCLC. Thus, we evaluated CTHRC1 functions in lung cancer cell migration and invasion. Consistent with the published effects of CTHRC1 on the invasive phenotype of NSCLC cells, CTHRC1 knockdown greatly decreased cell invasion and inhibited cell migration, whereas endogenous CTHRC1 overexpression significantly increased invasive ability.

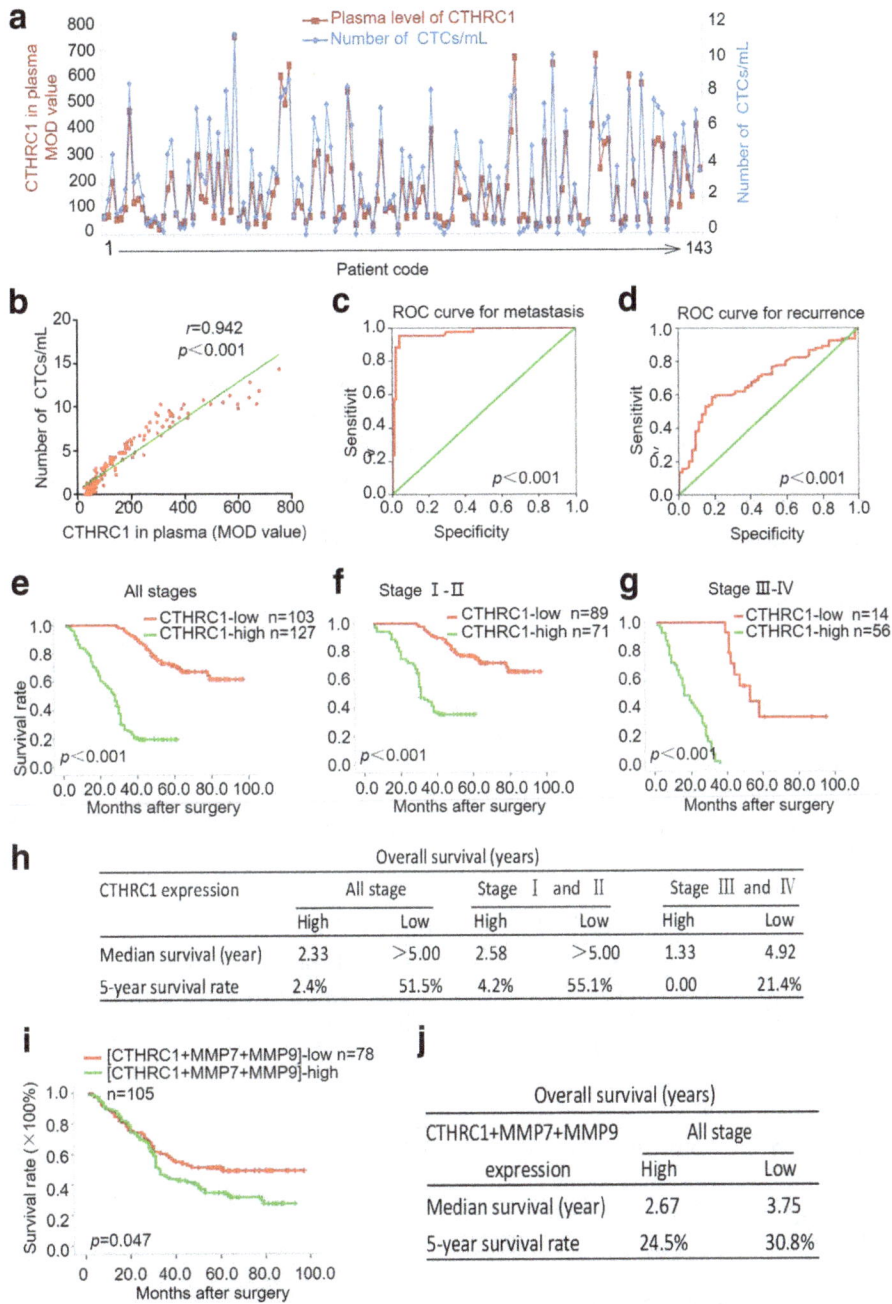

Fig. 7 Clinical relevance of CTHRC1 expression in NSCLC patients. **a, b** Circulating tumour cells (CTC) were detected using the NanoVelcro system. The CTHRC1 concentration positively correlated with the number of CTCs. **c, d** The cut-off value for CTHRC1 had optimal sensitivity and specificity for metastasis, with an area under the curve of 0.97 (95% CI: 0.941–1.000; $p < 0.001$), and optimal sensitivity and specificity for recurrence, with an area under the curve of 0.691 (95% CI: 0.604–0.788; $p < 0.001$). **e** IHC data indicating the post-surgery survival rate was significantly lower in the group of CTHRC1-high patients. **f, g** CTHRC1-low patients had much higher post-surgery survival rates, at both the early and late stages. **h** Summary of overall survival with high or low CTHRC1 expression. **i** Compared to low CTHRC1, MMP7 and MMP9 expression, the combined high expression of CTHRC1, MMP7 and MMP9 was associated with a significantly lower post-surgery survival rate. **j** Summary of overall survival with high or low combinatorial CTHRC1, MMP7 and MMP9 expression

Additionally, based on the IHC analysis of 230 clinical NSCLC specimens, CTHRC1 overexpression was significantly correlated with clinical stage, indicating CTHRC1 upregulation may facilitate NSCLC metastasis.

Tumour metastasis is initiated by a CTC sub-group that has been observed in patient blood. CTCs are used as a marker to predict disease progression in metastatic patients, including breast, colorectal and prostate cancers.

They are involved in metastatic spread to distant organs, leading to the formation of secondary sites of lung cancer [33]. Here, increased plasma levels of CTHRC1 were positively correlated with the presence of CTCs, suggesting plasma CTHRC1 attracts CTCs into circulation. However, the molecular mechanisms underlying tumour metastasis mediated by CTHRC1 require further investigation.

Proteolytic degradation of the stromal ECM is well known for its contribution to malignant invasion and metastasis [34, 35]. MMPs, as a family of zinc-dependent endopeptidases, are involved in degrading ECM and facilitating tumour invasion [11, 36, 37]. As shown in the present study, significantly higher expression of CTHRC1, MMP-7 and MMP-9 was observed in a cohort of NSCLC sera and surgically resected tumour tissues. CTHRC1 was positively correlated with MMP7 and MMP9 expression at both the protein and mRNA levels. MMP regulation, generally by hormones and cytokines, occurs primarily at the transcription level [38, 39]. MMPs are also regulated via the initiation of pro-MMP cleavage and proteolytic activity inhibition by specific inhibitors [40–42]. Our observations here indicate MMP7 and MMP9 may serve as the potential target genes of CTHRC1 in NSCLC, which may explain why CTHRC1 enhances NSCLC progression in vivo. However, it remains unclear whether the involvement of MMP7 and MMP9 in NSCLC progression is mechanistically regulated by CTHRC1.

CTHRC1, generally recognized as a secreted protein [19], was firstly confirmed in the nuclear localization of NSCLC cells. This builds the foundation for us to deeply explore the regulation mechanisms of CTHRC1 on MMP7 and MMP9. MMP7 and MMP9 expression is generally regulated via promoter binding sites for multiple transcription activators, such as AP-1 and β-catenin/TCF4 for MMP7 [43, 44] and AP-1, AP-2, NF-κB, and SP-1 for MMP9 [45, 46]. Based on previous findings from a luciferase-based ChIP assay, CTHRC1 binds to the MMP7 promoter (− 120 to + 50 bp) and MMP9 promoter (− 102 to + 31 bp and − 810 to − 510 bp). However, CTHRC1 does not contain DNA-binding sites [22].

Thus, CTHRC1 may cooperate with other transcription factors to bind to the promoters of downstream genes and initiate to their transcriptional activation. Sequence analysis revealed a potential binding site for AP-1 in the MMP7 promoter between nucleotide − 176 to + 50 bp. Two binding sites for NF-κB and AP-1 are also present in the MMP9 promoter between nucleotides − 164 to − 3 bp and − 690 to − 506 bp, respectively. Furthermore, AP-1/c-Jun depletion decreased the binding efficiency of CTHRC1 to the MMP7 promoter. Simultaneously, the knockdown of both NF-κB and AP-1/c-Jun suppressed CTHRC1 binding to the MMP9 promoter. In agreement with our hypothesis, c-Jun depletion downregulated

MMP7 expression, and knockdown of either NF-κB or c-Jun decreased MMP9 expression. However, whether the invasion mediated by CTHRC1 depends on MMP7 and MMP9 remains unclear.

The metalloproteinases MMP7 and MMP9 are overexpressed in NSCLC and other types of cancers and are strongly associated with poor prognosis [16, 47, 48]. An inhibitor of MMPs, including MMP7 and MMP9, was shown to suppress tumour metastasis [49]. Additionally, the application of MMP7 to colon cancer-bearing nude mice enhanced tumour metastasis [50] and MMP9-deficient mice were protected against tumour metastasis [14]. Consistent with these data, the enhanced tumour cell migration and invasion mediated by CTHRC1 overexpression was eradicated when either MMP7 or MMP9 was knocked down. Based on these data, CTHRC1-mediated invasion is MMP7- and MMP9-dependent.

In conclusion, our current systematic study identified CTHRC1 as a invasion-driving gene that promotes NSCLC progression by activating c-Jun/MMP7, c-Jun/MMP9 and NF-κB/MMP9 signalling; thus, therapeutic targeting of CTHRC1 may be a promising strategy to enhance the therapeutic effects of anticancer drugs against NSCLC. Additionally, CTHRC1 may serve as a sensitive predictor of the low 5-year overall survival in NSCLC and as an effective biomarker for evaluating the poor clinicopathological characteristics of NSCLC.

Conclusions

CTHRC1 promotes NSCLC invasion by upregulating MMP7 and MMP9. Targeting CTHRC1 may be beneficial for inhibiting NSCLC progression.

Abbreviations

ANTs: Non-tumour tissues; CTC: Circulating tumour cell; CTHRC1: Collagen triple helix repeat containing 1; ECM: Extracellular matrix; MMP-7: Matrix metalloproteinase 7; MMP-9: Matrix metalloproteinase 9; NSCLC: Non-small cell lung cancer

Acknowledgements

Not applicable.

Funding

This work was supported by grants from National Natural Science Foundation of China (30900650, 81372501, 81572260, 81773299, 81172232, 81570008, 81172564 and 31430030), Guangdong Natural Science Foundation (2011B031800025, S2012010008378, S2012010008270, S2013010015327, 2013B021800126, 20090171120070, 9451008901002146, 2013B021800126, 2014A030313052 and 2013B021800259), Guangdong Science and Technology Planning Program (2014 J4100132, 2015A020214010 and 2016A020215055) and Guangzhou Science and Technology Planning Program (201704020094, 2015ykzd07 and 16ykjc08). The funding body had no role in the design of the study and collection, analysis, and interpretation of data and in writing the manuscript.

Authors' contributions

ZK, WH, HZ, YW, YZ, XZ designed the study. YW, YL, YC, NJ, WJ, HW, ZW performed experiments. SL, YC, YS did the data analysis. HZ, WH, ZK, LW wrote the manuscript. All authors read and approved the final manuscript.

Competing interests

The authors declare that they have no competing interests.

Author details

[1]Department of Pathology, The First Affiliated Hospital, Sun Yat-sen University, No. 58, ZhongShan Second Road, Guangdong 510080, China. [2]Department of Gastrointestinal Surgery, The First Affiliated Hospital, Sun Yat-sen University, No. 58, ZhongShan Second Road, Guangdong 510080, China. [3]Department of Respiratory Medicine, The First Affiliated Hospital, Sun Yat-sen University, No. 58, ZhongShan Second Road, Guangdong 510080, China. [4]Department of Thoracic Surgery, The Central Hospital of Wuhan, No.26 Shenli Street, Jiang'an District, Wuhan 430014, Hubei Province, China. [5]Biomedical Engineering, The University of Texas at El Paso, El Paso, TX, USA. [6]Department of Molecular and Medical Pharmacology, Crump Institute for Molecular Imaging (CIMI), California NanoSystems Institute (CNSI), University of California, Los Angeles, 570 Westwood Plaza, California, Los Angeles 90095-1770, USA. [7]Guangdong Provincial Key Laboratory of Orthopedics and Traumatology, The First Affiliated Hospital, Sun Yat-sen University, No. 58, ZhongShan Second Road, Guangdong 510080, China.

References

1. Jemal A, Siegel R, Ward E, Hao Y, Xu J, Murray T, Thun MJ. Cancer statistics, 2008. CA Cancer J Clin. 2008;58(2):71–96.
2. Molina JR, Yang P, Cassivi SD, Schild SE, Adjei AA. Non-small cell lung cancer: epidemiology, risk factors, treatment, and survivorship. Mayo Clin Proc. 2008;83(5):584–94.
3. Reck M, Popat S, Reinmuth N, De Ruysscher D, Kerr KM, Peters S, Group EGW. Metastatic non-small-cell lung cancer (NSCLC): ESMO clinical practice guidelines for diagnosis, treatment and follow-up. Ann Oncol. 2014;25(Suppl 3):iii27–39.
4. Bremnes RM, Veve R, Hirsch FR, Franklin WA. The E-cadherin cell-cell adhesion complex and lung cancer invasion, metastasis, and prognosis. Lung Cancer. 2002;36(2):115–24.
5. Petty RD, Nicolson MC, Kerr KM, Collie-Duguid E, Murray GI. Gene expression profiling in non-small cell lung cancer: from molecular mechanisms to clinical application. Clin Cancer Res. 2004;10(10):3237–48.
6. Sandler AB. Molecular targeted agents in non-small-cell lung cancer. Clin Lung Cancer. 2003;5(Suppl 1):S22–8.
7. Friedl P, Wolf K. Tumour-cell invasion and migration: diversity and escape mechanisms. Nat Rev Cancer. 2003;3(5):362–74.
8. Friedl P, Alexander S. Cancer invasion and the microenvironment: plasticity and reciprocity. Cell. 2011;147(5):992–1009.
9. Foda HD, Zucker S. Matrix metalloproteinases in cancer invasion, metastasis and angiogenesis. Drug Discov Today. 2001;6(9):478–82.
10. Fingleton B. Matrix metalloproteinases: roles in cancer and metastasis. Front Biosci. 2006;11:479–91.
11. Stamenkovic I. Matrix metalloproteinases in tumor invasion and metastasis. Semin Cancer Biol. 2000;10(6):415–33.
12. Egeblad M, Werb Z. New functions for the matrix metalloproteinases in cancer progression. Nat Rev Cancer. 2002;2(3):161–74.
13. Wang FQ, So J, Reierstad S, Fishman DA. Matrilysin (MMP-7) promotes invasion of ovarian cancer cells by activation of progelatinase. Int J Cancer. 2005;114(1):19–31.
14. Itoh T, Tanioka M, Matsuda H, Nishimoto H, Yoshioka T, Suzuki R, Uehira M. Experimental metastasis is suppressed in MMP-9-deficient mice. Clin Exp Metastasis. 1999;17(2):177–81.
15. Dong QZ, Wang Y, Tang ZP, Fu L, Li QC, Wang ED, Wang EH. Derlin-1 is overexpressed in non-small cell lung cancer and promotes cancer cell invasion via EGFR-ERK-mediated up-regulation of MMP-2 and MMP-9. Am J Pathol. 2013;182(3):954–64.
16. Liu D, Nakano J, Ishikawa S, Yokomise H, Ueno M, Kadota K, Urushihara M, Huang CL. Overexpression of matrix metalloproteinase-7 (MMP-7) correlates with tumor proliferation, and a poor prognosis in non-small cell lung cancer. Lung Cancer. 2007;58(3):384–91.
17. Cox G, Jones JL, O'Byrne KJ. Matrix metalloproteinase 9 and the epidermal growth factor signal pathway in operable non-small cell lung cancer. Clin Cancer Res. 2000;6(6):2349–55.
18. Leinonen T, Pirinen R, Bohm J, Johansson R, Ropponen K, Kosma VM. Expression of matrix metalloproteinases 7 and 9 in non-small cell lung cancer. Relation to clinicopathological factors, beta-catenin and prognosis. Lung Cancer. 2006;51(3):313–21.
19. Pyagay P, Heroult M, Wang Q, Lehnert W, Belden J, Liaw L, Friesel RE, Lindner V. Collagen triple helix repeat containing 1, a novel secreted protein in injured and diseased arteries, inhibits collagen expression and promotes cell migration. Circ Res. 2005;96(2):261–8.
20. Tang L, Dai DL, Su M, Martinka M, Li G, Zhou Y. Aberrant expression of collagen triple helix repeat containing 1 in human solid cancers. Clin Cancer Res. 2006;12(12):3716–22.
21. Ma MZ, Zhuang C, Yang XM, Zhang ZZ, Ma H, Zhang WM, You H, Qin W, Gu J, Yang S, et al. CTHRC1 acts as a prognostic factor and promotes invasiveness of gastrointestinal stromal tumors by activating Wnt/PCP-rho signaling. Neoplasia. 2014;16(3):265–78. 278 e261-213
22. Chen YL, Wang TH, Hsu HC, Yuan RH, Jeng YM. Overexpression of CTHRC1 in hepatocellular carcinoma promotes tumor invasion and predicts poor prognosis. PLoS One. 2013;8(7):e70324.
23. Ke Z, He W, Lai Y, Guo X, Chen S, Li S, Wang Y, Wang L. Overexpression of collagen triple helix repeat containing 1 (CTHRC1) is associated with tumour aggressiveness and poor prognosis in human non-small cell lung cancer. Oncotarget. 2014;5(19):9410–24.
24. Park EH, Kim S, Jo JY, Kim SJ, Hwang Y, Kim JM, Song SY, Lee DK, Koh SS. Collagen triple helix repeat containing-1 promotes pancreatic cancer progression by regulating migration and adhesion of tumor cells. Carcinogenesis. 2013;34(3):694–702.
25. Hou M, Cheng Z, Shen H, He S, Li Y, Pan Y, Feng C, Chen X, Zhang Y, Lin M, et al. High expression of CTHRC1 promotes EMT of epithelial ovarian cancer (EOC) and is associated with poor prognosis. Oncotarget. 2015;6(34):35813–29.
26. Vu LT, Bui D, Le HT. Prevalence of cervical infection with HPV type 16 and 18 in Vietnam: implications for vaccine campaign. BMC Cancer. 2013;13:53.
27. Sun Y, Chen YS, Li SH, Lei YY, Xu D, Jiang N, Zhang Y, Cao J Ke ZF. NanoVelcro-captured CTC number concomitant with enhanced serum levels of MMP7 and MMP9 enables accurate prediction of metastasis and poor prognosis in patients with lung adenocarcinoma. Int J Nanomedicine. 2017;12:6399–412.
28. Shekhani MT, Forde TS, Adilbayeva A, Ramez M, Myngbay A, Bexeitov Y, Lindner V, Adarichev VA. Collagen triple helix repeat containing 1 is a new promigratory marker of arthritic pannus. Arthritis Res Ther. 2016;18:171.
29. Wang P, Wang YC, Chen XY, Shen ZY, Cao H, Zhang YJ, Yu J, Zhu JD, Lu YY, Fang JY. CTHRC1 is upregulated by promoter demethylation and transforming growth factor-beta1 and may be associated with metastasis in human gastric cancer. Cancer Sci. 2012;103(7):1327–33.
30. Vlodavsky I, Friedmann Y. Molecular properties and involvement of heparanase in cancer metastasis and angiogenesis. J Clin Invest. 2001; 108(3):341–7.
31. Hanahan D, Weinberg RA. Hallmarks of cancer: the next generation. Cell. 2011;144(5):646–74.
32. Morgensztern D, Ng SH, Gao F, Govindan R. Trends in stage distribution for patients with non-small cell lung cancer: a National Cancer Database survey. J Thorac Oncol. 2010;5(1):29–33.
33. Hou JM, Krebs M, Ward T, Sloane R, Priest L, Hughes A, Clack G, Ranson M, Blackhall F, Dive C. Circulating tumor cells as a window on metastasis biology in lung cancer. Am J Pathol. 2011;178(3):989–96.
34. Johnsen M, Lund LR, Romer J, Almholt K, Dano K. Cancer invasion and tissue remodeling: common themes in proteolytic matrix degradation. Curr Opin Cell Biol. 1998;10(5):667–71.
35. Butcher DT, Alliston T, Weaver VM. A tense situation: forcing tumour progression. Nat Rev Cancer. 2009;9(2):108–22.
36. Basset P, Okada A, Chenard MP, Kannan R, Stoll I, Anglard P, Bellocq JP, Rio MC. Matrix metalloproteinases as stromal effectors of human carcinoma progression: therapeutic implications. Matrix Biol. 1997;15(8–9):535–41.
37. Kenny HA, Kaur S, Coussens LM, Lengyel E. The initial steps of ovarian cancer cell metastasis are mediated by MMP-2 cleavage of vitronectin and fibronectin. J Clin Invest. 2008;118(4):1367–79.
38. Vincenti MP. The matrix metalloproteinase (MMP) and tissue inhibitor of metalloproteinase (TIMP) genes. Transcriptional and posttranscriptional regulation, signal transduction and cell-type-specific expression. Methods Mol Biol. 2001;151:121–48.

39. Ries C, Petrides PE. Cytokine regulation of matrix metalloproteinase activity and its regulatory dysfunction in disease. Biol Chem Hoppe Seyler. 1995; 376(6):345–55.
40. Chakraborti S, Mandal M, Das S, Mandal A, Chakraborti T. Regulation of matrix metalloproteinases: an overview. Mol Cell Biochem. 2003;253(1–2):269–85.
41. Crabbe T, O'Connell JP, Smith BJ, Docherty AJ. Reciprocated matrix metalloproteinase activation: a process performed by interstitial collagenase and progelatinase a. Biochemistry. 1994;33(48):14419–25.
42. Gomez DE, Alonso DF, Yoshiji H, Thorgeirsson UP. Tissue inhibitors of metalloproteinases: structure, regulation and biological functions. Eur J Cell Biol. 1997;74(2):111–22.
43. Gaire M, Magbanua Z, McDonnell S, McNeil L, Lovett DH, Matrisian LM. Structure and expression of the human gene for the matrix metalloproteinase matrilysin. J Biol Chem. 1994;269(3):2032–40.
44. Brabletz T, Jung A, Dag S, Hlubek F, Kirchner T. Beta-catenin regulates the expression of the matrix metalloproteinase-7 in human colorectal cancer. Am J Pathol. 1999;155(4):1033–8.
45. Ogawa K, Chen F, Kuang C, Chen Y. Suppression of matrix metalloproteinase-9 transcription by transforming growth factor-beta is mediated by a nuclear factor-kappaB site. Biochem J. 2004;381(Pt 2):413–22.
46. St-Pierre Y, Couillard J, Van Themsche C. Regulation of MMP-9 gene expression for the development of novel molecular targets against cancer and inflammatory diseases. Expert Opin Ther Targets. 2004;8(5):473–89.
47. Zheng S, Chang Y, Hodges KB, Sun Y, Ma X, Xue Y, Williamson SR, Lopez-Beltran A, Montironi R, Cheng L. Expression of KISS1 and MMP-9 in non-small cell lung cancer and their relations to metastasis and survival. Anticancer Res. 2010;30(3):713–8.
48. Thorns V, Walter GF, Thorns C. Expression of MMP-2, MMP-7, MMP-9, MMP-10 and MMP-11 in human astrocytic and oligodendroglial gliomas. Anticancer Res. 2003;23(5A):3937–44.
49. Naglich JG, Jure-Kunkel M, Gupta E, Fargnoli J, Henderson AJ, Lewin AC, Talbott R, Baxter A, Bird J, Savopoulos R, et al. Inhibition of angiogenesis and metastasis in two murine models by the matrix metalloproteinase inhibitor, BMS-275291. Cancer Res. 2001;61(23):8480–5.
50. Kioi M, Yamamoto K, Higashi S, Koshikawa N, Fujita K, Miyazaki K. Matrilysin (MMP-7) induces homotypic adhesion of human colon cancer cells and enhances their metastatic potential in nude mouse model. Oncogene. 2003; 22(54):8662–70.

9

Smokers' interest in a lung cancer screening programme

Samantha L. Quaife[1*], Charlotte Vrinten[1], Mamta Ruparel[2], Samuel M. Janes[2], Rebecca J. Beeken[1,3], Jo Waller[1] and Andy McEwen[1]

Abstract

Background: Following the recommendation of lung cancer screening in the US, screening committees in several European countries are reviewing the evidence for implementing national programmes. However, inadequate participation from high-risk groups poses a potential barrier to its effectiveness. The present study examined interest in a national lung cancer screening programme and modifiable attitudinal factors that may affect participation by smokers.

Methods: A population-based survey of English adults ($n = 1464$; aged 50–70 years) investigated screening intentions in different invitation scenarios, beliefs about lung cancer, early detection and treatment, worry about lung cancer risk, and stigma. Data on smoking status and perceived chances of quitting were also collected, but eligibility for lung screening in the event of a national programme was unknown.

Results: Intentions to be screened were high in all three invitation scenarios for both current (≥ 89%) and former (≥ 94%) smokers. However, smokers were less likely to agree that early-stage survival is good (43% vs. 53%; OR: 0.64, 0.46–0.88) or be willing to have surgery for an early stage, screen-detected cancer (84% vs. 94%; OR: 0.38, 0.21–0.68), compared with former smokers. Willingness to have surgery was positively associated with screening intentions; with absolute differences of 25% and 29%. Worry about lung cancer risk was also most common among smokers (48%), and one fifth of respondents thought screening smokers was a waste of NHS money.

Conclusions: A national lung cancer screening programme would be well-received in principle. To improve smokers' participation, care should be taken to communicate the survival benefits of early-stage diagnosis, address concerns about surgery, and minimise anxiety and stigma related to lung cancer risk.

Keywords: Lung cancer screening, Early detection, Screening uptake, Smoking, Attitudes, Behavioural science

Background

Lung cancer is the leading cause of cancer mortality worldwide and typically has a bleak prognosis [1]; partly because early diagnoses are infrequent [2]. Low-dose computed tomography (LDCT) screening offers a means of detecting disease early, and was shown by the US National Lung Screening Trial (NLST) to reduce the relative risk of lung cancer mortality by 20%, compared with chest X-ray, for high-risk adults screened annually over 3 years [3]. Screening is recommended by the US Preventive Services Task Force (USPSTF) for current smokers and recent ex-smokers (≤ 15 years since quitting) aged 55 to 80, who have accrued a 30 pack-year smoking history [4], and is funded by Medicare and Medicaid [5]. Implementation in the UK is under review by the National Screening Committee [6].

Crucial to the effectiveness of lung cancer screening is uptake by those at high risk. This will optimise the risk-benefit ratio as the majority (88%) of deaths prevented by the NLST were for participants scoring within the three highest risk quintiles [7]. However, enrolment into trials has been low, at less than 5% of all those invited in

* Correspondence: samantha.quaife@ucl.ac.uk
[1]Department of Behavioural Science and Health, University College London, Gower Street, London WC1E 6BT, UK
Full list of author information is available at the end of the article

the target age range, and biased toward those at lower risk. Current smoking status and low socioeconomic position (SEP) have predicted lower attendance across European and US trials [8–10]; the very factors associated with increased risk [11].

Surveys carried out in the community find smokers are more likely to express negative attitudes towards screening. One US population survey ($n = 2001$) found that, compared with former smokers, fewer current smokers were willing to be screened, believed early detection can increase survival, or anticipated agreeing to surgery for a screen-detected cancer [12]. In a US survey of ethnic minority groups, concerns about survival, radiation, financial cost, and the CT scan process predicted lower screening intentions [13]. More recently, an online US survey found that high perceived risk, low fear of CT scans and confidence in their accuracy, and the belief that early detection can improve prognosis, together predicted agreement to a LDCT scan [14]. In the UK, a mixed methods study of lower SEP communities suggested that fatalism about survival, risk, and treatment, and fear of an expected diagnosis may constitute important psychosocial deterrents for smokers [15]. Studies of trial non-participants have also implicated psychological deterrents, including emotional barriers such as fear, worry and avoidance [16, 17], fatalistic views and perceptions of low benefit in older age [18], and a lack of awareness that screening is beneficial for asymptomatic individuals [18]. Added to this is the potential role of social factors such as perceived stigmatisation of smoking [15, 19].

Characteristics of the invitation could also affect screening uptake. UK screening programmes for breast, colorectal and cervical cancer organise invitations through central NHS hubs, but there is good evidence that GP endorsement [20] and pre-scheduled appointments [21] improve uptake. The acceptability of these different invitation scenarios has not been studied for lung cancer screening.

This study aimed to: i) examine how screening intentions and perceptions of early detection of lung cancer might differ by smoking status, and ii) measure interest in, and acceptability of, an NHS lung cancer screening programme offered in different invitation scenarios.

Methods

A population-based sample of adults aged 50–70 years took part in the Attitudes, Behaviour and Cancer UK Survey (ABACUS) in April 2015. This age group was selected to represent individuals who could be eligible for, or approaching eligibility for, lung cancer screening according to the USPSTF criteria [4]. The survey was administered within the rolling Omnibus survey [22] carried out by TNS Research International, which uses

home-based computer-assisted, face-to-face interviews. Sampling points in England were selected using stratified random location sampling from the 2011 Census small area statistics [23], the Postcode Address File and Government Office Regions. At each sampling location, quotas were set for age, gender, children residing in the household, and employment status.

Measures

A brief, standardised description of lung cancer screening was provided and single-item questions were adapted from existing measures and studies, and piloted in cognitive interviews ($n = 15$), and an online survey ($n = 391$) prior to this study.

Lung cancer screening intentions

Participants were asked to rate their intention to be screened following three hypothetical invitation scenarios presented in the same order to all participants: i) an invitation from a national NHS programme, ii) a GP recommendation, and iii) an upcoming pre-scheduled appointment next month. These items were adapted from the colorectal cancer screening literature [24]. It was made clear to participants that there is currently no national lung cancer screening programme in England. Responses were on a five-point scale for the first two items ('yes definitely', 'yes probably', 'probably not', 'definitely not', 'not sure') and the third item ('very likely', 'likely', 'unlikely', 'very unlikely', 'not sure'). They were dichotomised for analysis as 'yes definitely/probably' vs. 'probably/definitely not', and 'very likely/likely' vs. 'very unlikely/unlikely'. Those answering 'not sure' or 'refused' on any of the three items were excluded.

Beliefs about lung cancer survival, early detection and screening

Two items were taken from the Awareness and Beliefs about Cancer (ABC) measure [25] concerning survival from cancer and lung cancer ('a diagnosis of cancer/lung cancer is a death sentence'). Response options were on a four-point scale dichotomised as 'strongly/tend to agree' vs. 'strongly/tend to disagree' for analysis. Participants could answer 'don't know' or 'refused', but these responses were excluded from analyses. Participants who had been diagnosed with cancer ($n = 127$) were not asked these questions.

Two items were adapted from Silvestri and colleagues' US survey [12] to assess beliefs about early-stage lung cancer: 'If lung cancer is detected early, what is the person's chance of surviving?' (response options on a three-point scale, dichotomised for analysis as 'good' vs. 'fair/poor') and 'If the screening test found that you had early-stage lung cancer, would you want to have the recommended surgery?' (responses were coded as 'yes definitely/probably' or 'probably/definitely not'). 'Not sure', 'don't know' or 'refused' responses were excluded.

The acceptability of a screening programme was also assessed ('Do you think lung cancer screening is a good idea?'), as well as opposition against screening targeted at smokers as an indicator of stigma ('Do you think that offering lung cancer screening to smokers is a waste of NHS money?') adapted from a validated cancer stigma scale [26]. Response options were 'yes' or 'no'; 'don't know' or 'refused' responses were excluded.

Worry about lung cancer risk

Frequency of worry about lung cancer risk was measured by asking, 'How often do you worry about your chance of getting lung cancer?'; adapted from Lerman's Cancer Worry Scale [27, 28]. Response options were 'never', 'occasionally', 'sometimes', 'often', 'very often', which were recoded as 'never' vs. 'at least occasionally' for analysis. Respondents who reported worry were asked, 'Would a clear lung CT scan reassure you?', to which they could respond 'yes' or 'no'. 'Don't know' and 'refused' responses were excluded from analyses.

Smoking

Smoking status was self-reported using the following two items from the ABC measure [25]. First, 'Do you smoke at all these days, either cigarettes (including hand-rolled ones), pipes or cigars?' and second, 'Have you ever regularly smoked cigarettes (including hand-rolled ones), pipes or cigars?'. Former smokers were therefore defined as individuals who had ever smoked tobacco regularly. We did not collect data on tobacco consumption or smoking duration and therefore could not determine likely screening eligibility status.

Current smokers were asked, 'How high would you rate your chances of giving up smoking for good?' on a scale adapted from the 'Motivation To Stop Scale' (MTSS) [29]. Responses were dichotomised as high ('extremely', 'very high', 'quite high') vs. low ('not very high', 'low' or 'very low') for analysis.

Demographics

Data on age, gender, ethnicity (White/Not White), marital status (i) married/cohabiting, ii) single/divorced/separated/widowed), and highest level of education (i) no formal qualifications, ii) CSEs/O-levels/equivalent, iii) A-levels/further education/equivalent, iv) Degree or higher) were collected. Cancer experience was assessed: 'Have any friends or family members that are close to you ever been diagnosed with cancer?' to which participants could answer 'yes' or 'no'.

Analyses

Descriptive frequencies were run to determine absolute levels of agreement. The associations between smoking status and agreement with each cancer belief and worry item were explored using chi-square analyses, and multi-variable logistic regression, adjusted for demographics and cancer experience. 'Don't know' ($\leq 6.9\%$) and 'refused' ($\leq 4.9\%$) responses were excluded from the respective analyses.

Chi-square and logistic regression analyses were also carried out to test for associations between demographics, smoking status, and screening intentions. Belief items associated with smoking status were then analysed to determine their association with screening intentions. Analyses of screening intentions excluded never smokers because they would not be eligible for lung cancer screening. Analyses also excluded cases answering 'not sure' ($\leq 2.5\%$) or 'refused' ($\leq 2.3\%$) on any one of the three intention items ($n = 44$). Further analyses tested for demographic differences between this group and the overall sample.

Finally, exploratory chi-square and logistic regression analyses tested for associations between quit confidence and the beliefs, lung cancer worry and screening intention variables among current smokers only. As multiple testing increases the type one error rate, a stringent significance threshold was set for the interpretation of all analyses ($p < .01$).

Results
Sample characteristics
In total, 1464 participants completed the survey. Participants were excluded if they did not report their smoking status ($n = 13$) or had been diagnosed with lung cancer ($n = 6$). The average age of the final sample was 60 years and there was good representation of different SEP (as indicated by education level; see Table 1). The majority were married or cohabiting (62%), and from a White ethnic background (93%). Experience of cancer through friends or family was commonly reported (70%).

Twenty two per cent of participants were current smokers, 26% were former smokers and 52% reported never having smoked. Current smokers had a lower level of education, and were less likely to be married (p's < .001). Most smokers (62%) rated their chances of stopping smoking as 'very low', 'low' or 'not very high'. Beyond age and smoking status, participants' likely eligibility in the event of a national lung cancer screening programme was unknown.

Compared with the main sample, current and former smokers answering 'don't know' or 'refused' on the intention items ($n = 44$; excluded from the intention analyses) did not differ in their sociodemographic characteristics.

Table 1 Characteristics of the sample by smoking status

	All (n = 1445)	Never smokers (n = 759)	Current smokers (n = 313)	Former smokers (n = 373)
Gender, % (n)				
Male	49.3 (712)	44.0 (334)[b]	55.9 (175)[b]	54.4 (203)[b]
Female	50.7 (733)	56.0 (425)	44.1 (138)	45.6 (170)
Age, mean (SD)	60.4 (6.3)	60.1 (6.3)	59.2 (6.3)	61.8 (6.1)
Marital status, % (n)				
Married/Cohabiting	61.7 (892)	65.3 (496)[b]	48.2 (151)[b]	65.7 (245)[b]
Single/Divorced/Separated/Widowed	38.3 (553)	34.7 (263)	51.8 (162)	34.3 (128)
Ethnicity, % (n)				
White	92.9 (1342)	89.3 (678)[b]	95.5 (299)[b]	97.9 (365)[b]
Not White	6.9 (100)	10.4 (79)	4.5 (14)	1.9 (7)
Refused	0.2 (3)	0.3 (2)	0.0 (0)	0.3 (1)
Education level, % (n)				
Degree	20.2 (292)	26.2 (199)[b]	10.2 (32)[b]	16.4 (61)[b]
A-levels/further/equivalent	22.6 (327)	24.0 (182)	16.9 (53)	24.7 (92)
CSEs/O-levels/equivalent	28.3 (409)	26.0 (197)	33.5 (105)	28.7 (107)
No formal qualifications	26.1 (377)	21.2 (161)	36.4 (114)	27.3 (102)
Don't know/Refused	2.8 (40)	2.6 (20)	2.9 (9)	2.9 (11)
Cancer experience, % (n)				
Yes (friends/family)	70.2 (1014)	68.8 (522)	69.0 (216)	74.0 (276)
No	28.2 (407)	30.0 (228)	29.1 (91)	23.6 (88)
Don't know/Refused	1.7 (35)	1.2 (9)	1.9 (6)	2.4 (9)
Quit confidence, % (n)				
Extremely high	–	–	4.2 (13)	–
Very high	–	–	10.2 (32)	–
Quite high	–	–	20.1 (63)	–
Not very high	–	–	21.7 (68)	–
Low	–	–	13.7 (43)	–
Very low	–	–	26.2 (82)	–
Don't know/Refused	–	–	3.8 (12)	–

% totals may not be exactly 100 due to rounding
[a] χ^2, $p < .01$, [b] χ^2, $p < .001$

Beliefs about lung cancer survival, early detection and screening

One in five respondents agreed that a cancer diagnosis is a death sentence, but this number doubled (48%) when the question concerned lung cancer (see Table 2). In relation to early-stage lung cancer, only half thought the chances of surviving were good, but 92% anticipated they would opt for surgery. Smokers were less likely to agree with these beliefs compared with former smokers (43% vs. 53%, $p = .01$; OR: 0.64, 0.46–0.88, and 84% vs. 94%, $p < .001$; OR: 0.38, 0.21–0.68 respectively).

The large majority of participants (97%) thought screening a good idea, across smoking groups. Using NHS money to screen smokers was perceived as a waste of NHS money by

21%, but most commonly by former (24%) and never smokers (22%) compared with current smokers (14%; OR: 0.45, 0.29–0.69; reference group was former smokers).

While there was a trend towards smokers with a lower perceived chance of stopping smoking endorsing more negative beliefs, there were no statistically significant associations in unadjusted analyses ($n = 301$; see Table 3). In adjusted analyses, smokers who perceived their chance of quitting as low were less likely to agree that early stage survival is good compared with those rating their chance of quitting as high (37% vs. 52%, $p = .02$; OR: 0.48, 0.29–0.82).

Worry about lung cancer risk

Worrying about risk of lung cancer at least occasionally was fairly common overall (31%; see Table 2). More

Table 2 Frequencies, chi-square analyses and multivariable logistic regression models[c], testing the associations between smoking status, beliefs and worry

	All (n = 1445)	Former smokers (reference)		Current smokers			Never smokers		
	% (n)	% (n)	OR	% (n)	OR	95% CI	% (n)	OR	95% CI
A diagnosis of cancer is a death sentence									
Strongly/tend to agree (vs. strongly/tend to disagree)	20.5 (257)	16.9[a] (53)	1.00	26.8[a] (75)	1.50	0.97–2.29	19.6[a] (129)	1.29	0.88–1.90
A diagnosis of lung cancer is a death sentence									
Strongly/tend to agree (vs. strongly/tend to disagree)	47.6 (582)	46.3 (138)	1.00	53.2 (149)	1.25	0.89–1.76	45.7 (295)	1.01	0.76–1.35
If lung cancer is detected early, what is the person's chance of surviving?									
Good (vs. fair/poor)	50.8 (689)	53.4 (189)	1.00	43.0 (125)	0.64	0.46–0.88	52.7 (375)	0.95	0.73–1.24
If the screening test found that you had early-stage lung cancer, would you want to have the recommended surgery?									
Yes definitely/probably (vs. definitely/probably not)	91.5 (1209)	93.9[b] (321)	1.00	84.3[b] (242)	0.38	0.21–0.68	93.4[b] (646)	0.99	0.56–1.75
Do you think that lung cancer screening is a good idea?									
Yes (vs. no)	97.1 (1354)	97.8 (352)	1.00	96.7 (294)	0.67	0.25–1.77	97.0 (708)	1.10	0.46–2.63
Do you think that offering screening to smokers is a waste of NHS money?									
Yes (vs. no)	20.7 (281)	23.9[a] (84)	1.00	14.2[a] (43)	0.45	0.29–0.69	21.9[a] (154)	0.92	0.67–1.27
How often do you worry about your chance of getting lung cancer?									
Very often to occasionally (vs. never)	30.6 (429)	28.7[b] (104)	1.00	47.9[b] (147)	2.38	1.70–3.33	24.4[b] (178)	0.81	0.60–1.10
Would a clear CT scan reassure you?[d]									
Yes (vs. no)	90.0 (385)	94.2 (97)	1.00	89.7 (130)	0.66	0.24–1.84	87.8 (158)	0.75	0.27–2.05

OR odds ratio, *95% CI* 95% confidence interval; n totals may not sum due to missing data
[a]χ^2, $p < .01$, [b] χ^2, $p < .001$
[c]adjusted for demographics and cancer experience
[d]asked of the subsample of participants reporting lung cancer worry (n = 429)

current smokers reported this worry (48%), compared with former smokers (29%; OR: 2.38, 1.70–3.33), and fewer never smokers compared with former smokers (24% vs. 29%, $p < .001$); although the latter association was not statistically significant in adjusted analyses (OR: 0.81, 0.60–1.10). Of the participants who worried about their risk ($n = 429$), 90% thought a clear CT scan would be reassuring, with no association with smoking status.

Lung cancer screening intentions

The large majority of current and former smokers intended to be screened for lung cancer (see Table 4). The proportion of intenders was highest if recommended by a GP (93% and 98%, for current and former smokers respectively), and was similar for the NHS (89% and 94% for current and former smokers) and upcoming appointment (89% and 94%) invitation scenarios.

Gender, age, ethnicity, level of education, marital status and cancer experience were not associated with screening intentions. Smoking status was associated with screening intentions in the GP invitation scenario only. Fewer current smokers (93%) than former (98%) smokers

intended to participate following a GP recommendation ($p < .01$; OR: 0.24, 0.09–0.65). Smokers' perceived chance of quitting smoking was not associated with their intentions to be screened.

Perceived survival from early-stage lung cancer was associated with screening intentions in the GP invitation scenario (see Table 4), with decreased odds for those thinking survival was poor or fair (94%), compared with good (98%, $p < .01$; OR: 0.23, 0.08–0.71). Anticipating not wanting surgery for a screen-detected early-stage lung cancer predicted a lower likelihood of intending to be screened in all three scenarios. Striking absolute differences in intentions were observed between the 'decline' and 'pro' surgery participants (26–29%; ORs: 0.04–0.14, $p < .001$).

Worrying about risk of lung cancer did not affect the odds of intending to be screened in any of the invitation scenarios. However, this group was predominantly comprised of individuals who worried sometimes or occasionally (85% of the current and former smokers reporting worry and included in the screening intention analyses).

There were too few cases to subdivide the frequency of worry by screening intentions for multivariate analysis.

Table 3 Frequencies, chi-square analyses, and multivariable logistic regression models[a], exploring associations between smokers' perceived chance of quitting, lung cancer beliefs and screening intentions

	High quit confidence (reference)		Low quit confidence		
	% (n)	OR	% (n)	OR	95% CI
A diagnosis of cancer is a death sentence					
Strongly/tend to agree (vs. strongly/tend to disagree)	25.5 (26)	1.00	28.2 (48)	1.23	0.68–2.24
A diagnosis of lung cancer is a death sentence					
Strongly/tend to agree (vs. strongly/tend to disagree)	50.0 (50)	1.00	53.8 (93)	1.14	0.68–1.92
If lung cancer is detected early, what is the person's chance of surviving?					
Good (vs. fair/poor)	51.9 (54)	1.00	37.3 (66)	0.48	0.29–0.82
If the screening test found that you had early-stage lung cancer, would you want to have the recommended surgery?					
Yes definitely/probably (vs. definitely/probably not)	88.0 (88)	1.00	81.3 (143)	0.58	0.27–1.24
Do you think that lung cancer screening is a good idea?					
Yes (vs. no)	96.3 (103)	1.00	96.8 (180)	1.11	0.29–4.20
Do you think that offering screening to smokers is a waste of NHS money?					
Yes (vs. no)	10.4 (11)	1.00	16.1 (30)	1.62	0.76–3.47
How often do you worry about your chance of getting lung cancer?					
Very often to occasionally (vs. never)	48.6 (52)	1.00	47.6 (90)	0.92	0.56–1.51
Would a clear CT scan reassure you?[b]					
Yes (vs. no)	92.2 (47)	1.00	87.6 (78)	0.48	0.13–1.84
NHS invitation					
Yes definitely/probably (vs. definitely/probably not)	93.2 (96)	1.00	86.4 (159)	0.55	0.22–1.37
GP recommendation					
Yes definitely/probably (vs. definitely/probably not)	94.3 (99)	1.00	92.0 (172)	0.82	0.29–2.29
Appointment next month					
Very likely/likely (vs. very unlikely/unlikely)	94.2 (98)	1.00	86.6 (161)	0.46	0.18–1.21

OR odds ratio; *95% CI* 95% confidence interval
[a]adjusted for demographics and cancer experience
[b]asked of the subsample of participants reporting lung cancer worry (n = 142)

The results of unadjusted Fisher's exact tests suggested that *infrequent worry* (i.e. occasionally or sometimes) was associated with higher screening intentions, whereas *frequent worry* (i.e. often or very often) was associated with lower intentions in the NHS invitation scenario (p = .01; results not reported).

Discussion

This is the first UK population-based study of older adults to investigate interest in, and perceptions of lung cancer screening, and to explore their association with smoking status. Most respondents thought screening a good idea and the majority of current and former smokers intended to be screened. However, positive intentions were at odds with frequently fatalistic perceptions of lung cancer. Negative beliefs about early-stage survival and surgery were particularly common among smokers, and associated with a lower likelihood of intending to be screened.

Based on intentions alone, these findings suggest that a UK national screening programme would be acceptable and well-attended; perhaps especially if recommended by a GP. These findings match the interest observed among a US population-based survey [12]. However, they are contrary to the low levels of screening uptake observed in the trial context [10]. The gap between intentions and behaviour is well-documented for health precautionary behaviours [30] suggesting these intentions may not be borne out in attendance. Cognitive, psychosocial or practical factors may subsequently determine whether intentions are enacted.

Beliefs about the screened disease could be an important factor. Perceptions of survival from lung cancer were frequently negative; even when early detection was specified. This is likely to reflect the poor prognosis lung cancer currently has, due largely to its late diagnosis. A deep-rooted lay interpretation might be that outcomes are universally poor, and there is evidence that early-stage survival is underestimated [31]. Notably, smokers

Table 4 Frequencies, chi-square analyses, and multivariable logistic regression models[c], exploring associations with lung cancer screening intentions among current and former smokers

	NHS invitation[d]			GP recommendation[d]			Appointment next month[e]		
	Intend % (n)	OR	95% CI	Intend % (n)	OR	95% CI	Intend % (n)	OR	95% CI
All (n = 642)	91.6 (588)	–	–	95.8 (615)	–	–	91.9 (590)	–	–
Gender									
Female	91.6 (261)	1.00	–	95.8 (273)	1.00	–	93.0 (265)	1.00	–
Male	91.6 (327)	1.06	0.59–1.90	95.8 (342)	1.01	0.44–2.33	91.0 (325)	0.78	0.42–1.44
Age	–	1.01	0.97–1.06	–	0.96	0.89–1.02	–	0.99	0.94–1.04
Marital status									
Married/Cohabiting	92.8 (347)	1.00	–	96.5 (361)	1.00	–	92.8 (347)	1.00	–
Single/Divorced/Widowed	89.9 (241)	0.69	0.26–1.24	94.8 (254)	0.60	0.26–1.39	90.7 (243)	0.69	0.37–1.27
Education level									
Degree	88.8 (79)	1.00		96.6 (86)	1.00	–	94.4 (84)	1.00	–
A-levels/further/equivalent	92.9 (130)	1.40	0.54–3.62	96.4 (135)	0.97	0.22–4.26	93.6 (131)	0.86	0.28–2.70
CSEs/O-levels/equivalent	92.5 (184)	1.55	0.64–3.73	96.5 (192)	1.24	0.31–5.04	91.0 (181)	0.68	0.24–1.93
No formal qualifications	91.6 (185)	1.35	0.56–3.24	95.0 (192)	1.04	0.27–4.08	92.1 (186)	0.84	0.29–2.42
Cancer experience									
Yes	92.3 (432)	1.00	–	96.4 (451)	1.00	–	93.2 (436)	1.00	–
No	89.9 (151)	0.67	0.36–1.26	94.0 (158)	0.53	0.23–1.23	88.1 (148)	0.48	0.26–0.89
Smoking status									
Former	93.7 (328)	1.00	–	98.3 (344)[a]	1.00	–	94.0 (329)	1.00	–
Current	89.0 (260)	0.67	0.36–1.24	92.8 (271)[a]	0.24	0.09–0.65	89.4 (261)	0.63	0.33–1.19
Early-stage survival									
Good	94.4 (289)	1.00	–	98.4 (301)[a]	1.00	–	94.4 (289)	1.00	–
Fair/Poor	89.4 (279)	0.46	0.24–0.87	93.9 (293)[a]	0.23	0.08–0.71	90.7 (283)	0.55	0.28–1.06
Early-stage surgery									
Yes definitely/probably	94.3 (512)[b]	1.00	–	98.7 (536)[b]	1.00	–	95.4 (518)[b]	1.00	–
Definitely/probably not	69.4 (43)[b]	0.14	0.07–0.28	74.2 (46)[b]	0.04	0.02–0.12	66.1 (41)[b]	0.09	0.04–0.20
Lung cancer worry									
Never	90.5 (364)	1.00	–	95.8 (385)	1.00	–	90.5 (364)	1.00	–
Occasionally to very often	93.7 (223)	1.68	0.88–3.20	96.2 (229)	1.44	0.60–3.46	94.5 (225)	1.80	0.91–3.57

OR odds ratio; 95% CI 95% confidence interval; n totals may not sum due to missing data
[a] χ^2, $p < .01$; [b] χ^2, $p < .001$
[c] adjusted for demographics, cancer experience and smoking status
[d] predicting yes definitely/probably vs. probably/definitely not
[e] predicting very likely/likely vs. very unlikely/unlikely

were the most negative. Fewer believed there is a good chance of surviving early-stage lung cancer, or that they would undergo surgery for a screen-detected cancer, mirroring the results of the US survey [12]. Smokers in this UK sample were more accepting of surgical treatment (84% vs. 56%), which could partly be due to differences in healthcare provision, as US smokers were more likely to be deterred by cost. Importantly, those holding negative beliefs about early-stage survival and surgery were less likely to intend to be screened, suggesting that negative perceptions of early detection could undermine smokers' screening intentions.

Smokers' greater pessimism about early-stage lung cancer may result from more negative experiences of the disease within their social networks. We adjusted for previous cancer experience, but did not assess the type. Alternatively, perhaps smokers in this relatively older age group have become increasingly fatalistic about their chances of surviving lung cancer because of their significant smoking history, such that screening and treatment are perceived as offering little promise. These feelings may be exacerbated by their tobacco dependence, especially if they feel unable to quit; important because a sizeable proportion of smokers (> 60%) rated their chances of quitting as low. While perceived chance of quitting was not associated with screening intention, this study provided preliminary evidence that lower perceptions of quitting could foster more negative perceptions of early detection for lung cancer. This hypothesis deserves further study.

Worry about risk of lung cancer was most prevalent among smokers; nearly half reported worrying at least occasionally. Overall, worry did not appear to affect the likelihood of intending to be screened among current and former smokers. However, subgroup analyses showed that *frequent worriers* actually had lower intentions to be screened, and that *infrequent worriers* had the highest intentions in the NHS invitation scenario. Although preliminary, these results are consistent with evidence for a curvilinear association [32]. Studies are needed to measure the constituent components of smokers' worry, including frequency, and to explore their effects on screening participation.

While many respondents worried about their risk of lung cancer, most believed they would find a clear screen reassuring. However, this belief may be irrelevant if screening is expected to lead to a lung cancer diagnosis, and smokers may therefore be less likely to anticipate reassurance. Previous data have shown smokers are more likely to delay symptomatic help-seeking [33] due to worry about what the doctor might find [34]. Studies have also warned that lung cancer screening could undermine motivation to stop smoking [35]. However, with the correct communication, screening offers the opportunity to both assist smoking cessation and raise symptom awareness. Research is needed which explores the psychological responses to different screening results to identify how best to communicate lung cancer risk to assist positive behaviour change.

Lung cancer screening would be the first cancer screening programme in the UK to select patients primarily using a behavioural risk factor. In this sample, nearly one fifth thought screening smokers would be a waste of NHS money, suggesting that the stigma attached to smoking may adversely affect the acceptability of a targeted programme. This finding also warns that the exclusion of never smokers could be a contentious issue as they can also develop lung cancer, and a quarter of never smokers reported worrying about this. Opposition to their exclusion should be addressed by carefully communicating why LDCT screening is only appropriate for those at high risk.

This study benefits from a large, population-based sample, with a higher proportion of smokers (22%) than was expected for this age group [36] and good representation of different SEP groups. The measurement of screening intentions was useful for exploring interest, but limited conclusions can be made about screening behaviour, because the two are not well-correlated [30].

This may have been exacerbated by the fact that the screening offer was hypothetical and social desirability bias may have inflated results. Furthermore, asking participants about multiple invitation scenarios may have led them to alter their response for subsequent scenarios relative to the previous scenarios. This method could have resulted in different invitation preferences compared to asking independent groups about each invitation scenario; although respondents could not alter their previous responses when interviewed. Alternative individual-level measures of SEP exist but education has been shown to be a good indicator in older samples [37]. Single-item, cross-sectional measures were chosen to minimise participant burden, but may have reduced the reliability of findings. For the same reason, we did not collect information on participants' smoking duration or history (i.e. pack years) which would have allowed us to determine their eligibility for lung cancer screening. We caution that not knowing the likely eligibility status of participants in our sample may reduce the generalisability of these findings to an eligible screening population in England, should a national screening programme be recommended.

Conclusions
The introduction of an NHS lung cancer screening programme appears to be acceptable to older UK adults, with most current and former smokers intending to be screened (upwards of 89% and 94%, respectively) especially if recommended by their GP. Smokers' greater pessimism about survival and treatment for early-stage cancer could help to explain their lower participation. Strategies aimed at engaging smokers with screening should focus on improving perceptions of the curability of early-stage disease and addressing concerns about surgical treatment. Communication throughout the screening process needs to be sensitively devised so that it is mindful of the existing stigma around smoking, and the anxiety smokers may have about their increased risk of lung cancer.

Abbreviations
ABACUS: Attitudes behaviour and cancer UK survey; ABC: Awareness and beliefs about cancer measure; GP: General practitioner; LDCT: Low-dose computed tomography; MTSS: Motivation to stop scale; NHS: National health service; SEP: Socioeconomic position; USPSTF: United States preventive services task force

Acknowledgements
The authors would like to acknowledge the substantial intellectual contribution made by Professor Jane Wardle who sadly passed away prior to publication, and is deeply missed by all of her co-authors, colleagues and students.

Funding
CV, JW and AM are funded by Cancer Research UK. The Attitudes, Behaviour and Cancer UK Survey (ABACUS) was funded by a Cancer Research UK programme grant (C1418/A14134). SLQ was funded by the Medical Research

Council (MR/K501268/1). RJB is supported by Yorkshire Cancer Research University Academic Fellowship funding. MR is funded by the Roy Castle Lung Cancer Foundation and a National Awareness and Early Diagnosis Initiative (NAEDI) project grant awarded by Cancer Research UK and a consortium of funders (Department of Health (England); Economic and Social Research Council; Health and Social Care R&D Division, Public Health Agency, Northern Ireland; National Institute for Social Care and Health Research, Wales; Scottish Government). SMJ is a Wellcome Trust Senior Fellow in Clinical Science and is supported by Rosetrees Trust, the Welton Trust, the Garfield Weston Trust and UCLH Charitable Foundation. This work was partially undertaken at UCLH/UCL who received a proportion of funding from the Department of Health's NIHR Biomedical Research Centre's funding scheme (SMJ). SMJ is funded by the Roy Castle Lung Cancer Foundation and is part of the CRUK Lung Cancer Centre of Excellence.

Authors' contributions

SLQ, CV, RJB, JW and AM contributed to the design of the study and measures, statistical analysis, data interpretation and writing of the manuscript. MR and SJ contributed to the interpretation of the data and writing of the manuscript. All authors read and approved the final manuscript.

Competing interests

SLQ, CV, MR, SMJ, RJB and JW have no competing interests to declare. AM has received travel funding, honorariums and consultancy payments from manufacturers of smoking cessation products (Pfizer Ltd., Novartis UK and GSK Consumer Healthcare Ltd) and hospitality from North51 who provide online and database services. AM also receives payment for providing training to smoking cessation specialists; receives royalties from books on smoking cessation and has a share in a patent of a nicotine delivery device. AM is an Associate of the New Nicotine Alliance (NNA) that works to foster greater understanding of safer nicotine products and technologies.

Author details

Department of Behavioural Science and Health, University College London, Gower Street, London WC1E 6BT, UK. [2]Lungs for Living Research Centre, UCL Respiratory, Division of Medicine, Rayne Building, University College London, 5 University Street, London WC1E 6JF, UK. [3]Leeds Institute of Health Sciences, University of Leeds, Worsley Building, Clarendon Way, Leeds LS2 9NL, UK.

References

1. Office for National Statistics. Statistical Bulletin Cancer Survival in England: Adults Diagnosed, 2008 to 2012, followed up to 2013. 2014. https://www.ons.gov.uk/peoplepopulationandcommunity/healthandsocialcare/conditionsanddiseases/bulletins/cancersurvivalinenglandadultsdiagnosed/2014-10-30. Accessed 13 Sept 2016.
2. Eastern Cancer Registration and Information Centre. Stage distribution of cancers diagnosed in 2009 in the East of England by cancer site and area of residence. 2009. http://www.ecric.nhs.uk/docs/ECRIC_incidenceXstage_2009.pdf. Accessed 13 Sept 2016.
3. National Lung Screening Trial Research Team, Aberle DR, Adams AM, Berg CD, Black WC, Clapp JD, Fagerstrom RM, Gareen IF, Gatsonis C, Marcus PM, Sicks JD. Reduced lung-cancer mortality with low-dose computed tomographic screening. N Engl J Med. 2011;365:395–409.
4. Moyer VA. Screening for lung cancer: U.S. preventive services task force recommendation statement. Ann Intern Med. 2014;160:330–8.
5. Centers for Medicare & Medicaid services. Decision memo for screening for lung cancer with low dose computed tomography (LDCT) (CAG-00439N). 2015. https://www.cms.gov/medicare-coverage-database/details/nca-decision-memo.aspx?NCAId=274. Accessed 13 Sept 2016.
6. UK National Screening Committee. The UK NSC recommendation on lung cancer screening in adult cigarette smokers. 2016. http://legacy.screening.nhs.uk/lungcancer. Accessed 13 Sept 2016.
7. Kovalchik SA, Tammemagi M, Berg CD, Caporaso NE, Riley TL, Korch M, Silvestri GA, Chaturvedi AK, Katki HA. Targeting of low-dose CT screening according to the risk of lung-cancer death. N Engl J Med. 2013;369:245–54.
8. National Lung Screening Trial Research Team, Aberle DR, Adams AM, Berg CD, Clapp JD, Clingan KL, Gareen IF, Lynch DA, Marcus PM, Pinsky PF. Baseline characteristics of participants in the randomized national lung screening trial. J Natl Cancer Inst. 2010;102:1771–9.
9. Hestbech MS, Siersma V, Dirksen A, Pedersen JH, Brodersen J. Participation bias in a randomised trial of screening for lung cancer. Lung Cancer. 2011;73:325–31.
10. McRonald FE, Yadegarfar G, Baldwin DR, Devaraj A, Brain KE, Eisen T, Holemans JA, Ledson M, Screaton N, Rintoul RC, Hands CJ, Lifford K, Whynes D, Kerr KM, Page R, Parmar M, Wald N, Weller D, Williamson PR, Myles J, Hansell DM, Duffy SW, Field JK. The UK lung screen (UKLS): demographic profile of first 88,897 approaches provides recommendations for population screening. Cancer Prev Res. 2014;7:362–71.
11. Parkin DM. 2. Tobacco-attributable cancer burden in the UK in 2010. Br J Cancer. 2011;105 Suppl 2: S6–S13,.
12. Silvestri GA, Nietert PJ, Zoller J, Carter C, Bradford D. Attitudes towards screening for lung cancer among smokers and their non-smoking counterparts. Thorax. 2007;62:126–30.
13. Jonnalagadda S, Bergamo C, Lin JJ, Lurslurchachai L, Diefenbach M, Smith C, Nelson JE, Wisnivesky JP. Beliefs and attitudes about lung cancer screening among smokers. Lung Cancer. 2012;77:526–31.
14. Cataldo JK. High-risk older smokers' perceptions, attitudes, and beliefs about lung cancer screening. Cancer Med. 2016;5:753–9.
15. Quaife SL, Marlow LAV, McEwen A, Janes SM, Wardle J. Attitudes towards lung cancer screening within socioeconomically deprived and heavy smoking communities: informing screening communication. Health Expect. 2016;384:1–11.
16. Patel D, Akporobaro A, Chinyanganya N, Hackshaw A, Seale C, Spiro SG, Griffiths C. Attitudes to participation in a lung cancer screening trial: a qualitative study. Thorax. 2012;67:418–25.
17. Ali N, Lifford KJ, Carter B, McRonald F, Yadegarfar G, Baldwin DR, Weller D, Hansell DM, Duffy SW, Field JK, Brain K. Barriers to uptake among high-risk individuals declining participation in lung cancer screening: a mixed methods analysis of the UK lung Cancer screening (UKLS) trial. BMJ Open. 2015;5:e008254.
18. van den Bergh KAM, Essink-Bot ML, van Klaveren RJ, de Koning HJ. Informed participation in a randomised controlled trial of computed tomography screening for lung cancer. Eur Respir J. 2009;34:711–20.
19. Carter-Harris L, Pham Ceppa D, Hanna N, Rawl SM. Lung cancer screening: what do long-term smokers know and believe? Health Expect. 2015;20:59–68.
20. Hewitson P, Ward AM, Heneghan C, Halloran SP, Mant D. Primary care endorsement letter and a patient leaflet to improve participation in colorectal cancer screening: results of a factorial randomised trial. Br J Cancer. 2011;105:475–80.
21. Bevan R, Rubin G, Sofianopoulou E, Patnick J, Rees CJ. Implementing a national flexible sigmoidoscopy screening program: results of the English early pilot. Endoscopy. 2015;47:225–31.
22. TNS. TNS CAPI Omnibus. 2006. http://www.tnsglobal.com/directory/service/omnibus-united-kingdom. Accessed 13 Sept 2016.
23. Central Statistics Office. Small area population statistics. 2011 http://census.cso.ie/sapmap/. Accessed 13 Sept 2016.
24. Wardle J, Williamson S, McCaffery K, Sutton S, Taylor T, Edwards R, Atkin W. Increasing attendance at colorectal cancer screening: testing the efficacy of a mailed, psychoeducational intervention in a community sample of older adults. Health Psychol. 2003;22:99–105.
25. Simon AE, Forbes LJL, Boniface D, Warburton F, Brain KE, Dessaix A, Donnelly M, Haynes K, Hvidberg L, Lagerlund M, Petermann L, Tishelman C, Vedsted P, Vigmostad MN, Wardle J, Ramirez AJ. An international measure of awareness and beliefs about cancer: development and testing of the ABC. BMJ Open. 2012;2:e001758.
26. Marlow LAV, Wardle J. Development of a scale to assess cancer stigma in the non-patient population. BMC Cancer. 2014;14:285.
27. Lerman C. Psychological and behavioral implications of abnormal mammograms. Ann Intern Med. 1991;114:657.

28. Lerman C, Kash K, Stefanek M. Younger women at increased risk for breast cancer: perceived risk, psychological well-being, and surveillance behavior. J Natl Cancer Inst Monogr. 1994;16:171–6.

29. Kotz D, Brown J, West R. Predictive validity of the motivation to stop scale (MTSS): a single-item measure of motivation to stop smoking. Drug Alcohol Depend. 2013;128:15–9.

30. Sheeran P. Intention—behavior relations: a conceptual and empirical review. Eur Rev Soc Psychol. 2002;12:1–36.

31. Mazieres J, Pujol J, Kalampalikis N, Bouvry D, Quoix E, Filleron T, Targowla N, Jodelet D, Milia J, Milleron B. Perception of lung cancer among the general population and comparison with other cancers. J Thorac Oncol. 2015;10:420–5.

32. Vrinten C, Waller J, von Wagner C, Wardle J. Cancer fear: facilitator and deterrent to participation in colorectal Cancer screening. Cancer Epidemiol Biomark Prev. 2015;24:400–5.

33. Friedemann Smith C, Whitaker KL, Winstanley K, Wardle J. Smokers are less likely than non-smokers to seek help for a lung cancer 'alarm' symptom. Thorax. 2016;71:659–61.

34. Quaife SL, McEwen A, Janes SM, Wardle J. Smoking is associated with pessimistic and avoidant beliefs about cancer: results from the international Cancer benchmarking partnership. Br J Cancer. 2015;112:1799–804.

35. Zeliadt SB, Heffner JL, Sayre G, Klein DE, Simons C, Williams J, Reinke LF, Au DH. Attitudes and perceptions about smoking cessation in the context of lung Cancer screening. JAMA Intern Med. 2015;175:1530–7.

36. Office for National Statistics. Chapter 1 - Smoking (General Lifestyle Survey Overview - a report on the 2011 General Lifestyle Survey). 2013. http://www.ons.gov.uk/ons/dcp171776_302558.pdf (accessed: 06/01/2015). Accessed 13 Sept 2016.

37. Grundy E, Holt G. The socioeconomic status of older adults: how should we measure it in studies of health inequalities? J Epidemiol Community Heal. 2001;55:895–904.

10

Bexarotene inhibits the viability of non-small cell lung cancer cells via slc10a2/PPARγ/PTEN/mTOR signaling pathway

Xinghao Ai[1,2†], Feng Mao[2†], Shengping Shen[2], Yang Shentu[2], Jiejun Wang[1*] and Shun Lu[2*]

Abstract

Background: Thirty to 40 % of non-small cell lung cancer (NSCLC) patients developed higher hypertriglyceridemia in the process of treatment with bexarotene. And bioinformatics studies discovered that the expression of slc10a2 was increased in high-grade hypertriglyceridemia patients. So, we will explore the mechanism which may involve in this process.

Methods: We constructed slc10a2 overexpressed A549 cells and H1299 cells as cell models, normal A549 cells and H1299 cells as control. Then we explored the effects of slc10a2 on A549 cells and H1299 cells behaviors, including proliferation, invasion and apoptosis. The expression of apoptotic related genes and anti-cancer genes also been detected.

Results: We found that the proliferation and migration were inhibited and the apoptosis of NSCLC cells was accelerated by bexarotene. In addition, overexpressed slc10a2 in NSCLC cells can further suppress the proliferation and migration, and promote apoptosis under the treatment of bexarotene. On the contrary, the opposite results were obtained after slc10a2 gene was silenced in NSCLC cells treated with bexarotene. Moreover, the expression of caspase 3, caspase 7, PTEN, P21, P53, LKB1, TSC2 were increased and the expression of Bcl-2, cyclin D1, c-FLIP were declined in NSCLC cells and slc10a2 overexpressed NSCLC cells with the treatment of bexarotene, and the opposite situations were seen after slc10a2 gene was silenced in NSCLC cells. The further studies revealed the increased expression of slc10a2 activated the expression of peroxisome proliferator-activated receptor γ (PPARγ), then up-regulated PTEN expression and down-regulated mTOR expression.

Conclusion: These results suggest that bexarotene inhibits the viability of lung cancer cells via slc10a2/PPARγ/PTEN/mTOR signaling pathway.

Keywords: Non-small cell lung cancer, A549 cells, H1299 cells, Bexarotene, slc10a2, PPARγ

Background

The incidence of lung cancer is rapidly increasing in the world, and it has become the first leading cause of cancer death, especially in China [1]. Non-small cell lung cancer (NSCLC) is the most common type of lung cancer, accounting for almost 80% [2]. In clinic trials, bexarotene showed both satisfactory safety and promising efficacy for the treatment of advanced NSCLC patients [3, 4]. However 30–40%

of the patients appeared to be more sensitive to bexarotene treatment and developed higher hypertriglyceridemia. Interestingly, survival analysis in high-grade hypertriglyceridemia patients revealed significantly longer survival compared to the patients in the control, low-grade hypertriglyceridemia and middle-grade hypertriglyceridemia groups [5, 6].

Bexarotene (Scheme 1) is a synthetic retinoid modulator of retinoid X receptors (RXRs), it can selectively bind and activate RXRs [2], which include (RXRα, RXRβ, and RXRγ) [7], and play a critical role in cellular growth modulation, activation of apoptosis, induction of differentiation. It has been widely explored as potential target for cancer therapies for several years [8, 9]. The expression of RXRs was

* Correspondence: jiejunw@csco.org.cn; shun_lu@hotmail.com
†Equal contributors
[1]Department of Medical Oncology, Changzheng Hospital, The Second Military Medical University, Shanghai 200433, China
[2]Lung Tumor Clinical Medical Center, Shanghai Chest Hospital, Shanghai Jiao Tong University, Shanghai 200030, China

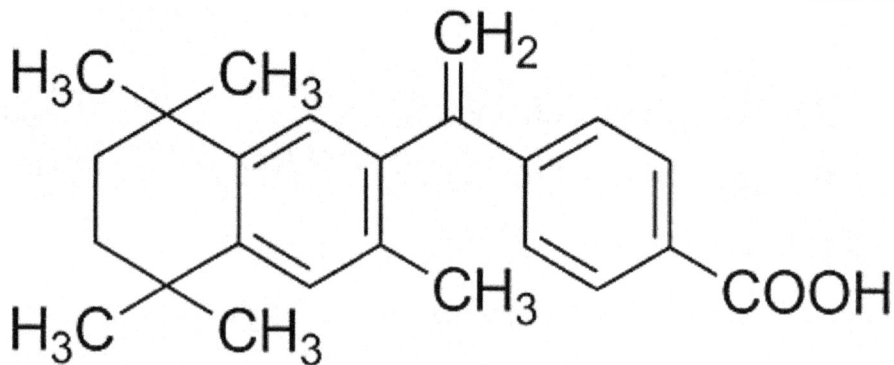

Scheme 1 The chemical structure of bexarotene

reduced in some NSCLC biopsy specimens, and increased RXRs expression has been associated with an increased survival in NSCLC patients [10].

Slc10a2 is a member of solute carrier family 10 of the sodium/bile acid co-transporter apical sodium-dependent bile acid transporter (ABST) [11], which plays a key role in the enterohepatic circulation through its reabsorption of bile acids from the ileum and indirectly conduces to cholesterol homoeostasis [12, 13]. ASBT is able to inhibit the concentration of plasma triglyceride and increase the concentration of HDL (high-density lipoprotein) cholesterol [14], and now it has aroused much concern as a drug target for the pharmacological treatment of hypercholesterolaemia [15, 16].

The goal of this study is to explore the role of slc10a2 in the treatment of NSCLC with bexarotene. We hypothesis that bexarotene inhibits the viability of NSCLC cells (e.g. A549 cells and H1299 cells) via increasing the expression of slc10a2. In this study, we have successfully constructed slc10a2 overexpressed A549 cells and H1299 cells, and the proliferation, apoptosis, migration behaviors were detected in slc10a2 overexpressed A549 cells and H1299 cells respectively. Moreover, we also explored the expression of apoptosis genes, anti-apoptosis genes, tumor suppressor genes in slc10a2 overexpressed A549 cells and H1299 cells. Furthermore, the possible mechanism which involved in this process was discovered.

Methods
Materials
Bexarotene was obtained from Aladdin (Shanghai, China). Cell Counting Kit-8 was ordered from Dojindo (Japan). Cell culture plates and Transwell plates were ordered from Corning (NY, USA). Crystal violet was obtained from Beyotime (Haimen, China). Annexin V/fluorescein isothiocyanate (FITC) apoptosis detection kit was obtained from Beyotime biotech company (China). Gentamicin, Fetal bovine serum, glutamine, and RPMI 1640 medium were purchased from Thermo Fisher Scientific (Waltham, MA, USA). The primary antibodies including slc10a2,

PPARγ, mTOR and PTEN (Abcam, Cambridge, UK), GAPDH (Thermo, Walteham, Washington, USA). The pcDNA3 and pcDNA3-slc10a2 plasmid, slc10a2-shRNA, GW9662 were obtained from Shanghai Funeng Biological Technology, Co., LTD.

Cell lines
The human NSCLC cell lines A549 cells (CRM-CCL-185™) and H1299 cells (CRL-5803™) was obtained from American Type Culture Collection (Rockville, MD). Cells were maintained in RPMI 1640 media plus 10% fetal bovine serum, 1% glutamine and 0.05 mg/ml gentamycin sulfate at 37 °C and 5% CO_2.

The construction of slc10a2 overexpressed A549 cells and H1299 cells
Before transfection, A549 cells and H1299 cells were seeded into 6-well plate at a density of 2×10^6 cells/well, after cells grow above 80% areas, A549 cells were transfected with 8 mg pcDNA3-slc10a2 plasmid using Lipofect2000 transfection Reagent according to manufacturer's instructions, pcDNA3 treatment as control. The transfection medium was replaced by regular growth medium after 5 h transfection, and at each time point, the cells were used to observation using inverted fluorescence microscope.

Proliferation assay
A549 cells, H1299 cells and slc10a2 overexpressed A549 cells, H1299 cells were seeded in a 96-well plate, 5×10^3 cells per well. After 12 h culture, the cultured medium was replaced by conditional medium, which was added with bexarotene, bexarotene in combination with slc10a2-shRNA, bexarotene in combination with GW9662 respectively. At indicated time point, ten microliter CCK-8 was added each well and continually incubated for 4 h. Then the optical density (OD) value (450 nm) was determined by an enzyme-linked immunosorbent assay plate reader (Bioreader).

Transwell migration assay

A549 cells and slc10a2 overexpressed A549 cells were starved for 12 h, then resuspended in serum-free medium, and adjusted to 1×10^6 cells/ml. One hundred microliters of A549cells or slc10a2 overexpressed A549 cells were placed in the upper chamber of Transwell plates. Serum-free RPMI 1640 medium with bexarotene, bexarotene in combination with slc10a2-shRNA, was added to the lower chamber respectively, RPMI 1640 medium as control. Prior to the addition of cells suspension, preheated serum free RPMI 1640 medium (300 μl) was added to the upper chamber. After 24 h incubation, the invaded cells were collected from lower chambers, then stained with crystal violet.

Apoptosis assay

The apoptosis of A549 cells, H1299 cells and slc10a2 overexpressed A549 cells, H1299 cells was analyzed using the Apoptosis Detection Kit according to the manufacturer's instructions. Cells were seeded in 6-well plate (1×10^5 cells/well) with different medium, including RPMI 1640 medium plus bexarotene, RPMI 1640 medium plus bexarotene in combination with slc10a2-shRNA for 2 days. At indicated times, cells were digested then resuspended in 300 μL binding buffer solution which containing 5 ul Annexin V-FITC and 5 ul PI solution, then incubated in the dark for 20 min at room temperature. Finally flow cytometry (FACScan; BD Biosciences) was used to analyzed the apoptotic rate of each kind of cells.

RT quantitative-PCR analysis

The total RNA of A549 cells and H1299 cells were isolated by using RNeasy kit according to the manufacturer's protocol (Qiagen, Valencia, CA). Briefly, total RNA (1 μg) was used as a template to prepare cDNA (Invitrogen), and was amplified by Platinum SYBR Green qPCR SuperMix-UDG (Invitrogen). A master mix was prepared for each PCR reaction, which included Platinum SYBR Green qPCR SuperMix-UDG, forward primer, reverse primer, and 10 ng of template cDNA. PCR was performed with the following thermocycling conditions: An initial 5 min at 95 °C, followed by 40 cycles of 95 °C for 30 s, 55 °C for 30 s and 72 °C for 30 s. [17] The forward and backward primer sequences for Bcl-2 was 5'-CCGATCAGTGGGAGCTGAAGAA-3'(sense) and 5'-GCCACAGGATGTTCTCGTCA-3'(antisense), cyclin D1:5'-CAAGGCCTGAACCTGAGGAG-3'(sense) and 5 '-CTTGGGGTCCATGTTCTGCT-3'(antisense), c-FLIP :5'-GAGTGCCGGCTATTGGACTT-3'(sense) and 5'-G CGCTTCTCTCCTACACCTC-3'(antisense), Caspase-3:5'-GCGGTTGTAGAAGTTAATAAAGGT-3'(sense) and 5'-TACCAGACCGAGATGTCATTCC-3'(antisense), Caspase-7:5'-CGTGGGAACGGCAGGAAGT-3'(sense) and 5'-CG

GGTGGTCTTGATGGATCG-3'(antisense), PTEN:5'-CAG-GATACGCGCTCGGC-3'(sense) and 5'-TCAGGAGAAGC CGAGGAAGA-3'(antisense), P21:5'-AGTCAGTTCCTTG TGGAGCC-3'(sense) and 5'-CATTAGCGCATCACAGT CGC-3'(antisense), P53:5'-GTGCTCAAGACTGGCGCTA AA-3'(sense) and 5'-CAGTCTGGCCAATCCAGGGAAG-3'(antisense), LKB1:5'-GACCTGCTGAAAGGGATGCT-3'(sense) and 5'-GACCTGCTGAAAGGGATGCT-3'(antisense), TSC2:5'-TCTGAACATGTGGTCCGCAG-3'(sense) and 5'-TCTGAACATGTGGTCCGCAG-3'(antisense).

Western blot

A549 cells and H1299 cells were treated with 1 mM, 5 mM, 10 mM bexarotene for 24 h, then the cells were harvested, then total protein from tissue or cell was extracted using radioimmunoprecipitation lysis buffer containing 1 mM phenylmethanesulfonylfluoride and the protein concentration was determined using the Bradford method (Beyotime Institute of Biotechnology, Nantong, China) according to the manufacturer's instructions. Proteins (20 μg) were separated by 10% SDS-PAGE and transferred onto a nitrocellulose membrane. After blocking with 5% non-fat milk for 1 h at 4 °C, then membrane was incubated with the primary antibody at 4 °C overnight. Membranes were washed 3 times with 0.25% PBST and then incubated with the peroxidase-conjugated secondary antibody for 2 h at room temperature. After washed 3 times, the specific protein bands were detected using the enhanced chemiluminescence reagents [18].

Statistical analysis

All data were expressed as mean ± S.D. Differences between the groups were analyzed using one-way analysis of variance (ANOVA) using SPSS 13.0 (SPSS Inc, Chicago, IL, USA). p-values less than 0.05 were considered statistically significant.

Results

The construction of slc10a2 overexpressed NSCLC cells

As shown in Fig. 1a, after 24 h treatment with pcDNA3.1-slc10a2 plasmid in 293 T cells, the 293 T cells had successfully transfected with slc10a2 gene, and efficiency of transfection is about 92%. Then the supernatant of virus was added to A549 cells, after this slc10a2 overexpressed A549 cells were successfully constructed (Fig. 1b). Similarly we also used this method to construct slc10a2 overexpressed H1299 cells (data not show). The western blot results further demonstrated that the expression of slc10a2 was obviously higher in transfected group than control group (Fig. 1c). And the expression of slc10a2 was declined after treated with slc10a2-shRNA in A549 cells, this result suggests slc10a2-shRNA can effectively prohibit the expression of slc10a2 in A549 cells (Fig. 1d). In addition, slc10a2-

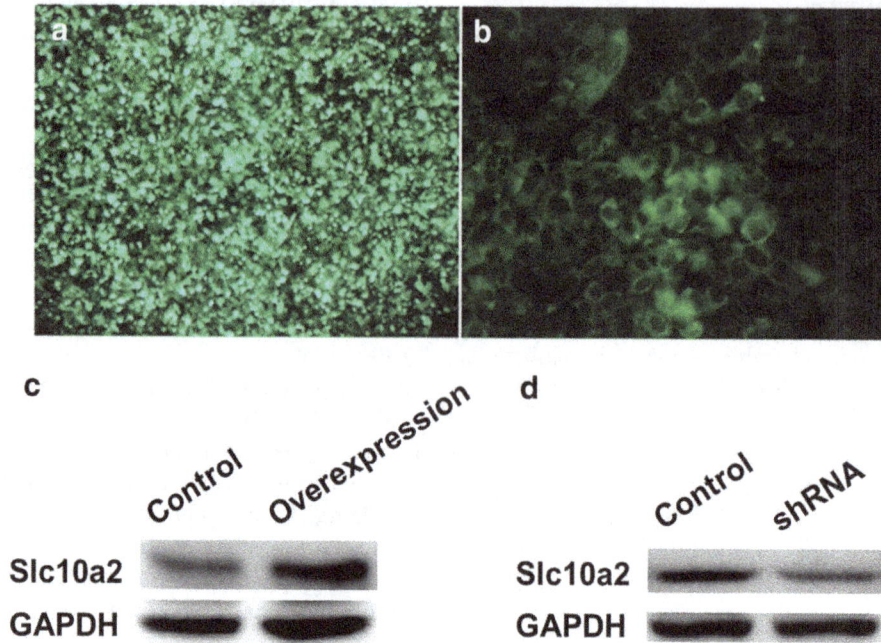

Fig. 1 The construction and identification of slc10a2 overexpressed A549 cells. **a** The immunofluorescence staining showed slc10a2 gene had successfully transfected into 293 T cells; **b** The immunofluorescence staining showed slc10a2 overexpressed A549 cells were successfully constructed; **c** The expression of slc10a2 was significant higher in slc10a2 overexpressed A549 cells than in A549 cells; **d** Slc10a2-shRNA can effectively inhibit the expression of slc10a2 in A549 cells. All experiments were repeated 3 times

shRNA also can significantly inhibit the expression of slc10a2 in H1299 cells (data not show).

Slc10a2 plays an important role in the proliferation of NSCLC cells with the treatment of bexarotene

As Fig. 2 showed, in comparison to the control group (without any treatment), bexarotene can inhibit the proliferation of A549 cells on day 3 and day 4. And the proliferation of slc10a2 overexpressed A549 cells was significantly prohibited with the treatment of bexarotene on both day 3 and day 4. However, the proliferation of A549 cells was increased when co-treated with bexarotene and slc10a2-shRNA at all of the detected time points. Moreover, the same results can be seen

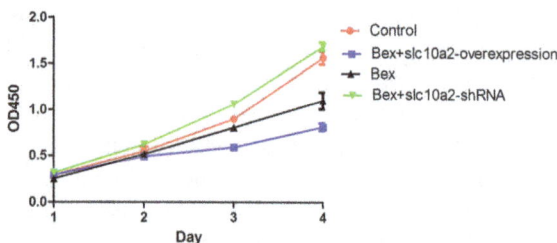

Fig. 2 The proliferation of A549 cells treated with bexarotene, bexarotene + slc10a2-shRNA, bexarotene + slc10a2-overexpression respectively. A549 cells without treatment as control. All experiments were repeated 3 times

in H1299 cells (Additional file 1: Figure S1A). These results suggest slc10a2 involve in the process of bexarotene inhibits the proliferation of NSCLC cells.

Slc10a2 plays an important role in the invasion of NSCLC cells with the treatment of bexarotene

Transwell invasion test showed that (Fig. 3), the migration of A549 cells was decreased with the treatment of bexarotene for 24 h when compared with control group, the similar situation was discovered in slc10a2 overexpressed A549 cells treated with bexarotene. While the migration of A549 cells was increased when co-treated with bexarotene and slc10a2-shRNA. It reveals that slc10a2 involve in the process of bexarotene inhibits the invasion of NSCLC cells.

Slc10a2 plays an important role in the apoptosis of NSCLC cells with the treatment of bexarotene

As shown in Fig. 4a, in comparison to the control group (Fig. 4d), there is no significant difference in apoptosis rate between 0.1 mM bexarotene treated group and control group. However, the apoptosis rate in 1 mM and 10 mM bexarotene treated groups was obviously higher than control group. In addition, the apoptosis rate of slc10a2 overexpressed A549 cells treated with 1 mM and 10 mM bexarotene was significantly increased than in

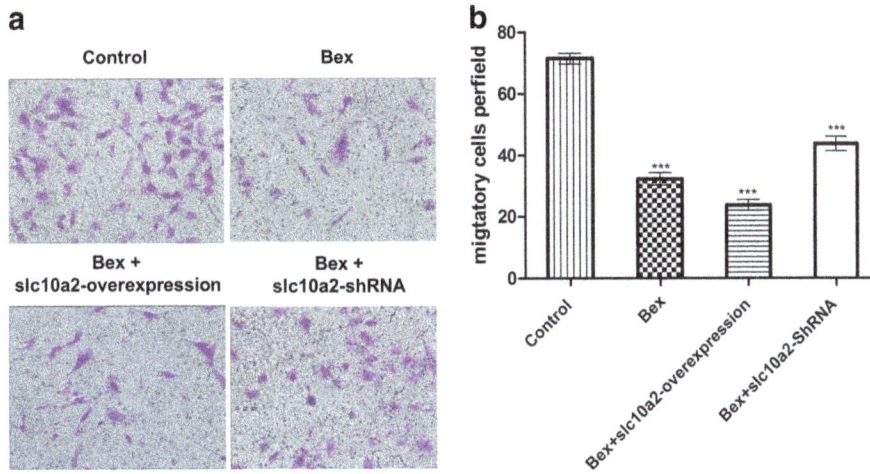

Fig. 3 The effects of slc10a2 on invasion of A549 cells treated with bexarotene. **a** The invasion behavior of A549 cells treated with bexarotene, bexarotene + slc10a2-shRNA, bexarotene + slc10a2-overexpression respectively, A549 cells without any treatment as control group. **b** The quantification of migratory A549 cells treated with bexarotene, bexarotene + slc10a2-shRNA, bexarotene + slc10a2-overexpression respectively. All experiments were repeated 3 times. ***$p < 0.001$

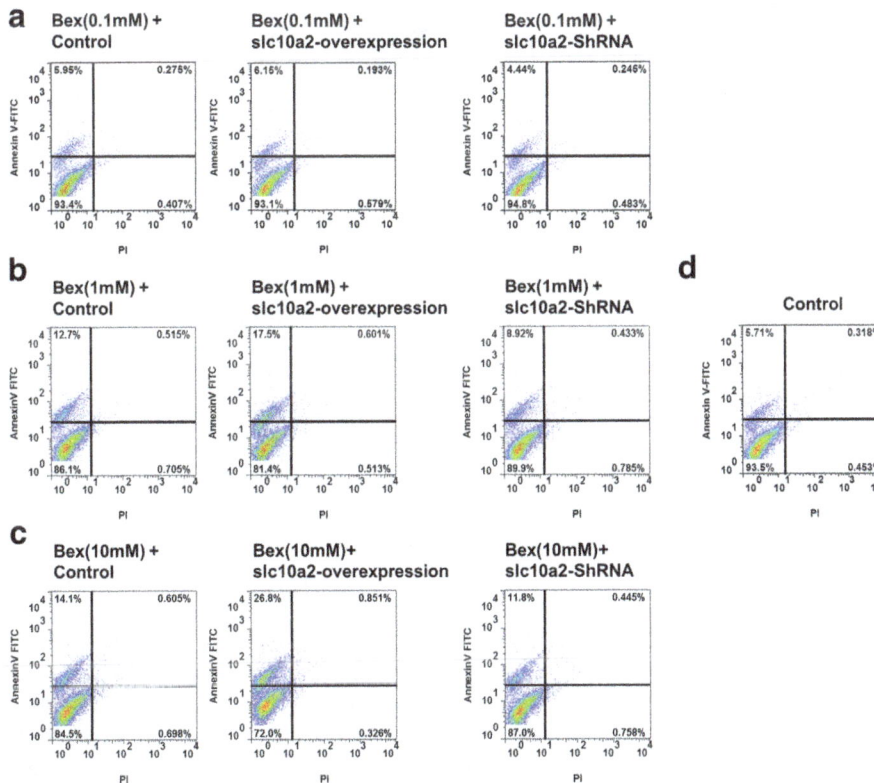

Fig. 4 The effects of slc10a2 on apoptosis of A549 cells treated with bexarotene. **a** The apoptosis rate of A549 cells treated with 0.1 mM bexarotene, overexpressed slc10a2 in combination with 0.1 mM bexarotene, slc10a2-shRNA in combination with 0.1 mM bexarotene respectively; **b** The apoptosis rate of A549 cells treated with 1 mM bexarotene, overexpressed slc10a2 in combination with 1 mM bexarotene, slc10a2-shRNA in combination with 1 mM bexarotene respectively; **c** The apoptosis rate of A549 cells treated with 10 mM bexarotene, overexpressed slc10a2 in combination with 10 mM bexarotene, slc10a2-shRNA in combination with 10 mM bexarotene respectively, A549 cells without any treatment as control group (**d**). All experiments were repeated 3 times

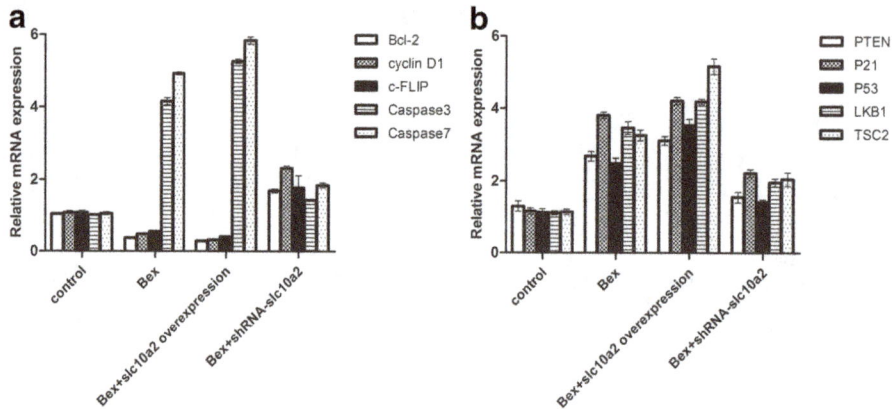

Fig. 5 The effects of slc10a2 on expression of apoptosis related genes in A549 cells treated with bexarotene. **a** The expression of apoptotic related genes Bcl-2, cyclin D1, c-FLIP, caspase 3, caspase 7 in A549 cells treated with bexarotene, overexpressed slc10a2 in combination with bexarotene, slc10a2-shRNA in combination with bexarotene respectively, A549 cells without any treatment as control group. **b** The expression of tumor suppressor genes PTEN, P21, P53, LKB1, TSC2 in A549 cells treated with bexarotene, overexpressed slc10a2 in combination with bexarotene, slc10a2-shRNA in combination with bexarotene respectively, A549 cells without any treatment as control group. All experiments were repeated 3 times

A549 cells, and it distinctly declined in A549 cells after treated with slc10a2-shRNA in combination with bexarotene when compared to the bexarotene single treated group (Fig. 4b and c). Moreover, the apoptosis of H1299 cells was significant increased when H1299 cells treated with 10 mM bexarotene + slc10a2-overexpression, and it

decreased when H1299 cells treated with 10 mM bexarotene + shRNA-slc10a2 (Additional file 1: Figure S1B).

Slc10a2 plays an important role in tumor suppressor with the treatment of bexarotene

As shown in Fig. 5 and Additional file 2: Figure S2, after A549 cells and H1299 cells treated with bexarotene for 24 h, the expression of apoptotic related genes caspase 3, caspase 7, and tumor suppressor genes PTEN, P21, P53, LKB1 and TSC2 were significantly increased ($p < 0.05$) and the expression of anti-apoptotic genes bcl 2, cyclin D1, c-FLIP were decreased ($p < 0.05$). Similarly, the same situations were observed in slc10a2 overexpressed A549 cells and H1299 cells. While, the expression of caspase 3, caspase 7, PTEN, P21, P53, LKB1 and TSC2 were reduced ($p < 0.05$) and the expression of bcl 2, cyclin D1, c-FLIP were increased ($p < 0.05$) when A549 cells and H1299 cells were co-treated with bexarotene and slc10a2-shRNA.

Slc10a2 via PPARγ plays an important role in the proliferation of NSCLC cells with the treatment of bexarotene

According to the aforementioned, we have demonstrated that slc10a2 plays an important role in the proliferation of A549 cells with the treatment of bexarotene, how can the slc10a2 effect in this process. As Fig. 6a showed, by comparison, the proliferation of A549 cells was inhibited when treated with bexarotene on both day 3 and day 4. However, we found that GW992 (selective PPARγ antagonist) can shortened the proliferative inhibition effects of bexarotene. The proliferation rate of A549 cells was higher in bexarotene in combination with GW9662 treated group than the bexarotene treated group on day

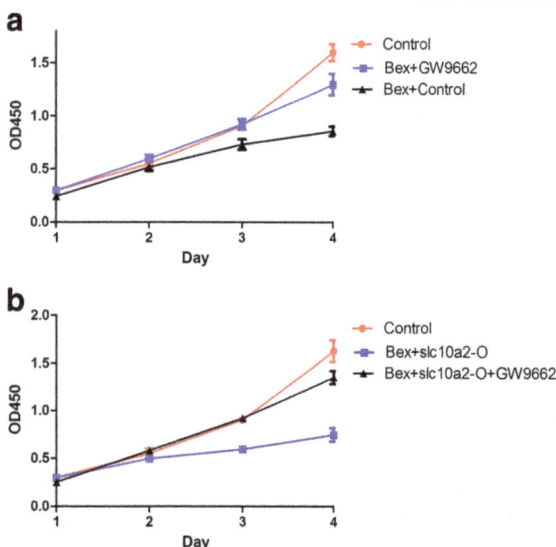

Fig. 6 Slc10a2 via PPARγ plays an important role in the proliferation of A549 cells with the treatment of bexarotene. **a** The proliferation rate of A549 cells treated with bexarotene, bexarotene in combination with GW9662 respectively, A549 cells without any treatment as control group. **b** The proliferation rate of slc10a2 overexpressed A549 cells treated with bexarotene, bexarotene in combination with GW9662 respectively, A549 cells without any treatment as control group. All experiments were repeated 3 times

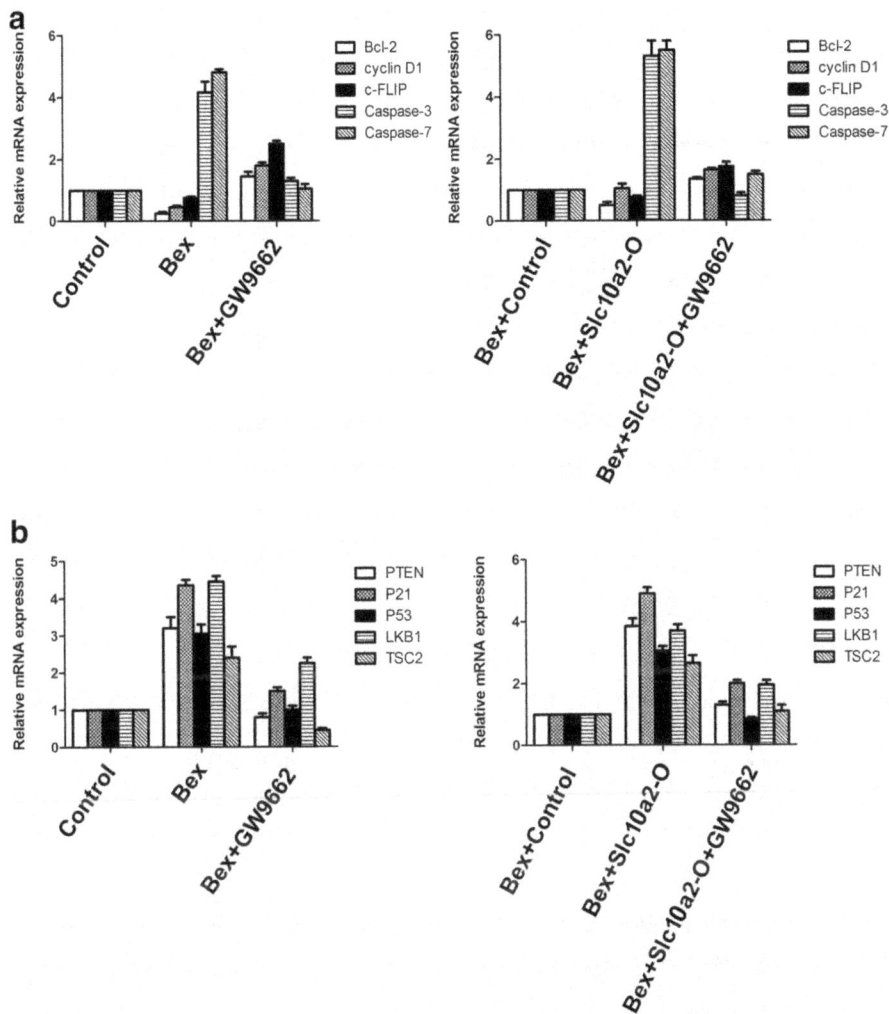

Fig. 7 Slc10a2 via PPARγ plays an important role in tumor suppressor with the treatment of bexarotene. **a** The expression of apoptotic related genes Bcl-2, cyclin D1, c-FLIP, caspase 3, caspase 7 in A549 cells and slc10a2 overexpressed A549 cells when treated with bexarotene, bexarotene in combination with GW9662 respectively; **b** The expression of tumor suppressor genes PTEN, P21, P53, LKB1, TSC2 in A549 cells and slc10a2 over-expressed A549 cells when treated with bexarotene, bexarotene in combination with GW9662 respectively. A549 cells without any treatment as control group. All experiments were repeated 3 times

3 and day 4. Furthermore, a similar result was found in slc10a2 overexpressed A549 cells (Fig. 6b).

Slc10a2 via PPARγ plays an important role in tumor suppressor with the treatment of bexaroten

We further explored whether slc10a2 via PPARγ plays an important role in tumor suppressor with the treatment of bexarotene. As shown in Fig. 7 and Additional file 3: Figure S3 after A549 cells, H1299 cells or slc10a2 overexpressed A549 cells, H1299 cells treated with bexarotene, the expression of apoptotic genes caspase 3, caspase 7, and tumor suppressor genes PTEN, P21, P53, LKB1 and TSC2 were significantly increased ($p < 0.05$) and the expression of anti-apoptotic genes bcl 2, cyclin D1, c-FLIP were reduced ($p < 0.05$). While, the expression of caspase 3, caspase 7, PTEN, P21, P53, LKB1 and TSC2 were

declined ($p < 0.05$) and the expression of bcl 2, cyclin D1, c-FLIP were increased ($p < 0.05$) when A549 cells, H1299 cells or slc10a2 overexpressed A549 cells, H1299 cells were co-treated with bexarotene and GW9662.

Bexarotene inhibits the viability of NSCLC cells via slc10a2/PPARγ/PTEN/mTOR signaling pathway

As shown in Fig. 8a, b and Additional file 4: Figure S4, the western blotting and RT-PCR results showed the expression of slc10a2 was gradually enhanced with the increase of bexarotene's concentrations from 1 mM to 10 mM. Also the expression of PPARγ was increased with the increase of bexarotene's concentrations. Additionally, the expression of slc10a2 can be reduced in Bex + GW9662 treated group. Moreover the expression of PTEN was increased in bexarotene treated group

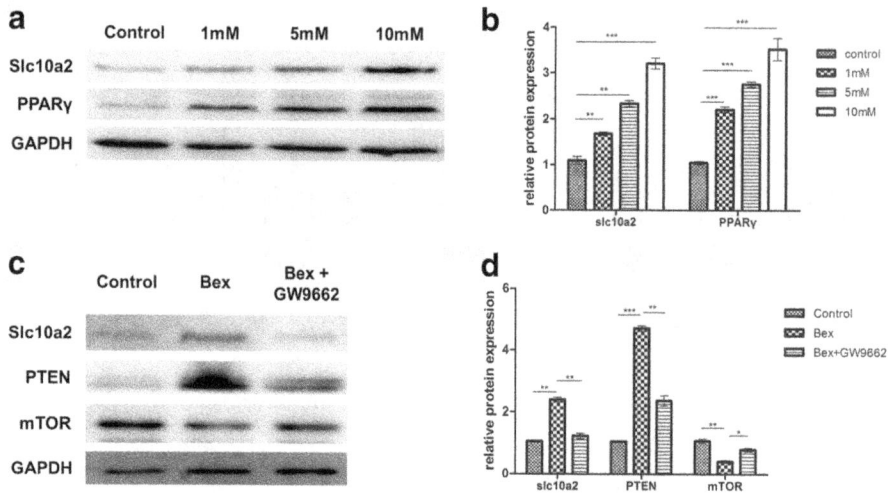

Fig. 8 Bexarotene inhibits the viability of A549 cells via slc10a2/PPARγ/PTEN/mTOR signaling pathway. **a** The expression of slc10a2 and PPARγ in A549 cells treated with 1 mM, 5 mM, 10 mM bexarotene respectively. **b** The quantification of slc10a2 and PPARγ expression in A549 cells treated with 1 mM, 5 mM, 10 mM bexarotene respectively. **c** The expression of slc10a2, PTEN, mTOR in A549 cells treated with bexarotene, bexarotene + GW9662 respectively. **d** The quantification of slc10a2, PTEN, mTOR expression in A549 cells treated with bexarotene, bexarotene + GW9662. All experiments were repeated 3 times. *$p < 0.05$, **$p < 0.01$

when compared to the control group, while it can be inhibit when A549 cells treated with bexarotene and GW9662. On the contrary, the expression of mTOR was suppressed by bexarotene, and this inhibition effects can be shortened by GW9662 (Fig. 8c, d).

Discussion

Three types of PPARs have been identified: alpha, gamma, and delta, they are a group of nuclear receptor proteins which function as transcription factors regulating the expression of genes [19]. Among the three phenotypes, PPARγ has been attracting tremendous attention, the previous studies revealed that PPARγ plays essential roles in the regulation of cellular differentiation, development, and metabolism (carbohydrate, lipid, protein), and tumorigenesis [20, 21].

A mass of studies have demonstrated that PPARγ agonists via inhibiting the expression of cyclinD1, cyclinB, cyclinE, CDK4 and CDK2 and increasing the expression of CDKN1A to prevent cell cycle from G1 to S phase to prohibit tumor cells proliferation [22–26]. In this study we found that bexarotene worked as a PPARγ agonists, which was capable of enhancing the expression of PPARγ, then the expression of cyclinD1 was suppressed and the proliferation of A549 cells was prohibited, these results were consistent with the previous studies.

The activation of PPARγ can induce tumor cell apoptosis via several different pathways. PPARγ agonists was able to up-regulate pro-apoptotic protein BAX and BAD expression, and then induced glioma cells apoptosis through releasing cytochrome C and activating the activation of caspase [27]. Li et al. reported the activation of

PPARγ was associated with a decrease of the expression of Bcl-2 and increase of the expression of P53 in human melanoma cell line A375 cells [28]. Similarly, we found that the expression of anti-apoptotic proteins Bcl-2, cyclin D1 and c-FLIP was reduced whereas the expression of apoptotic proteins caspase-3, caspase-7 and tumor suppressor gene PTEN, P21, P53, LKB1, TSC2 were accelerated in A549 cells with the treatment of bexarotene, which was associated with the activation of PPARγ through enhancing the expression of slc10a2, resulting in promoting the apoptosis of A549 cells.

Moreover, the activation of PPARγ can reduce the invasion ability of tumor cells. Thiazolidinedione (TZD) is a synthetic agonist of PPARγ, which contains troglitazone, pioglitazone and rosiglitazone [29]. Willson et al. discovered that after adrenocortical cancer cell lines H295R cells co-cultured with pioglitazone and rosiglitazone, the expression of MMP-2 which play an important role in cell migration was reduced, and the migration of H295R cells was significantly declined [30]. Also Galli et al. found that TZD can effectively inhibit tumor cell invasion, after pancreatic cancer cell treated with TZD for 24 h, the activity and transcriptional level of MMP-2 were declined [31]. And in this study, the migration ability of A549 cells was significantly shortened after treated with bexarotene, whereas the migration of A549 cells was distinctly accelerated after with the treatment of bexarotene in combination with GW9662.

PI3K/Akt/mTOR signaling pathway exists in almost all mammals, it regulates cell growth mainly through controlling the protein synthesis. PTEN as a negative regulator of this pathway via suppressing the expression of

PI3K and Akt. Patel et al. revealed that PPARγ can combined with peroxisome proliferator responsive element 1 (PPRE1) and PPRE2, the upstream gene of PTEN, and increased the expression of PTEN then induced phosphorylation of Akt decreased, cells differentiation and apoptosis [32]. And it has been preclinically showed that deficiency of TSC2 or PTEN expression induces impaired PI3K/Akt/mTOR activation, suggesting that mTOR overexpression with the loss of PTEN plays a key role in the development and progression of pancreatic neuroendocrine tumors [33]. In this study, we discovered that bexarotene accelerated the expression of PPARγ through enhancing the expression of slc10a2, also the expression of PPARγ was promoted, while the expression of mTOR was declined, thus the viability of A549 cells was suppressed. Finally this study has some limitations, for example, PPAR agonist bexarotene induces PPARγ and slc10a2 in a dose dependent manner, but the effects of bexarotene on PPARα, PPARβ/δ expression we don't explore. We have clarified limitations in the discussion section, and we will explore the effects of bexarotene on PPARα, PPARβ/δ expression in our future study.

Conclusion

In this study we found that bexarotene can suppress the proliferation, migration, and promote the apoptosis of NSCLC cells. Moreover, we demonstrated that this effects owned to the increased expression of PPARγ via enhancing the expression of slc10a2, then up-regulated the expression of PTEN and down-regulated the expression of mTOR, thus increased the expression of apoptotic genes and anti-cancer genes, and reduced the expression of anti-apoptotic genes to suppress the proliferation of NSCLC cells and promote the apoptosis of NSCLC cells [34].

Additional files

Additional file 1: Figure S1. (A) The proliferation of H1299 cells treated with bexarotene, bexarotene + shRNA-slc10a2, bexarotene + slc10a2-overexpression respectively, H1299 cells without treatment as control. (B) The apoptosis of H1299 cells treated with bexarotene, bexarotene + shRNA-slc10a2, bexarotene + slc10a2-overexpression respectively, H1299 cells without treatment as control. All experiments were repeated 3 times. (TIFF 739 kb)

Additional file 2: Figure S2. (A) The expression of apoptotic related genes Bcl-2, cyclin D1, c-FLIP, caspase 3, caspase 7 in H1299 cells treated with bexarotene, overexpressed slc10a2 in combination with bexarotene, slc10a2-shRNA in combination with bexarotene respectively. (B) The expression of tumor suppressor genes PTEN, P21, P53, LKB1, TSC2 in H1299 cells treated with bexarotene, overexpressed slc10a2 in combination with bexarotene, slc10a2-shRNA in combination with bexarotene respectively, H1299 cells without any treatment as control group. All experiments were repeated 3 times. (TIFF 516 kb)

Additional file 3: Figure S3. (A) The expression of apoptotic related genes Bcl-2, cyclin D1, c-FLIP, caspase 3, caspase 7 in H1299 cells when

treated with bexarotene, bexarotene in combination with GW9662 respectively. (B) The expression of apoptotic related genes Bcl-2, cyclin D1, c-FLIP, caspase 3, caspase 7 in slc10a2 overexpressed H1299 cells when treated with bexarotene, bexarotene in combination with GW9662 respectively. (C) The expression of tumor suppressor genes PTEN, P21, P53, LKB1, TSC2 in H1299 cells when treated with bexarotene, bexarotene in combination with GW9662 respectively. (D) The expression of tumor suppressor genes PTEN, P21, P53, LKB1, TSC2 in slc10a2 overexpressed H1299 cells when treated with bexarotene, bexarotene in combination with GW9662 respectively. H1299 cells without any treatment as control group. All experiments were repeated 3 times. (TIFF 882 kb)

Additional file 4: Figure S4. The expression of slc10a2 in A549 cells treated with 1 mM, 5 mM, 1 0 mM bexarotene respectively, A549 cell without treatment as control. (TIFF 68 kb)

Abbreviations
ANOVA: One-way analysis of variance; CCK-8: Cell Counting Kit-8; HDL: High-density lipoprotein; NSCLC: Non-small cell lung cancer; PPAR: Peroxisome proliferator-activated receptor; PPRE: Peroxisome proliferator responsive element; RXRs: Retinoid X receptors; TZD: Thiazolidinedione

Acknowledgements
Not applicable

Funding
This work was supported by Major Key Project of Shanghai Chest Hospital Science & Technology foundation (2014YZDC10600). The funding source has no role in the study design, analysis, or interpretation of the data, writing of the manuscript, or the decision to submit the manuscript for publication.

Authors' contributions
Prof. SL designed this study; Prof. YST gave final approval of the version to be published; XHA wrote and revised this paper; FM made substantial contributions to acquisition of data, analysis and interpretation of data, SPS and JJW performed experiments and collected data. All authors have read and approved the manuscript.

Competing interests
The authors declare that they have no competing interests.

References
1. Zheng R, Zeng H, Zhang S, Fan Y, Qiao Y, Zhou Q, et al. Lung cancer incidence and mortality in China, 2010. Thoracic Cancer. 2016;7(1):94–99.
2. Hermann TW, Yen W-C, Tooker P, Fan B, Roegner K, Negro-Vilar A, et al. The retinoid X receptor agonist bexarotene (Targretin) synergistically enhances the growth inhibitory activity of cytotoxic drugs in non-small cell lung cancer cells. Lung Cancer. 2005;50:9–18.
3. Rizvi NA, Marshall JL, Dahut W, Ness E, Truglia JA, Loewen G, et al. A phase I study of LGD1069 in adults with advanced cancer. Clin Cancer Res. 1999;5:1658–64.
4. Miller VA, Benedetti FM, Rigas JR, Verret AL, Pfister DG, Straus D, et al. Initial clinical trial of a selective retinoid X receptor ligand, LGD1069. J Clin Oncol. 1997;15:790–5.
5. Luo W, Schork NJ, Marschke KB, Ng S-C, Hermann TW, Zhang J, et al. Identification of polymorphisms associated with hypertriglyceridemia and prolonged survival induced by bexarotene in treating non-small cell lung cancer. Anticancer Res. 2011;31:2303–11.
6. Blumenschein GR, Khuri FR, von Pawel J, Gatzemeier U, Miller WH, Jotte RM, et al. Phase III trial comparing carboplatin, paclitaxel, and bexarotene with carboplatin and paclitaxel in chemotherapy-naive patients with advanced or metastatic non–small-cell lung cancer: SPIRIT II. J Clin Oncol. 2008;26:1879–85.

7. Malik SM, Collins B, Pishvaian M, Ramzi P, Marshall J, Hwang J. A phase I trial of bexarotene in combination with docetaxel in patients with advanced solid tumors. Clin Lung Cancer. 2011;12:231–6.

8. Tang X-H, Gudas LJ. Retinoids, retinoic acid receptors, and cancer. Annu Rev Pathol. 2011;6:345–64.

9. Dawson MI, Xia Z. The retinoid X receptors and their ligands. Biochim Biophys Acta. 2012;1821:21–56.

10. Brabender J, Metzger R, Salonga D, Danenberg KD, Danenberg PV, Hölscher AH, et al. Comprehensive expression analysis of retinoid acid receptors and retinoid X receptors in non-small cell lung cancer: implications for tumor development and prognosis. Carcinogenesis. 2005;26(3):525–30.

11. Wong MH, Rao PN, Pettenati MJ, Dawson PA. Localization of the ileal sodium-bile acid cotransporter gene (SLC10A2) to human chromosome 13q33. Genomics. 1996;33:538–40.

12. Dawson PA. Role of the intestinal bile acid transporters in bile acid and drug disposition. Drug transporters: Springer; Handb Exp Pharmacol. 2011; (201):169–203.

13. Kosters A, Karpen SJ. Bile acid transporters in health and disease. Xenobiotica. 2008;38:1043–71.

14. Paresh PC, Peter WS. Resveratrol promotes degradation of the human bile acid transporter ASBT (SLC10A2). Biochem J. 2014;459:301–12.

15. Kitayama K, Nakai D, Kono K, van der Hoop AG, Kurata H, de Wit EC, et al. Novel non-systemic inhibitor of ileal apical Na$^+$-dependent bile acid transporter reduces serum cholesterol levels in hamsters and monkeys. Eur J Pharmacol. 2006;539:89–98.

16. West KL, McGrane M, Odom D, Keller B, Fernandez ML. SC-435, an ileal apical sodium-codependent bile acid transporter inhibitor alters mRNA levels and enzyme activities of selected genes involved in hepatic cholesterol and lipoprotein metabolism in Guinea pigs. J Nutr Biochem. 2005;16:722–8.

17. Liu ZY, Wang JY, Liu HH, Ma XM, Wang CL, Zhang XP, et al. Retinoblastoma protein-interacting zinc-finger gene 1 (RIZ1) dysregulation in human malignant meningiomas. Oncogene. 2013;32:1216.

18. Qiu Z, Dyer KD, Xie Z, Rådinger M, Rosenberg HF. GATA transcription factors regulate the expression of the human eosinophil-derived neurotoxin (RNase 2) gene. J Biol Chem. 2009;284:13099–109.

19. Michalik L, Auwerx J, Berger JP, Chatterjee VK, Glass CK, Gonzalez FJ, et al. International Union of Pharmacology. LXI. Peroxisome proliferator-activated receptors. Pharmacol Rev. 2006;58:726–41.

20. Berger J, Moller DE. The mechanisms of action of PPARs. Annu Rev Med. 2002;53:409–35.

21. Feige JN, Gelman L, Michalik L, Desvergne B, Wahli W. From molecular action to physiological outputs: peroxisome proliferator-activated receptors are nuclear receptors at the crossroads of key cellular functions. Prog Lipid Res. 2006;45:120–59.

22. Nagamine M, Okumura T, Tanno S, Sawamukai M, Motomura W, Takahashi N, et al. PPARγ ligand-induced apoptosis through a p53-dependent mechanism in human gastric cancer cells. Cancer Sci. 2003;94:338–43.

23. Baek SJ, Wilson LC, Hsi LC, Eling TE. Troglitazone, a peroxisome proliferator-activated receptor γ (PPARγ) ligand, selectively induces the early growth Response-1 gene independently of PPARγ. A novel mechanism for its anti-tumorigenic activity. J Biol Chem. 2003;278:5845–53.

24. Ricote M, Li AC, Willson TM, Kelly CJ, Glass CK. The peroxisome proliferator-activated receptor-γ is a negative regulator of macrophage activation. Nature. 1998;391:79–82.

25. Han S, Sidell N, Fisher PB, Roman J. Up-regulation of p21 gene expression by peroxisome proliferator-activated receptor γ in human lung carcinoma cells. Clin Cancer Res. 2004;10:1911–9.

26. Koga H, Sakisaka S, Harada M, Takagi T, Hanada S, Taniguchi E, et al. Involvement of p21WAF1/Cip1, p27Kip1, and p18INK4c in troglitazone-induced cell-cycle arrest in human hepatoma cell lines. Hepatology. 2001; 33:1087–97.

27. Zander T, Kraus JA, Grommes C, Schlegel U, Feinstein D, Klockgether T, et al. Induction of apoptosis in human and rat glioma by agonists of the nuclear receptor PPARγ. J Neurochem. 2002;81:1052–60.

28. Li Y, Meng Y, Li H, Li J, Fu J, Liu Y, et al. Growth inhibition and differentiation induced by peroxisome proliferator activated receptor gamma ligand rosiglitazone in human melanoma cell line A375. Med Oncol. 2006;23:393–402.

29. Lehmann JM, Moore LB, Smith-Oliver TA, Wilkison WO, Willson TM, Kliewer SA. An antidiabetic thiazolidinedione is a high affinity ligand for peroxisome proliferator-activated receptor γ (PPARγ). J Biol Chem. 1995;270:12953–6.

30. Ferruzzi P, Ceni E, Tarocchi M, Grappone C, Milani S, Galli A, et al. Thiazolidinediones inhibit growth and invasiveness of the human adrenocortical cancer cell line H295R. J Clin Endocrinol Metab. 2005;90:1332–9.

31. Galli A, Ceni E, Crabb DW, Mello T, Salzano R, Grappone C, et al. Antidiabetic thiazolidinediones inhibit invasiveness of pancreatic cancer cells via PPARγ independent mechanisms. Gut. 2004;53:1688–97.

32. Patel L, Pass I, Coxon P, Downes CP, Smith SA, Macphee CH. Tumor suppressor and anti-inflammatory actions of PPARγ agonists are mediated via upregulation of PTEN. Curr Biol. 2001;11:764–8.

33. Han X, Ji Y, Zhao J, Xu X, Lou W. Expression of PTEN and mTOR in pancreatic neuroendocrine tumors. Tumor Biol. 2013;34:2871–9.

34. Ai X, Lu S. PUB061 Bexarotene inhibits the viability of A549 cells via slc10a2/ PPARγ/PTEN/mTOR signaling pathway. J Thorac Oncol. 2015;10:761–90.

11

Signaling protein signature predicts clinical outcome of non-small-cell lung cancer

Bao-Feng Jin[1†], Fan Yang[2†], Xiao-Min Ying[3†], Lin Gong[1], Shuo-Feng Hu[3], Qing Zhao[1], Yi-Da Liao[2], Ke-Zhong Chen[2], Teng Li[1], Yan-Hong Tai[4,7], Yuan Cao[4], Xiao Li[2], Yan Huang[1], Xiao-Yan Zhan[1], Xuan-He Qin[1], Jin Wu[1], Shuai Chen[1], Sai-Sai Guo[1], Yu-Cheng Zhang[1], Jing Chen[1], Dan-Hua Shen[5], Kun-Kun Sun[5], Lu Chen[6], Wei-Hua Li[1], Ai-Ling Li[1], Na Wang[1], Qing Xia[1], Jun Wang[2*] and Tao Zhou[1*] (iD)

Abstract

Background: Non-small-cell lung cancer (NSCLC) is characterized by abnormalities of numerous signaling proteins that play pivotal roles in cancer development and progression. Many of these proteins have been reported to be correlated with clinical outcomes of NSCLC. However, none of them could provide adequate accuracy of prognosis prediction in clinical application.

Methods: A total of 384 resected NSCLC specimens from two hospitals in Beijing (BJ) and Chongqing (CQ) were collected. Using immunohistochemistry (IHC) staining on stored formalin-fixed paraffin-embedded (FFPE) surgical samples, we examined the expression levels of 75 critical proteins on BJ samples. Random forest algorithm (RFA) and support vector machines (SVM) computation were applied to identify protein signatures on 2/3 randomly assigned BJ samples. The identified signatures were tested on the remaining BJ samples, and were further validated with CQ independent cohort.

Results: A 6-protein signature for adenocarcinoma (ADC) and a 5-protein signature for squamous cell carcinoma (SCC) were identified from training sets and tested in testing sets. In independent validation with CQ cohort, patients can also be divided into high- and low-risk groups with significantly different median overall survivals by Kaplan-Meier analysis, both in ADC (31 months vs. 87 months, HR 2.81; $P < 0.001$) and SCC patients (27 months vs. not reached, HR 9.97; $P < 0.001$). Cox regression analysis showed that both signatures are independent prognostic indicators and outperformed TNM staging (ADC: adjusted HR 3.07 vs. 2.43, SCC: adjusted HR 7.84 vs. 2.24). Particularly, we found that only the ADC patients in high-risk group significantly benefited from adjuvant chemotherapy ($P = 0.018$).

Conclusions: Both ADC and SCC protein signatures could effectively stratify the prognosis of NSCLC patients, and may support patient selection for adjuvant chemotherapy.

Keywords: Adenocarcinoma, Non-small-cell lung cancer, Prognosis, Protein signature, Squamous cell carcinoma

Background

Lung cancer is the most common cause of cancer-related mortality worldwide, and approximately 80% cases are non-small-cell lung cancer (NSCLC) mainly including adenocarcinomas (ADC) and squamous cell carcinomas (SCC) [1, 2]. The tumor-node-metastasis (TNM) staging system is currently adopted to predict prognosis and guide treatment decisions for patients with NSCLC [3, 4]. However, the current staging system is not always accurate [5, 6]. After complete surgical resection of NSCLC, about 30% pathologic stage IA patients die of relapse within five years, while nearly 50% of stage IIA and 24% stage IIIA patients can survive [6].

To improve the outcome prediction of NSCLC, tremendous efforts have been made to identify prognostic markers. Based on gene microarray analysis, many groups have identified different gene signatures [7–19]. These signatures were usually identified on fresh or frozen tissue samples, the mixture of stroma, tumor and

* Correspondence: jwangmd@yahoo.com; tzhou@ncba.ac.cn
†Equal contributors
2Department of Thoracic Surgery, People's Hospital, Peking University, Beijing 100044, China
1State Key Laboratory of Proteomics, Institute of Basic Medical Sciences, China National Center of Biomedical Analysis, Beijing 100850, China
Full list of author information is available at the end of the article

normal cells. In addition, mRNA levels in gene-based signatures are not always consistent with protein expression levels. Until now, this approach has not yielded a signature that could be applied in NSCLC clinical practice [13]. On the other hand, the management of cancer patients is still mainly guided based on combinations of clinicopathological features, including prognostic markers derived from careful histopathological analysis of tumors. For breast cancer, the combination of three protein markers, oestrogen receptor (ER), progesterone receptor (PR) and human epidermal growth factor receptor 2 (HER2), has been successfully utilized for clinical decision making and the use of this framework has contributed to the steady decline in the mortality of breast cancer patients. For lung cancer, numerous signaling proteins have been identified as abnormal in cancer development and progression [1, 20–22], and many of them have been reported to be correlated with clinical outcome of NSCLC [23]. However, none of them could provide adequate accuracy in clinical application. Based on these proteins, we attempt to identify a multi-protein signature to improve the prognosis prediction of NSCLC.

In this study, we performed an immunohistochemistry (IHC) analysis of 75 signaling proteins in paraffin-embedded surgical specimens of NSCLCs. These proteins represent the most important signaling pathways involved in cancer development [20, 21, 24]. Using random forest algorithm (RFA) and support vector machines (SVM), we successfully identified a 6-protein signature for ADC and a 5-protein signature for SCC that accurately predicted prognosis of ADC and SCC respectively.

Methods
Study design
The objective of this study was to identify signaling protein signature for NSCLC prognosis. Patients were eligible to enter the study if they underwent complete resection of invasive NSCLC at People's Hospital of Peking University in Beijing (BJ) and Southwest Hospital of Chongqing (CQ) between January, 2004, and December, 2010. Information on the clinical variables and follow-up data were obtained from a prospectively maintained database of individual hospitals. We then excluded the patients who received any treatment prior to resection, received epidermal growth factor receptor tyrosine kinase inhibitor (EGFR TKI), died within 30 days of resection, or had no follow-up information. In total, 211 samples of patients from BJ hospital and 173 samples of patients from CQ hospital who fulfilled the inclusion criteria were collected for our study. The protocols of this study were approved by the Institutional Review Board of People's Hospital and Southwest Hospital. Written consent for the use of the resected tissue for research purposes was obtained at time of surgery.

We assessed the expression levels of 75 signaling proteins via immunohistochemistry (IHC) on BJ samples. BJ samples were randomly partitioned into training (2/3 samples) and testing (1/3 samples) sets. Random forest algorithm and support vector machines were employed to identify prognostic signatures. Since previous studies have suggested fundamental differences between ADC and SCC regarding their molecular make-ups [2, 25], we separately identified the signature for ADC and SCC patients. CQ cohort was used for independent validation.

Selection of IHC markers
To create the panel of IHC markers, we started with all of the 1027 proteins in "pathways in cancer" (Entry No. map05200) and "non-small cell lung cancer" (Entry No. map05223) of KEGG (Kyoto Encyclopedia of Genes and Genomes) pathway database. After searching NCBI Gene database using gene IDs and the related articles in PubMed ("See all citations in PubMed" under item "Bibliography" in the webpages), we found that 765 of 1027 candidates were associated with prognosis of cancer. After further filtering with "IHC" and "FFPE" and checking the existing literature, we found that 103 of the 765 proteins had been tested with IHC assay on FFPE samples in prognosis analysis.

We then purchased antibodies against all these 103 proteins and tested them by Western blot and immunofluorescence analysis. Seventy-four antibodies against 74 different proteins/phospho-proteins were found with high specificity/sensitivity and were used in our subsequent study. These 74 proteins/phospho-proteins plus CUEDC2, a potential oncogene that we identified and studied extensively [26–29], were the final members of the IHC marker panel. Schematic diagram of IHC marker selection is depicted in Additional file 1: Figure S1.

Tissue microarray
All hematoxylin and eosin (H&E) slides were centrally reviewed at Department of Pathology in People's Hospital according to the histopathological classification system adopted by the World Health Organization (WHO) to confirm tumor type and differentiation grade. Tissue microarrays were prepared as previously described [30]. Representative areas of each tissue sample were identified and carefully marked on H&E-stained sections. Core-tissue specimens (2 mm in diameter) were punched from the corresponding individual donor tissue blocks and rearranged in recipient blocks using a trephine apparatus (SuperBioChips Laboratories, Seoul, Korea) [31].

IHC analysis
IHC staining was performed and evaluated as previously described [32]. The consecutive 4-μm-thick sections of

tissue array were cut and mounted on glass slides. The slides were baked at 60 °C for 2 h prior to the high-throughput IHC procedure. The arrays were deparaffinized via sequential washing with xylene, graded ethanol and water. Antigens were retrieved (or not) for 15 min at 95 °C (see Additional file 1: Table S1 for detail). Endogenous peroxidase was blocked with 3% H_2O_2 for 30 min. Nonspecific staining was blocked using 10% normal goat serum (in 1× PBS) for 1 h at room temperature. The slides were incubated overnight at 4 °C with various antibodies (diluted in 1× PBS, see Additional file 1: Table S1 for dilution). The enhancing step, incubation with the secondary antibody (1 h at room temperature) and the diaminobenzidine (DAB) substrate (5 min at room temperature) were all performed following the protocol of ABC kit (Vector Laboratories, Burlingame, CA). Hematoxylin was used as a counterstain in the last step. The slides were then rinsed, cleared and mounted. The staining of each antibody was optimized based on negative and positive controls. For complete data of optimal antibody dilutions and assay conditions, see Additional file 1: Table S1. The flurescent images and Western blot results for specificity/sensitivity validation of each antibody are deposited in Clinical Research Database (CRD, see http://202.38.152.246:81/crd2/frontend/www/, username: nsclc, password: nsclcnsclc).

Semiquantative analysis of the immunostained slides was performed using a modified histochemical scoring (H-score) system to assess both the intensity of the staining and the percentage of positively-stained cells, as previously described [32]. Briefly, for the intensity, a score of 0 to 3 (corresponding to negative, weak, moderate or strong staining) was recorded. The scoring was normalized with controls. In addition, the percentage of positively-stained cells at each intensity was estimated. The H-score was calculated as 1 × (weak %) + 2 × (moderate %) + 3 × (strongly stained %). All slides were concurrently evaluated by three certified pathologists (Y.H.T., D.H.S and K.K.S), blinded to clinical data, to improve the accuracy of the results. The evaluation was repeated under multi-headed microscope if there was a discrepancy between the pathologists in the interpretation of the slides until consensus was achieved. All the digital images and the results of IHC evaluation are deposited in CRD.

Data process of protein expression profiles
The expression score of each protein was processed for further analysis. Missing values were replaced with the median score of the respective protein in all tumors (see Supplementary methods for the details). The ratio of the expression score of each protein in a single sample to the mean score of that protein was calculated. The expression level was then quantified as log_{10} (expression ratio). To avoid zeros in the logarithm, a score of 0.01 was added to all scores. For independent validation, missing values were replaced with the median score. The expression profiles were processed as described above.

Signature identification and model development
The patients were grouped according to the survival status at three years for modeling. Two-thirds of ADC and SCC patients from BJ cohort were assigned as training sets by computer-generated random numbers. Random forest algorithm was used to identify protein signatures in the training sets [33]. The procedure was implemented using the R varSelRF package with parameters "ntree = 5000, ntreeIterat = 2000, vars.drop.frac = 0.2", which was built upon the randomForest package [34, 35]. The set of proteins with the smallest out-of-bag error rate among all the forests were returned and selected as signatures.

After signatures were identified, SVM was employed to develop the classification models in the training sets. The radial basis function (RBF) kernel was chosen for SVM training. The parameters C and γ for RBF kernel were tuned using the grid search strategy [36]. The parameter C was tuned from 2^{-5} to 2^{15} with the step of 2^2. The parameter γ was tuned from 2^3 to 2^{-15} with the step of 2^{-2}. During the training phase, the performance of SVM was evaluated using 5-fold cross-validation accuracy. The classification model was trained using SVM with the optimal C and γ. All the procedure was implemented using libSVM, a library for support vector machines [36].

To analyze the robustness of our signatures, enrichment analysis was performed. Ten thousand training sets were generated from BJ ADC and BJ SCC patients respectively, by randomly partitioning BJ ADC and BJ SCC patients into training set and testing set for 10,000 times. Each training set involved 2/3 ADC or SCC patients. A signature was identified on each training set using random forest algorithm. For each protein, the fraction of the signatures containing the protein (i.e. percentage of subsets) in all 10,000 subsets in ADC or SCC patients from BJ cohort was calculated. The proteins were sorted in descending order of the percentages.

Statistical analysis
Overall survival (OS) from the time of resection was chosen as the primary endpoint since it is verifiable through multiple sources and less subject to interpretation bias [14]. Differences in survival between patients with good and poor prognosis and between patients treated with adjuvant chemotherapy or not were analyzed using Kaplan-Meier analysis and the two-sided log-rank test. Related covariates in this study were compared with clinical outcome using univariate and multivariate Cox regression analysis. A Wald likelihood ratio

test was performed to assess statistical significance. For all statistical tests, a two-sided α of 0.05 was regarded as statistically significant. The analyses were performed in the R programming language (version 3.0.2).

Results
Patient characteristics
In this study, 211 patients who fulfilled the inclusion criteria from Beijing People's Hospital were used as the training and testing sets (BJ cohort) (Table 1). A total of 173 patients from Chongqing Southwest Hospital were used as the independent validation cohort (CQ cohort) (Table 1). All the samples are resected tissues from patients underwent surgery at TNM stages I-IIIA. Of the

Table 1 Clinical-pathological characteristics of non-small-cell lung cancer patients

Variable	All patients (n = 384)	BJ cohort (n = 211)	CQ cohort (n = 173)
Age			
≤60	151 (39.32%)	73 (34.60%)	78 (45.09%)
>60	233 (60.68%)	138 (65.40%)	95 (54.91%)
Gender			
Male	270 (70.31%)	135 (63.98%)	135 (78.03%)
Female	114 (29.69%)	76 (36.02%)	38 (21.97%)
Smoking index (pack years)			
Never smokers	142 (36.98%)	94 (44.55%)	48 (27.75%)
Light smokers (< 20)	41 (10.68%)	26 (12.32%)	15 (8.67%)
Heavy smokers (≥20)	183 (47.65%)	88 (41.71%)	95 (54.91%)
Unknown	18 (4.69%)	3 (1.42%)	15 (8.67%)
Histology			
Adenocarcinoma	206 (53.65%)	122 (57.82%)	84 (48.55%)
Squamous cell carcinoma	178 (46.35%)	89 (42.18%)	89 (51.45%)
Follow-up (months; median; IQR)	58 (22–75)	59 (19–74)	56 (29–76)
Deaths	175 (45.57%)	93 (44.07%)	82 (47.40%)
Differentiation grade			
Well	75 (19.53%)	45 (21.33%)	30 (17.34%)
Moderate	140 (36.46%)	67 (31.75%)	73 (42.20%)
Poor	138 (35.94%)	98 (46.45%)	40 (23.12%)
Unknown	31 (8.07%)	1 (0.47%)	30 (17.34%)
Pathologic stage			
I	188 (48.96%)	95 (45.02%)	93 (53.76%)
II	101 (26.30%)	47 (22.28%)	54 (31.21%)
III	95 (24.74%)	69 (32.70%)	26 (15.03%)
Adjuvant chemotherapy			
No	141 (36.72%)	100 (47.39%)	41 (23.70%)
Yes	243 (63.28%)	111 (52.61%)	132 (76.30%)

Data are number (%), unless otherwise stated. IQR = interquartile range

total cases, 63% (243 of 384) patients received adjuvant platinum-based doublet chemotherapy. The median duration of follow-up was 58 months (interquartile range, 22 to 75), and during the follow-up period, 175 patients died (Table 1). Because previous studies have suggested fundamental differences between ADC and SCC regarding their molecular make-ups [2, 25], we separately identified the prognostic signature for ADC and SCC patients based on the expression levels of the detected signaling proteins.

Identification of the ADC signature
In our experiments, all the antibodies used were commercially available and were validated by Western blot and immunofluorescence analysis (Additional file 1: Table S1). Using IHC, we investigated the expression levels of 75 signature protein candidates in BJ cohort (Additional file 1: Table S1). To make the detailed staining and clinical information of each case accessible to the public, we developed a clinical research database (CRD) and all the results were deposited in it (http://202.38.152.246:81/crd2/frontend/www/, username: nsclc, password: nsclcnsclc). Two thirds of ADC patients from BJ cohort were randomly assigned as the training set, and the remaining 1/3 as the testing set (Fig. 1, BJ cohort). We performed signature discovery using random forest algorithm on the training set. The identified signature of ADC comprised six proteins: c-SRC, Cyclin E1, TTF1, p65, CHK1, and JNK1. We developed a classification model with the 6-protein signature using SVM algorithm (Additional file 1: Tables S2 and S3). For each patient, the model was used to calculate a prognosis score, which represents the combined information of the six proteins in the signature.

The performance of the ADC signature in the training set was evaluated by receiver-operating characteristic (ROC) analysis. The value of area under the ROC curve (AUC) of the signature on training set was 0.967 (Fig. 2a), indicating that the signature accurately predicted the prognosis in the training set. Based on the ROC curve, the optimal cutoff point of the prognosis score was calculated as 0.710 to separate good and poor prognosis. A patient with a prognosis score smaller than 0.710 was classified into poor-prognosis group; otherwise, the patient was classified into good-prognosis group. In the training set, the good-prognosis group showed a three-year survival of 91.9% (95% CI, 81.7 to 96.6%) and 11.1% (95% CI, 1.9 to 29.8%) in the poor-prognosis group in Kaplan-Meier analysis (HR 14.54; 95% CI, 6.35 to 33.31; $P < 0.001$, Fig. 2b).

We next evaluated the prognostic performance of this 6-protein signature in the testing set. The result indicated that the ADC signature was strongly associated with overall survival of these patients. Kaplan-Meier

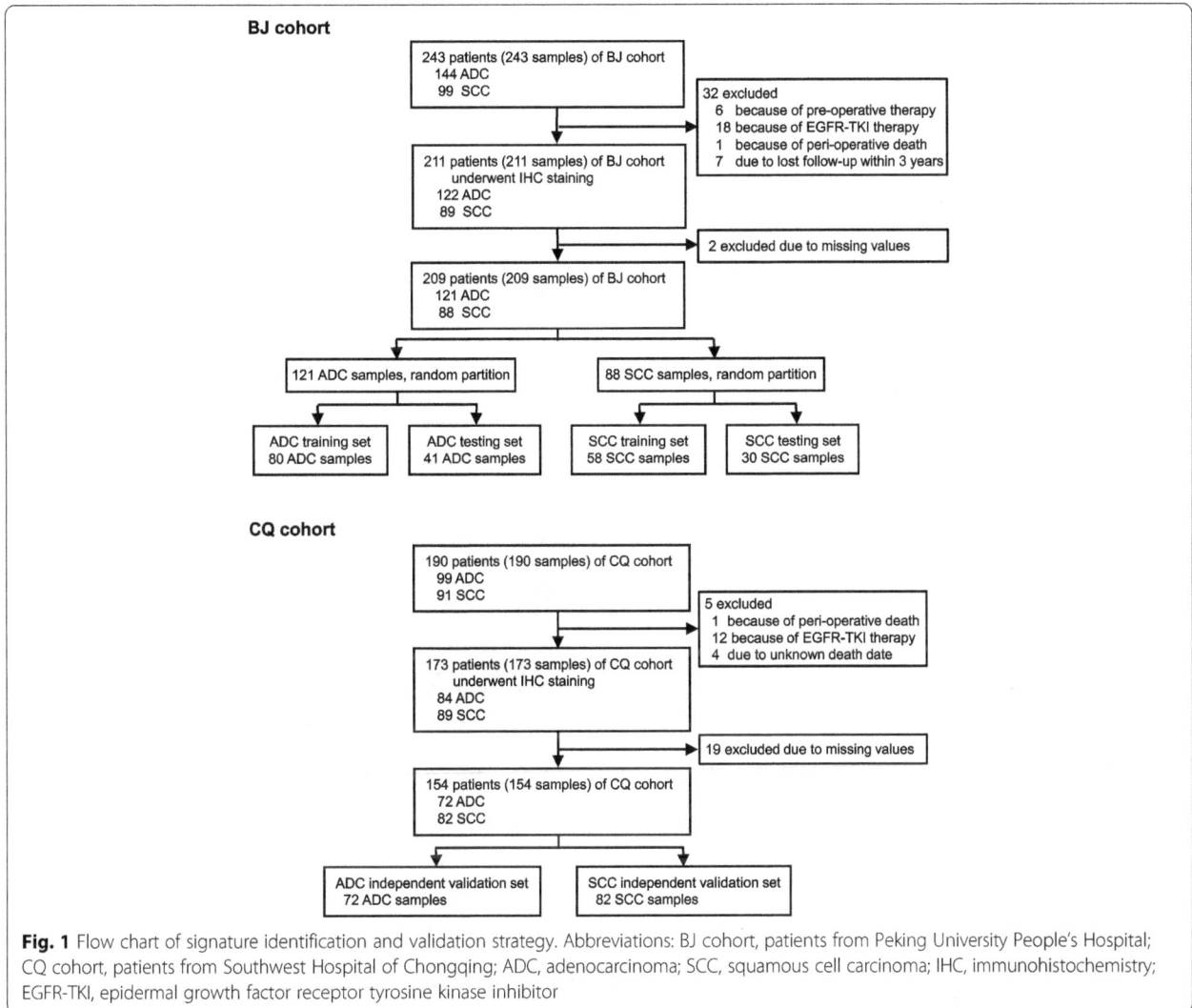

Fig. 1 Flow chart of signature identification and validation strategy. Abbreviations: BJ cohort, patients from Peking University People's Hospital; CQ cohort, patients from Southwest Hospital of Chongqing; ADC, adenocarcinoma; SCC, squamous cell carcinoma; IHC, immunohistochemistry; EGFR-TKI, epidermal growth factor receptor tyrosine kinase inhibitor

analysis showed a three-year overall survival of 96.0% (95% CI, 74.8 to 99.4%) in good-prognosis group, but just 37.5% (95% CI, 15.4 to 59.8%) in poor-prognosis group (HR 7.67; 95% CI, 3.96 to 39.34; $P < 0.001$, Fig. 2c).

The prognosis score distribution, prognosis prediction, three-year survival status and the expression profile of the signature proteins of the ADC patients from BJ cohort are summarized in Fig. 2d. The comparison of the prognosis score distribution (top panel) and the three-year survival data (middle panel) indicated that the 6-protein signature accurately predicted the three-year survival of patients. Particularly, in the distribution of prognosis scores, the top part (32%) and the bottom part (15%) are completely correct in predicting three-year survival, suggesting that the prognosis score is a reliable predictor for prognosis. The expression profile of the six signature proteins was shown in the bottom panel.

Independent validation of the ADC signature

To further verify the performance of the ADC signature, we used another cohort (CQ cohort) of ADC patients as an independent validation set (Fig. 1, CQ cohort). Kaplan-Meier analysis showed a significant difference in overall survival between the predicted good- and poor-prognosis groups (HR 2.81; 95% CI, 1.65 to 6.05; $P < 0.001$; Fig. 2e). The good-prognosis group had a three-year survival of 97.3% (95% CI, 82.3 to 99.6%), and the poor-prognosis group had a rate of 42.9% (95% CI, 26.4 to 58.3%; Fig. 2e). The prognosis score distribution, prognosis prediction, the survival status, and the expression profile of the six signature proteins of CQ cohort were presented in Fig. 2f. These results further demonstrated the effectiveness of the 6-protein signature in the prognosis prediction of ADC patients.

We compared the prognostic value of ADC signature with that of clinical risk factors, including pathologic stage, age, tumor size, smoking index, and chemotherapy,

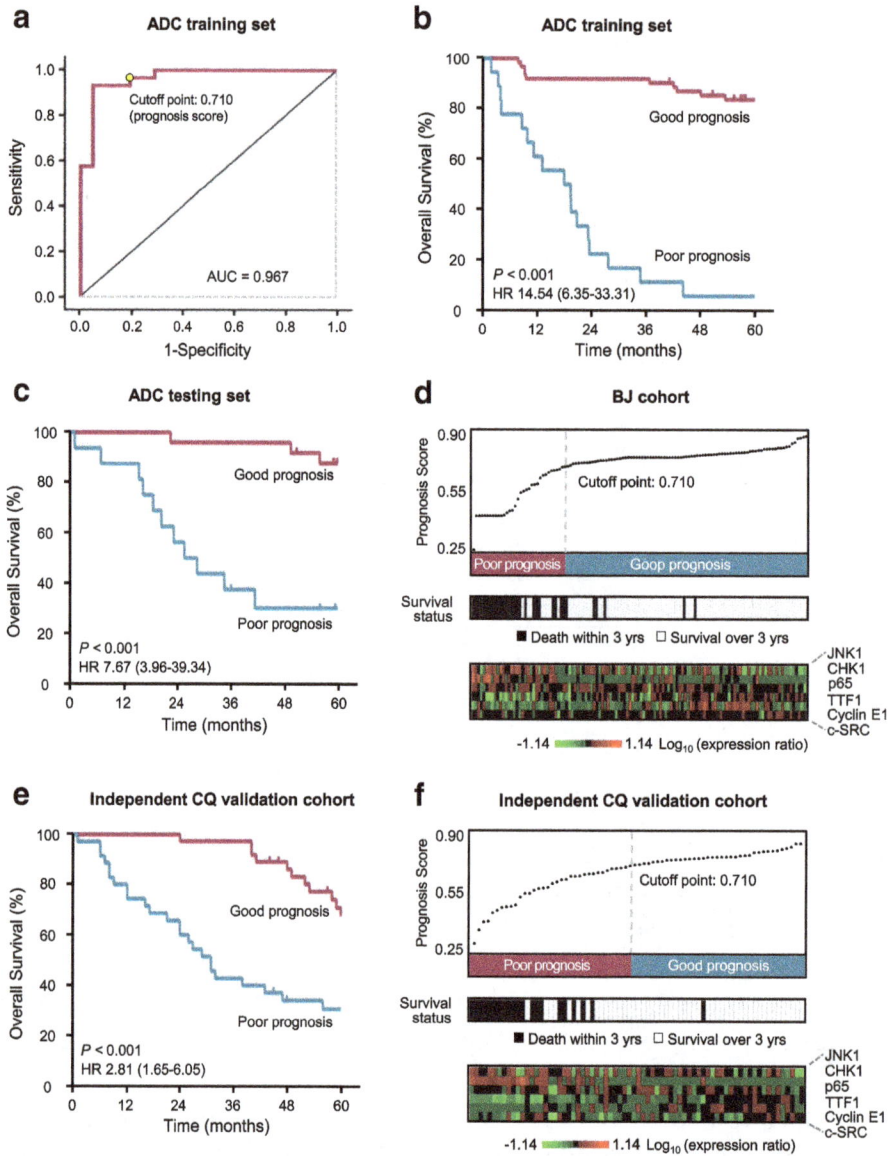

Fig. 2 Identification and validation of the 6-protein signature for adeno-carcinoma (ADC). **a** The ROC curve of the ADC training set. The cutoff point of prognosis scores is shown. **b-c** Patients of the training set (**b**) and testing set (**c**) were classified into poor- and good-prognosis groups using the 6-protein ADC signature. The Kaplan-Meier estimates of overall survival for the two predicted prognosis groups are shown. (**d**) The prognosis score distribution, prognosis prediction using the ADC signature, the three-year survival status and the expression profile of the 6-protein signature proteins were summarized on ADC patients of BJ cohort. Each column represents an individual patient. **e** ADC patients of the independent CQ validation cohort were classified into poor- and good-prognosis groups using the 6-protein ADC signature. The Kaplan-Meier survival curves for the two prognosis groups are shown. **f** The prognosis score distribution, prognosis prediction using the signature, the three-year survival status and the expression profile of the 6-protein signature proteins of CQ ADC patients are shown

by both univariate and multivariate Cox regression analysis in independent CQ cohort. The univariate analysis indicated that the 6-protein signature is a better prognostic predictor of three-year overall survival (HR 2.89; 95% CI, 1.52 to 5.48; $P = 0.001$) than the pathologic stage (HR 2.43; 95% CI, 1.64 to 3.60; $P < 0.001$), although both of them are statistically significant (Table 2). The multivariate analysis further showed that the 6-protein signature is an independent

predictor (HR 3.07; 95% CI, 1.29 to 7.32; $P = 0.011$) after adjusting for the above risk factors (Table 2).

Identification and independent validation of the SCC signature

Using a similar procedure as in the discovery of the ADC signature, we also identified a protein signature for SCC with BJ cohort (Table 1; Fig. 1; CRD; Additional file 1: Tables S4 and S5). The SCC signature is distinct from the

Table 2 Cox regression analysis of overall survival in the independent CQ validation cohort

Histology	Variable	Univariate analysis		Multivariate analysis	
		HR(95% CI)	P value	HR(95% CI)	P value
ADC	Six-protein signature[a]	2.89 (1.52–5.48)	0.001	3.07 (1.29–7.32)	0.011
	Stage[b]	2.43 (1.64–3.60)	< 0.001	2.43 (1.46–4.03)	0.001
	Age > 60 years	1.33 (0.70–2.53)	0.390	1.37 (0.65–2.87)	0.413
	Tumor size	1.09 (0.91–1.30)	0.341	1.02 (0.84–1.24)	0.880
	Smoking index	1.01 (0.99–1.03)	0.425	0.99 (0.97–1.01)	0.426
	Chemotherapy	1.09 (0.52–2.30)	0.816	1.50 (0.61–3.67)	0.379
SCC	Five-protein signature[a]	10.84 (4.15–28.31)	< 0.001	7.84 (2.88–21.31)	< 0.001
	Stage[b]	2.85 (1.78–4.57)	< 0.001	2.24 (1.26–3.99)	0.006
	Age > 60 years	1.73 (0.86–3.50)	0.127	1.48 (0.70–3.14)	0.307
	Tumor size	1.15 (1.00–1.32)	0.058	1.02 (0.85–1.23)	0.838
	Smoking index	1.00 (0.99–1.01)	0.994	1.00 (0.98–1.02)	0.659
	Chemotherapy	1.23 (0.56–2.71)	0.615	1.45 (0.55–3.83)	0.452

ADC, adenocarcinoma; SCC, squamous cell carcinoma; HR, hazard ratio
[a]Compared with low-risk group. [b]Modeled as a continuous variable

ADC signature and consists of five proteins: EGFR, p38α, AKT1, SOX2, and E-cadherin. An ROC analysis on the training set showed an AUC value of 0.913 and the optimal cutoff point of the prognosis score was 0.597 (Fig. 3a). With this cutoff point, the prognosis prediction of the 5-protein SCC signature in the training set showed a three-year survival of 96.2% (95% CI, 75.7 to 99.5%) in good-prognosis group and 25.0% (95% CI, 11.8 to 40.7%) in poor-prognosis group (HR 11.65; 95% CI, 3.65 to 16.41; $P < 0.001$, Fig. 3b).

The evaluation result of this signature on the testing set indicated that it was strongly associated with overall survival of SCC patients. The three-year overall survival in good-prognosis group was 72.7% (95% CI, 37.1 to 90.3%) and 15.8% (95% CI, 3.9 to 34.9%) in poor-prognosis group (HR 3.51; 95% CI, 1.39 to 7.73; $P = 0.008$; Fig. 3c). The patients with low prognosis scores had significantly more death events than those with high scores, indicating that the SCC signature effectively predicted prognosis (Fig. 3d).

We further used the SCC patients from CQ cohort for independent validation (Fig. 1, CQ cohort). A significant difference in overall survival between the predicted good- and poor-prognosis groups was shown by Kaplan-Meier analysis (HR 9.97; 95% CI, 4.46 to 17.99; $P < 0.001$; Fig. 3e). 97.6% (95% CI, 83.9 to 99.7%) of the patients in good-prognosis group survived at least three years, but only 29.3% (95% CI, 16.4 to 43.4%) of the patients in poor-prognosis group did so (Fig. 3e). Figure 3f showed the prognosis score distribution, prognosis prediction, the survival status, and the expression profile of the five proteins in CQ cohort. Notably, in the distribution of prognosis scores, the top part (50%) and the bottom part (20%) are completely correct in predicting

the three-year survival. These results showed that the 5-protein SCC signature accurately predicted the prognosis of patients of CQ cohort. Cox regression analysis further showed that the SCC signature is an independent prognostic factor and has a greater prognostic power than TNM staging system (Table 2).

Both signatures distinguish between good and poor prognosis within TNM stages

We next investigated whether our signatures could be used to further distinguish between poor- versus good-prognosis groups in each TNM stage (stage I, II, or IIIA). Using the combined samples of the ADC patients from BJ and CQ cohorts, we found that the 6-protein ADC signature could clearly divide the patients into poor- and good-prognosis groups within each stage (Additional file 1: Figure S2 A to C. HR 6.1; 95% CI, 1.81 to 20.27; $P < 0.0001$ for Stage I; HR 3.59; 95% CI, 1.72 to 7.51; $P = 0.0007$ for Stage II; and HR 2.96; 95% CI, 1.43 to 6.11; $P = 0.015$ for Stage IIIA). Similarly, the 5-protein SCC signature also markedly classified SCC patients into good- and poor-prognosis groups within each stage (Additional file 1: Figure S2 D to F. HR 7.36; 95% CI, 2.76 to 19.68; $P < 0.0001$ for Stage I; HR 7.27; 95% CI, 3.28 to 16.08; $P < 0.0001$ for Stage II; and HR 5.13; 95% CI, 2.56 to 10.29; $P = 0.0020$ for Stage IIIA). Taken together, these results indicate that both the ADC and SCC signatures can distinguish between good and poor prognosis within each stage.

Predicted poor-prognosis ADC patients benefited from adjuvant chemotherapy

According to the American Society of Clinical Oncology (ASCO) guidelines, adjuvant chemotherapy is recommended

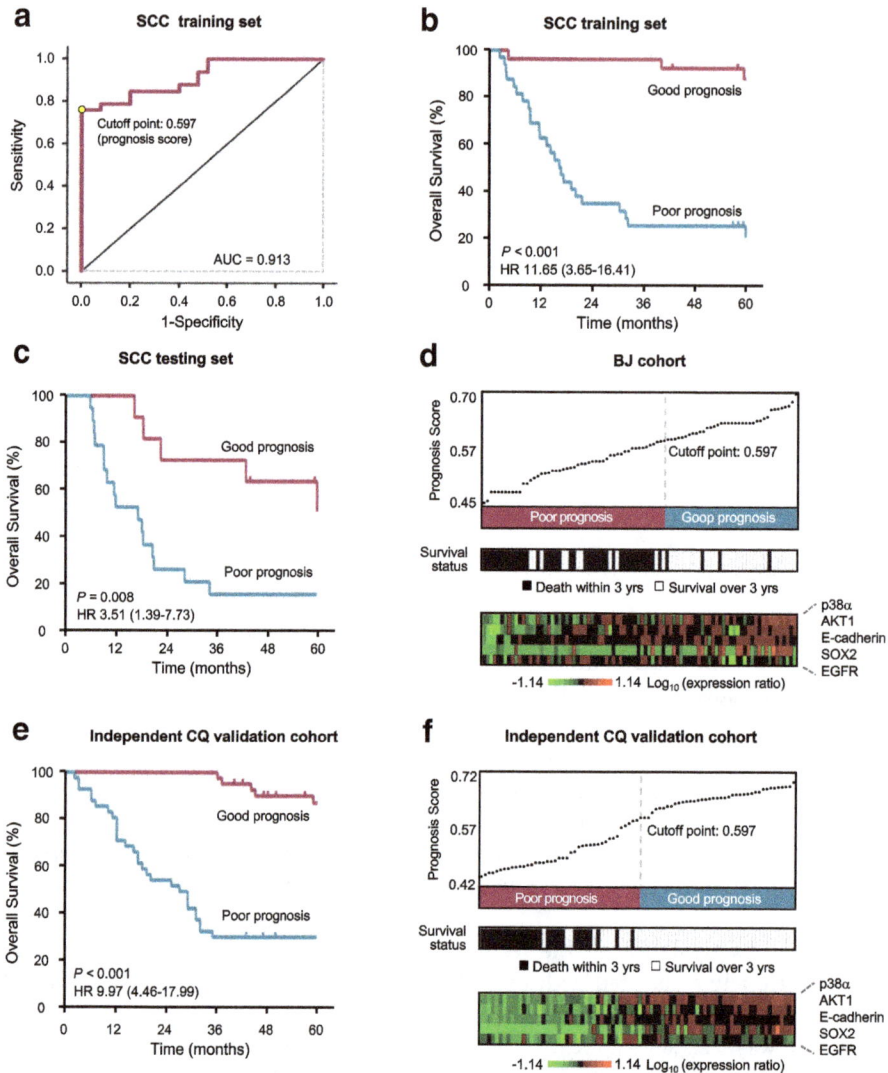

Fig. 3 Identification and validation of the 5-protein signature for squamous cell carcinoma (SCC). **a** The ROC curve of the SCC training set. The cutoff point of prognosis scores is shown. **b-c** Patients of the training set (**b**) and testing set (**c**) were classified into poor- and good-prognosis groups using the 5-protein SCC signature. The Kaplan-Meier estimates of overall survival for the two predicted prognosis groups are shown. **d** The prognosis score distribution, prognosis prediction using the signature, the three-year survival status and the expression profile of the 5-protein signature proteins were summarized on SCC patients of BJ cohort. Each column represents an individual patient. **e** SCC patients of the independent CQ validation cohort were classified into poor- and good-prognosis groups using the 5-protein SCC signature. The Kaplan-Meier survival curves for the two prognosis groups are shown. **f** Prognosis score distribution, prognosis prediction using the SCC protein signature, patient survival status and the expression profile of the 5-protein signature proteins of CQ SCC patients are shown

for routine use in stage II and IIIA patients [37]. Reports also showed that adjuvant chemotherapy can improve overall survival of NSCLCs in stage IB [38, 39]. However, only a small portion of these patients gain benefit in terms of 5-year survival [40]. To test whether our protein signatures are valuable in selecting patients for adjuvant chemotherapy, we did an exploratory analysis of the predictive value of our prognostic signatures of NLCSCs in stage IB, II and IIIA. For the good-prognosis group classified by the ADC signature, adjuvant chemotherapy did not significantly prolong overall survival of the patients (HR 0.99; 95% CI, 0.40 to 2.46; $P = 0.987$;

Fig. 4a). However, for the poor-prognosis group, adjuvant chemotherapy significantly improved survival (HR 0.51; 95% CI, 0.24 to 0.86; $P = 0.018$; Fig. 4b).

We further assessed the capacity of 6-protein ADC and 5-protein SCC signatures to predict benefit from adjuvant therapy when the different stages are analyzed separately. In ADC, we found that adjuvant chemotherapy did not significantly prolong overall survival in either good-prognosis group classified by the ADC signature or poor-prognosis group in stage IB (Additional file 1: Figure S3 A to D). But significant benefit from adjuvant therapy was observed for

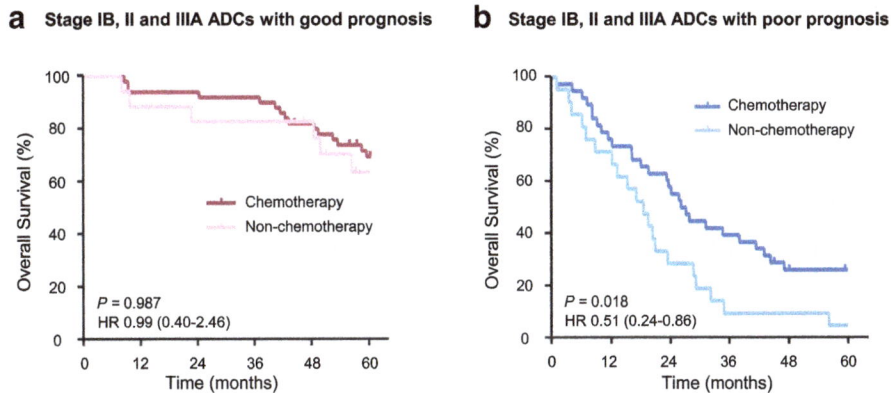

Fig. 4 Analysis of adjuvant chemotherapy benefit based on the 6-protein adenocarcinoma (ADC) signature. Kaplan-Meier estimates of overall survival for the patients at stages IB, II and IIIA with or without adjuvant chemotherapy in the good-prognosis (**a**) and poor-prognosis (**b**) group was analyzed

the poor-prognosis group in stage II and stage IIIA (Additional file 1: Figure S3 E and F. HR 0.36; 95% CI, 0.15 to 0.90; $P = 0.0134$ for Stage II; HR 0.183; 95% CI, 0.02 to 1.56; $P = 0.0003$ for Stage IIIA).

For SCC, we performed similar analysis in all patients or patients within different stages, and did not observe any significant benefit in either good- or poor-prognosis groups. (Additional file 1: Figure S4 and Additional file 1: Figure S5).

Permutation validation and enrichment analysis

The optimal signature proteins were identified using random forest algorithm (RFA) through a large number iterations of signature building and evaluation. RFA is an ensemble learning method composing of thousands of decision trees [33]. In this study, the decision trees were built with patients and proteins selected randomly and independently. RFA can avoid over-fitting and yield small number protein-contained signatures that retain a high predictive accuracy [41]. Permutation analysis showed the efficacy of RFA in our study (Fig. 5a and b). The performances of ADC and SCC signatures were among the top 2.68% and 1.82% in 10,000 randomly generated protein combinations respectively. For each protein, we calculated the percentage of the signatures containing this protein in 10,000 signatures identified using RFA from 10,000 randomly partitioned training sets. The six proteins of the ADC signature are present on the top 15 most highly enriched proteins (Fig. 5c). Especially, the proteins c-SRC, TTF1 and CHK1 are ranked in the top 3. Meanwhile, the five proteins of the SCC signature are among the top five proteins (Fig. 5d). The high frequencies of our signature proteins demonstrated the robustness and the low bias of our signatures.

Discussion

IHC is currently the most practical method of assessing the expression levels of prognostic and predictive protein

biomarkers in tumor cells [42, 43]. Due to the heterogeneity of protein expressions in tumors, the IHC scoring system used in this study considered both the intensity of the staining (richness) and the percentage of positively-stained tumor cells (evenness). We examined the expression levels of 75 signaling proteins representing the most important pathways involved in cancer development (Additional file 1: Table S1). Based on the expression scores of these proteins in lung cancer tissues, we calculated a prognostic score using the SVM algorithm-based model for each patient (Figs. 2 and 3). This score represents the combined information of the expression levels of the signature proteins, 6 proteins for ADC and 5 proteins for SCC. As shown in the distribution of prognosis scores (Fig. 2d and f; Fig. 3d and f), the higher prognostic score indicates more chance of good survival. The results indicated that the prognostic scores might be actionable in the NSCLCs prognosis.

The successful identification of the signatures with excellent performances strongly suggests that NSCLCs at different stages are featured by their specific signaling status, which is represented by expression levels of certain signaling proteins [41, 42]. The good performance of the signatures owed to three important aspects: selection of signaling proteins that play pivotal roles in lung cancer development, reliable and accurate assessment of protein expression levels with IHC staining that distinguishes cancer cells from stromal cells, and the implementation of high-efficient signature identification methods: random forest algorithm and SVM computation.

The prognostic signatures with excellent performance were identified from 75 signaling proteins. The selection of the proteins was based on their known importance in cancer development and prognosis prediction, and availability and suitability of a corresponding antibody for paraffin-embedded tissues. Although these proteins show some prognostic values, however, none of them

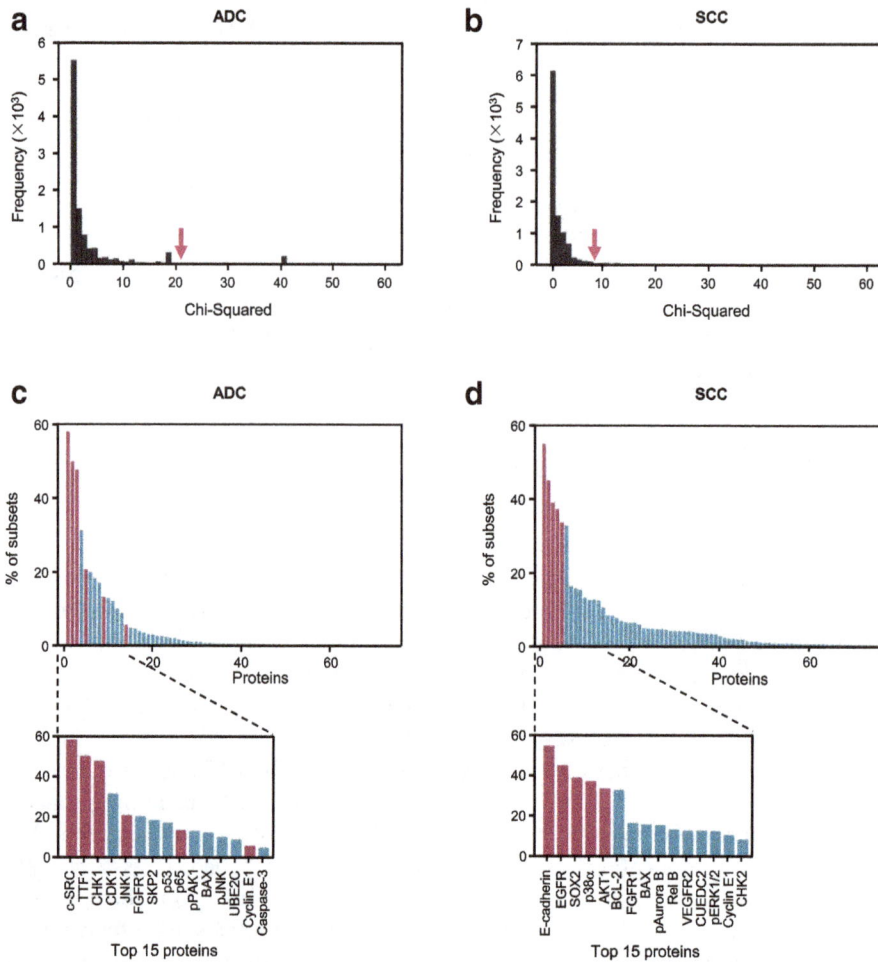

Fig. 5 Permutation validation and enrichment analysis. In permutation validation, ten thousand protein combinations were generated randomly. The model with each combination was trained on the training set using SVM. The ability of each combination to separate the testing set into good- and poor-prognosis groups was evaluated using the log-rank test. Histograms of the χ^2 value from the log-rank test on ADC testing set (**a**) and SCC testing set (**b**) were illustrated. The x axis indicates the χ^2 value. A larger χ^2 value indicates a lower P value and a more statistically significant ability to separate the testing set. The y axis shows the frequency and higher values indicate a larger fraction of the population. The performance of the ADC/SCC signature is marked with a red arrow. In enrichment analysis, ten thousand signatures were identified on 10,000 randomly partitioned training sets using random forest algorithm. For each protein, the fraction of the signatures containing the protein (i.e. percentage of subsets) in ADC (**c**) and SCC (**d**) patients from BJ cohort was calculated. A zoom-in on the 15 most enriched proteins is also shown. Each column corresponds to a protein, the signature proteins are denoted in red

individually predicts accurately in clinical practice [5, 43], as CQ Zhu et al. summarized. Using a signature of multiple proteins will likely overcome the limitation of single protein as prognostic predictors because the multiple-protein signature may reflect the heterogeneity of tumourigenesis. In this study, we identified the signatures with multiple proteins which have effective prognostic values in NSCLCs. Both 6-protein ADC signature and 5-protein SCC signature performed much better than each of the signature protein (Additional file 1: Figure S6 and Additional file 1: Figure S7). We noticed that the ADC signature does not include some top ranked proteins. One possible reason is that these proteins have functional redundancies with some ADC signature proteins. For

example, CDK1 correlates with CHK1 in regulating G2/M transition and SKP2 is also a key regulator of cell cycle [44, 45]. The inclusion of these redundant proteins in the signature will limit its ability to reflect the contribution of multiple important pathways to the complexity of cancer.

Over-treating with adjuvant chemotherapy of cancer patients is a major concern. Only a survival advantage of 5.4% was found in Lung Adjuvant Cisplatin Evaluation meta-analysis [40]. Therefore, it is necessary to develop more accurate tool for identifying patients most likely to benefit from adjuvant chemotherapy. The ADC prognostic signature in this study can identify a poor-prognosis subset from stage II-IIIA patients who could benefit from adjuvant chemotherapy. Meantime, the ADC signature also showed that the good-prognosis patients do not benefit from adjuvant chemotherapy. Hence, using ADC signature to identify patients for the treatment may spare the patients with good prognosis from adjuvant chemotherapy and avoid over-treatment of lung cancer patients.

The signatures identified in the study not only provide a tool for better prognosis prediction, but also help to reveal novel roles of the signature proteins in the development of lung cancer (Additional file 1: Table S6). For example, the upregulation of JNK1 and CHK1 are known to promote breast cancer metastasis [46]. Our study suggests that they might play similar roles in lung cancer metastasis, as the majority of ADC patients with poor prognosis had high JNK1 and CHK1 expression levels, whereas most ADC patients with good prognosis had low CHK1 expression. As we have identified several patients with good prognosis but high JNK1 expression, low CHK1 expression may have a dominant effect on tumor progression, possibly by promoting metastasis (Fig. 2d and f). Further studies will help to determine how these signature proteins cooperate to regulate NSCLC progression.

Conclusions

To our knowledge, this is one of the best identification of protein signatures that precisely predict the prognosis of NSCLC patients. Both signatures contain only a small number of proteins, six for ADC and five for SCC. This makes the application of the signatures more practical in routine clinical application. However, a prospective study with larger sample size cohorts from multiple centers, especially including non-Asian cohorts, will be needed to further validate the performance of the signatures. Nevertheless, our study demonstrated that signaling protein signatures are obviously valuable in prognosis prediction of lung cancer.

Abbreviations

ADC: Adenocarcinoma; ASCO: American Society of Clinical Oncology; AUC: Area under the curve; BJ: Beijing; CI: Confidence interval; CQ: Chongqing; CRD: Clinical research database; H&E: Hematoxylin and eosin; HR: Hazard ratio; IHC: Immunohistochemistry; NSCLC: Non-small-cell lung cancer; OS: Overall survival; RBF: Radial basis function; RFA: Random forest algorithm; ROC: Receiver-operating characteristic; SCC: Squamous cell carcinoma; SVM: Support vector machines; TNM: Tumor-node-metastasis

Acknowledgments
We thank all the patients and their families for their participation. We thank Dr. XM Zhang, Dr. ZG Liu for discussion and critical reading of the manuscript, and thank Dr. XW Bian for providing tissue samples and clinical information of patients.

Funding
This work was supported by grants from China National High Technology Research and Development Program (2014AA020612 and 2014AA020602),

National Key Technology R&D Program of China (2015BAK45B01), China National Basic Research Program (2013CB910802), China National Natural Science Foundation (81521064 and 81025010) and Frontier technology of Beijing Municipal Science and Technology Commission (Z141100000214003) and National Science and Technology Major Project (No. 2016ZX08011007). The funding organizations had no role in the design and conduct of the study, collection, management, analysis, and interpretation of the data; or preparation or review of the final manuscript.

Authors' contributions
Conception and design: BF J, F Y, XM Y, J W, T Z. Financial support: BF J, F Y, XM Y, J W, T Z. Administrative support: J W, T Z. Provision of study materials or patient information: F Y, J W, L C. Collection and assembly of data: L G, Q Z, J C, YH T, YD L, X L, KZ C, Y C, T L, XY Z, XH Q, J W, S C, SS G, YC Z, DH S, KK S, BF J. Data analysis and interpretation: XM Y, SF H, WH L, AL L, Q X, F Y, BF J, T Z. Manuscript writing: BF J, XM Y, F Y, T Z. All authors read and approved the final manuscript.

Competing interests
The authors declare that they have no competing interests.

Author details
State Key Laboratory of Proteomics, Institute of Basic Medical Sciences, China National Center of Biomedical Analysis, Beijing 100850, China. ₁Department of Thoracic Surgery, People's Hospital, Peking University, Beijing 100044, China. ³Computational Medicine Laboratory, Beijing Institute of Basic Medical Sciences, Beijing 100850, China. ⁴The 90th Hospital of Jinan, Jinan 250031, China. ⁵Department of Pathology, People's Hospital, Peking University, Beijing 100044, China. ⁶Institute of Pathology, Southwest Cancer Center, Southwest Hospital, Chongqing 400038, China. ⁷Department of Pathology, The 307th Hospital of Chinese PLA, Beijing 100071, China.

References
1. Schiller JH, Gandara DR, Goss GD, Vokes EE. Non-small-cell lung cancer: then and now. J Clin Oncol. 2013;31:981–3.
2. Campbell JD, Alexandrov A, Kim J, Wala J, Berger AH, Pedamallu CS, et al. Distinct patterns of somatic genome alterations in lung adenocarcinomas and squamous cell carcinomas. Nat Genet. 2016;48:607–16.
3. Goldstraw P. New staging system: how does it affect our practice? J Clin Oncol. 2013;31:984–91.
4. Rusch VW, Crowley J, Giroux DJ, Goldstraw P, Im J-G, Tsuboi M, et al. The IASLC lung cancer staging project: proposals for the revision of the N descriptors in the forthcoming seventh edition of the TNM classification for lung cancer. J Thorac Oncol. 2007;2:603–12.
5. Crosbie PAJ, Shah R, Summers Y, Dive C, Blackhall F. Prognostic and predictive biomarkers in early stage NSCLC: CTCs and serum/plasma markers. Transl Lung Cancer Res. 2013;2:382–97.
6. Rusch VW, Asamura H, Watanabe H, Giroux DJ, Rami-Porta R, Goldstraw P, et al. The IASLC lung cancer staging project: a proposal for a new international lymph node map in the forthcoming seventh edition of the TNM classification for lung cancer. J Thorac Oncol. 2009;4:568–77.
7. Yanagisawa K, Tomida S, Shimada Y, Yatabe Y, Mitsudomi T, Takahashi T. A 25-signal proteomic signature and outcome for patients with resected non-small-cell lung cancer. J Natl Cancer Inst. 2007;99:858–67.
8. Lu Y, Lemon W, Liu P-Y, Yi Y, Morrison C, Yang P, et al. A gene expression signature predicts survival of patients with stage I non-small cell lung cancer. PLoS Med. 2006;3:e467.
9. Raz DJ, Ray MR, Kim JY, He B, Taron M, Skrzypski M, et al. A multigene assay is prognostic of survival in patients with early-stage lung adenocarcinoma. Clin Cancer Res. 2008;14:5565–70.
10. Roepman P, Jassem J, Smit EF, Muley T, Niklinski J, van de Velde T, et al. An immune response enriched 72-gene prognostic profile for early-stage non-small-cell lung cancer. Clin Cancer Res. 2009;15:284–90.
11. Beer DG, Kardia SLR, Huang C-C, Giordano TJ, Levin AM, Misek DE, et al. Gene-expression profiles predict survival of patients with lung adenocarcinoma. Nat Med. 2002;8:816–24.

12. Yu S-L, Chen H-Y, Chang G-C, Chen C-Y, Chen H-W, Singh S, et al. MicroRNA signature predicts survival and relapse in lung cancer. Cancer Cell. 2008;13:48–57.

13. Subramanian J, Simon R. Gene expression-based prognostic signatures in lung cancer: ready for clinical use? J Natl Cancer Inst. 2010;102:464–74.

14. Kratz JR, He J, Van Den Eeden SK, Zhu Z-H, Gao W, Pham PT, et al. A practical molecular assay to predict survival in resected non-squamous, non-small-cell lung cancer: development and international validation studies. Lancet Lond Engl. 2012;379:823–32.

15. Zhu Z-H, Sun B-Y, Ma Y, Shao J-Y, Long H, Zhang X, et al. Three immunomarker support vector machines-based prognostic classifiers for stage IB non-small-cell lung cancer. J Clin Oncol. 2009;27:1091–9.

16. Director's Challenge Consortium for the Molecular Classification of Lung Adenocarcinoma, Shedden K, JMG T, Enkemann SA, Tsao M-S, Yeatman TJ, et al. Gene expression-based survival prediction in lung adenocarcinoma: a multi-site, blinded validation study. Nat Med. 2008;14:822–7.

17. Boutros PC, Lau SK, Pintilie M, Liu N, Shepherd FA, Der SD, et al. Prognostic gene signatures for non-small-cell lung cancer. Proc Natl Acad Sci U S A. 2009;106:2824–8.

18. Chen H-Y, Yu S-L, Chen C-H, Chang G-C, Chen C-Y, Yuan A, et al. A five-gene signature and clinical outcome in non-small-cell lung cancer. N Engl J Med. 2007;356:11–20.

19. Zhu C-Q, Ding K, Strumpf D, Weir BA, Meyerson M, Pennell N, et al. Prognostic and predictive gene signature for adjuvant chemotherapy in resected non-small-cell lung cancer. J Clin Oncol. 2010;28:4417–24.

20. Oxnard GR, Binder A, Jänne PA. New targetable oncogenes in non-small-cell lung cancer. J Clin Oncol. 2013;31:1097–104.

21. Stella GM, Luisetti M, Pozzi E, Comoglio PM. Oncogenes in non-small-cell lung cancer: emerging connections and novel therapeutic dynamics. Lancet Respir Med. 2013;1:251–61.

22. Berger AH, Brooks AN, Wu X, Shrestha Y, Chouinard C, Piccioni F, et al. High-throughput phenotyping of lung cancer somatic mutations. Cancer Cell. 2016;30:214–28.

23. Zhang B, Zheng A, Hydbring P, Ambroise G, Ouchida AT, Goiny M, et al. PHGDH defines a metabolic subtype in lung adenocarcinomas with poor prognosis. Cell Rep. 2017;19:2289–303.

24. Kim J, Hu Z, Cai L, Li K, Choi E, Faubert B, et al. CPS1 maintains pyrimidine pools and DNA synthesis in KRAS/LKB1-mutant lung cancer cells. Nature. 2017;546:168–72.

25. Herbst RS, Heymach JV, Lippman SM. Lung cancer. N Engl J Med. 2008;359: 1367–80.

26. Pan X, Zhou T, Tai Y-H, Wang C, Zhao J, Cao Y, et al. Elevated expression of CUEDC2 protein confers endocrine resistance in breast cancer. Nat Med. 2011;17:708–14.

27. Gao Y-F, Li T, Chang Y, Wang Y-B, Zhang W-N, Li W-H, et al. Cdk1-phosphorylated CUEDC2 promotes spindle checkpoint inactivation and chromosomal instability. Nat Cell Biol. 2011;13:924–33.

28. Zhang P-J, Zhao J, Li H-Y, Man J-H, He K, Zhou T, et al. CUE domain containing 2 regulates degradation of progesterone receptor by ubiquitin-proteasome. EMBO J. 2007;26:1831–42.

29. Chen Y, Wang S-X, Mu R, Luo X, Liu Z-S, Liang B, et al. Dysregulation of the miR-324-5p-CUEDC2 axis leads to macrophage dysfunction and is associated with colon cancer. Cell Rep. 2014;7:1982–93.

30. Gustavson MD, Rimm DL, Dolled-Filhart M. Tissue microarrays: leaping the gap between research and clinical adoption. Pers Med. 2013;10:441–51.

31. Zlobec I, Koelzer VH, Dawson H, Perren A, Lugli A. Next-generation tissue microarray (ngTMA) increases the quality of biomarker studies: an example using CD3, CD8, and CD45RO in the tumor microenvironment of six different solid tumor types. J Transl Med. 2013;11:104.

32. McCarty KS, Miller LS, Cox EB, Konrath J, McCarty KS. Estrogen receptor analyses. Correlation of biochemical and immunohistochemical methods using monoclonal antireceptor antibodies. Arch. Pathol. Lab. Med. 1985;109:716–21.

33. Breiman L. Random Forests. Mach Learn. 2001;45:5–32.

34. Diaz-Uriarte R. GeneSrF and varSelRF: a web-based tool and R package for gene selection and classification using random forest. BMC Bioinformatics. 2007;8:328.

35. Liaw A, Wiener M. Classification and regression by RandomForest. R News. 2001;2(3):18–22.

36. Chang C-C, Lin C-J. LIBSVM: a library for support vector machines. ACM Trans Intell Syst Technol. 2011;2(27):1–27.

37. Pisters KMW, Evans WK, Azzoli CG, Kris MG, Smith CA, Desch CE, et al. Cancer Care Ontario and American Society of Clinical Oncology adjuvant chemotherapy and adjuvant radiation therapy for stages I-IIIA resectable non small-cell lung cancer guideline. J Clin Oncol. 2007;25:5506–18.

38. Dediu M. Adjuvant chemotherapy in stage IB NSCLC: implication of the new TNM staging system. Memo - mag. Eur. Med. Oncologia. 2011;4:16–8.

39. Morgensztern D, Du L, Waqar SN, Patel A, Samson P, Devarakonda S, et al. Adjuvant chemotherapy for patients with T2N0M0 NSCLC. J Thorac Oncol. 2016;11:1729–35.

40. Pignon J-P, Tribodet H, Scagliotti GV, Douillard J-Y, Shepherd FA, Stephens RJ, et al. Lung adjuvant cisplatin evaluation: a pooled analysis by the LACE collaborative group. J Clin Oncol. 2008;26:3552–9.

41. Díaz-Uriarte R, Alvarez de Andrés S. Gene selection and classification of microarray data using random forest. BMC Bioinformatics. 2006;7:3.

42. Jacquemier J, Ginestier C, Rougemont J, Bardou V-J, Charafe-Jauffret E, Geneix J, et al. Protein expression profiling identifies subclasses of breast cancer and predicts prognosis. Cancer Res. 2005;65:767–79.

43. Zhu C-Q, Shih W, Ling C-H, Tsao M-S. Immunohistochemical markers of prognosis in non-small cell lung cancer: a review and proposal for a multiphase approach to marker evaluation. J Clin Pathol. 2006;59:790–800.

44. Krämer A, Mailand N, Lukas C, Syljuåsen RG, Wilkinson CJ, Nigg EA, et al. Centrosome-associated Chk1 prevents premature activation of cyclin-B-Cdk1 kinase. Nat Cell Biol. 2004;6:884–91.

45. Liao Y-J, Bai H-Y, Li Z-H, Zou J, Chen J-W, Zheng F, et al. Longikaurin a, a natural ent-kaurane, induces G2/M phase arrest via downregulation of Skp2 and apoptosis induction through ROS/JNK/c-Jun pathway in hepatocellular carcinoma cells. Cell Death Dis. 2014;5:e1137.

46. Wang Y, Shenouda S, Baranwal S, Rathinam R, Jain P, Bao L, et al. Integrin subunits alpha5 and alpha6 regulate cell cycle by modulating the chk1 and Rb/E2F pathways to affect breast cancer metastasis. Mol Cancer. 2011;10:84.

12

Aggregation of lipid rafts activates c-met and c-Src in non-small cell lung cancer cells

Juan Zeng, Heying Zhang, Yonggang Tan, Cheng Sun, Yusi Liang, Jinyang Yu and Huawei Zou[*]

Abstract

Background: Activation of c-Met, a receptor tyrosine kinase, induces radiation therapy resistance in non-small cell lung cancer (NSCLC). The activated residual of c-Met is located in lipid rafts (Duhon et al. Mol Carcinog 49:739-49, 2010). Therefore, we hypothesized that disturbing the integrity of lipid rafts would restrain the activation of the c-Met protein and reverse radiation resistance in NSCLC. In this study, a series of experiments was performed to test this hypothesis.

Methods: NSCLC A549 and H1993 cells were incubated with methyl-β-cyclodextrin (MβCD), a lipid raft inhibitor, at different concentrations for 1 h before the cells were X-ray irradiated. The following methods were used: clonogenic (colony-forming) survival assays, flow cytometry (for cell cycle and apoptosis analyses), immunofluorescence microscopy (to show the distribution of proteins in lipid rafts), Western blotting, and biochemical lipid raft isolation (purifying lipid rafts to show the distribution of proteins in lipid rafts).

Results: Our results showed that X-ray irradiation induced the aggregation of lipid rafts in A549 cells, activated c-Met and c-Src, and induced c-Met and c-Src clustering to lipid rafts. More importantly, MβCD suppressed the proliferation of A549 and H1993 cells, and the combination of MβCD and radiation resulted in additive increases in A549 and H1993 cell apoptosis. Destroying the integrity of lipid rafts inhibited the aggregation of c-Met and c-Src to lipid rafts and reduced the expression of phosphorylated c-Met and phosphorylated c-Src in lipid rafts.

Conclusions: X-ray irradiation induced the aggregation of lipid rafts and the clustering of c-Met and c-Src to lipid rafts through both lipid raft-dependent and lipid raft-independent mechanisms. The lipid raft-dependent activation of c-Met and its downstream pathways played an important role in the development of radiation resistance in NSCLC cells mediated by c-Met. Further studies are still required to explore the molecular mechanisms of the activation of c-Met and c-Src in lipid rafts induced by radiation.

Keywords: Lipid rafts, Mesenchymal-epithelial transition factor (c-met), C-Src, Radiation resistance, NSCLC

Background

Radiotherapy alone or combined with chemotherapy is the foundation for treating various solid tumors. However, radiation resistance greatly limits the curative effect of radiotherapy, which becomes one of the most important reasons for local recurrence and metastasis. Therefore, reversing the resistance of radiotherapy and increasing the radiosensitivity become the toughest challenge in cancer treatment.

Lipid rafts are special microdomains in the plasma membrane that influence cell proliferation, apoptosis, angiogenesis, immunity, cell polarity, and membrane fusion

[1, 2]. c-Met, a receptor tyrosine kinase located in lipid rafts, promotes cancer cell migration and invasion and mediates resistance to current anticancer therapies, including radiotherapy. Studies have demonstrated that the activated residual of c-Met is located in lipid rafts [3, 4]. c-Src, a type of non-receptor tyrosine kinase, plays a vital role in a number of diverse cell signaling pathways, including cellular proliferation, cell cycle control, apoptosis, tumor progression, metastasis, and angiogenesis [5]. c-Src participates in radiation resistance [6] and might be the bridge to the activation of the downstream signaling pathway of c-Met. Whether and how lipid rafts are involved in the radio-resistance of non-small cell lung cancer (NSCLC) mediated by c-Met has not been established. We reveal here that disturbing lipid raft integrity inhibits the activation

* Correspondence: zouhwsj@126.com
The First Oncology Department, Shengjing Hospital affiliated with China Medical University, Shenyang 110004, China

of c-Met and its downstream pathways, increases the sensitivity of NSCLC cells to radiotherapy, enhances the therapeutic ratio, and thus provides a new strategy to address the radio-resistance of NSCLC cells.

Methods

Cell lines, reagents and instruments

Human NSCLC cell line A549 (catalogue number: TCHu150) was obtained from the Cell Bank of the Chinese Academy of Sciences and H1993 (catalogue number: ATCC®CRL-5909™) was obtained from the American Type Culture Collection (ATCC). Methyl-β-cyclodextrin (MβCD) was purchased from Meilun Biotechnology (Dalian, Liaoning, China). Antibodies against c-Met, c-Src and β-actin were purchased from Wanlei Biotechnology (Shenyang, Liaoning, China). Antibodies against phosphorylated (p)-c-Met and p-c-Src were obtained from Bioss Inc. (Woburn, Massachusetts, USA). Anti-flotillin-1 antibody was obtained from Boster Biotechnology (Pleasanton, CA, USA). Fluorescein isothiocyanate-conjugated-anti-cholera toxin subunit B was purchased from Sigma (St. Louis, Missouri, USA). Horseradish peroxidase-conjugated specific goat anti-rabbit secondary antibody, Cy3-labeled goat anti-rat c-Met antibody, Cy3-labeled goat anti-rat c-Src antibody, phenylmethanesulfonyl fluoride (PMSF), radioimmunoprecipitation assay (RIPA) lysis buffer, SDS, trypsin and a cell cycle analysis kit were purchased from Beyotime Biotechnology (Shanghai, China). A cell apoptosis analysis kit was purchased from Nanjing Keygen Biotechnology (Nanjing, Jiangsu, China).

The following instruments were used: a linear particle accelerator used for human radiotherapy (Clinac 600C/D; ONCOR-PLUS, Siemens, Germany); a flow cytometer (C6; BD Biosciences, Franklin lakes, New Jersey, USA); a low-temperature refrigerated centrifuge (H-2050R; Xiangyi Company, Changsha, Hunan, China); a dual-gel vertical protein electrophoresis apparatus (DYCZ-24DN; Beijing Liuyi Biotech, Beijing, China); a gel imaging system (WD-9413B; Beijing Liuyi Biotech, Beijing, China); a fluorescence microscope (BX3; Olympus, Japan); and a Beckman SW40 rotor (Beckman Coulter GmbH, Unterschleissheim-Lohhof, Germany).

Cell culture and treatment

A549 and H1993 cells were cultured in DMEM supplemented with 10% fetal bovine serum (FBS) at 37 °C under 5% carbon dioxide conditions. Cells were routinely subcultured in a monolayer, digested with 0.25% trypsin and stopped with DMEM when the cells covered 90% of the culture bottle. Then, the cells were cultured in FBS-free medium for another 24 h and prepared for various treatments.

MβCD is a cyclic polysaccharide containing a hydrophobic cavity that enables the extraction of cholesterol from cell membranes [7]. Cholesterol is the main component of lipid rafts. Therefore, MβCD is widely used as a lipid raft inhibitor. In this study, MβCD was dissolved in DMEM and used at final concentrations of 5 and 10 mM. In the experimental groups, cells were pretreated with MβCD for 1 h before irradiation. Control cells were treated with equal volumes of DMEM. As previous studies have shown, the survival fraction of A549 cells decreases when treated with increasing doses of X-ray irradiation (e.g., 0, 1, 2, 4, 6 and 8 Gy). This time, we exposed A549 and H1993 cells to conventional X-ray (0, 4, 8, 12 Gy; 3 Gy per min) emitted by a linear particle accelerator used for human radiotherapy operated at 6 MV and room temperature to obtain a proper radiation dose for our study.

Clonogenic survival assays

Clonogenic survival assays described by Franken et al. [8] were used to evaluate the proliferative ability of irradiated A549 and H1993 cells. Briefly, cells were treated with either DMEM (control) or MβCD (5 or 10 mM) for 1 h followed by X-ray irradiation to a discontinuous rising dose of 0, 4, 8 and 12 Gy, and then cells were counted. Every 200 cells were seeded in a 35-mm dish at 37 °C under 5% carbon dioxide conditions and incubated for 30 days to allow macroscopic colony formation. Colonies were fixed with 4% paraformaldehyde for 20 min and then stained with Wright-Giemsa stain for 5 to 8 min. The number of colonies formed in each group was counted, and colonies containing approximately 50 viable cells were considered representative of clonogenic cells. The clonogenic fraction was calculated using these formulas: colony-plating efficiency (PE) = (number of colonies/number of seeded cells) × 100%; survival fraction (SF) = (PE of MβCD treated cells/PE of control cells) × 100%.

Flow cytometry assays

Cell cycle and apoptosis analysis were performed with flow cytometry assays. Cells at a density of 2×10^6/ml were exposed to either control DMEM or 5 or 10 mM MβCD for 1 h followed by X-ray irradiation (8 Gy) or control irradiation (0 Gy) then cultured in fresh DMEM. Cells were harvested and fixed in ice-cold 70% ethanol (4 °C) after being cultured for 4, 8, or 24 h. For cell cycle assays, after staining with 25 µl propidium iodide (PI, 100 µg/ml), the samples were incubated with 10 µl RNase A for 30 min in the dark at 37 °C. Cell apoptosis assays were performed with 5 µl PI for 15 min in the dark at 37 °C after mixing with 5 µl Annexin V-FITC. Cell cycle and apoptosis were evaluated by flow cytometry (C6; BD Biosciences, Franklin lakes, New Jersey, USA), and the data were analyzed with BD Accuri C6 Software 1.0.264.21.

Immunofluorescence microscopy

Cells were plated on Lab-Tek chamber slides. After treatment with MβCD or control for 1 h followed by irradiation at 0 or 8 Gy, cells were fixed with 4% paraformaldehyde at 37 °C for 15 min, permeabilized with 0.5% Triton-X 100 after washing with PBS three times and then blocked with goat serum for 15 min. For lipid raft staining, cells were incubated with 0.05 mg/ml fluorescein isothiocyanate-conjugated-anti-cholera toxin subunit B for 1 h. For c-Met and c-Src staining, cells were incubated with anti-c-Met (Cy3-labeled) or anti-c-Src (Cy3-labeled) for 1 h then washed and blocked. 4′,6-Diamidine-2′-phenylindole dihydrochloride (DAPI) was used to stain the nuclei. Imaging was performed via fluorescence microscopy.

Western immunoblotting analysis

Western immunoblotting analysis was performed as previously described [9]. Briefly, A549 cells were treated with indicated reagents (DMEM or 10 mM MβCD for 1 h followed by irradiation at 0 or 8 Gy) then washed with ice-cold PBS three times and lysed in RIPA lysis buffer containing 50 mM Tris-HCl (pH 7.4), 150 mM NaCl, 1% NP-40, and 0.1% SDS. Then, samples were centrifuged at 12000 rpm at 4 °C for 10 min in a low-temperature refrigerated centrifuge, and the supernatants were retained as protein lysates. For immunoblotting, 40 μg of protein lysates were subjected to electrophoresis on 4 to 10% SDS gels transferred to PVDF membranes, and blocked with 5% (w/v) skim milk in Tris-buffered saline-Tween 20 (0.05%, v/v; TTBS) for 1 h at 37 °C. Membranes were incubated overnight at 4 °C with primary antibodies against c-Met, p-c-Met, c-Src, p-c-Src and β-actin. After the overnight incubation, membranes were incubated with the appropriate horseradish peroxidase-conjugated specific goat anti-rabbit secondary antibody for 45 min and then washed with TTBS six times. The blots were developed by enhanced chemiluminescence followed by exposure to film, and the optical density values of target blots were analyzed with Gel-Pro-Analyzer software.

Biochemical lipid raft isolation

Biochemical lipid raft isolation was performed following established protocols [10, 11]. Briefly, all steps were performed at 4 °C. Cells were plated at a density of 1×10^7 cells in six 100-mm plates. Treated and untreated cells were washed twice with cold PBS, scraped into 2 ml of TNE solution [0.5% Triton-X-100, 1 mM PMSF, 150 mM NaCl, and 1 mM EDTA] and incubated for 40 min. The samples were scraped and homogenized completely by passing through a 5-ml needle 40 times. Homogenates were mixed with 2 ml of 90% (w/v) sucrose and placed at the bottom of a 15-ml ultracentrifuge tube. A 5–35% (w/v) discontinuous sucrose gradient was formed above

the homogenate-sucrose mixture with a 4-ml layer of 35% sucrose followed by a 4-ml layer of 5% sucrose by adding sucrose solution along the tube wall gently and slowly while avoiding any shake during the whole process. Next, samples were centrifuged at 39000 rpm at 4 °C for 20 h in a Beckman SW40 rotor. Twelve 1-ml gradient fractions were collected from the top of the gradient. Each fraction with no MβCD treatment and no irradiation was separated via SDS-PAGE and established the expression of flotillin-1, c-Met, p-c-Met, c-Src, p-c-Src by Western blot analysis. Fractions 2–6 were determined to be lipid raft fractions due to the presence of the lipid raft-specific protein flotillin-1 (Fig. 1). Then, we examined the total expression of c-Met, p-c-Met, c-Src, and p-c-Src in fractions 2–6 treated with either control DMEM or 10 mM MβCD for 1 h followed by irradiation to dose at 0 or 8 Gy.

Statistical analysis

Student's t-tests were performed utilizing the statistical software in GraphPad Prism version 5.0. Values of $P < 0.05$ were considered statistically significant. All the data expressed in our study are the mean ± SD from at least three independent experiments.

Results

MβCD suppressed proliferation of A549 and H1993 cells with or without X-ray irradiation

MβCD was used to disrupt lipid rafts in cell membranes via depletion of cholesterol from the plasma membrane [12]. To assess a potential role for MβCD in suppressing proliferation, we exposed A549 and H1993 cells pretreated with either DMEM or MβCD to a rising dose of X-ray irradiation (0, 4, 8 and 12 Gy, respectively). The results of clonogenic survival assays were shown in Additional file 1: Table S1 and Additional file 2: Table S2 and Fig. 2. Within each cell line and each pretreatment group, there was a radiation dose-dependent decrease in colony-plating efficiency (PE) showing that higher radiation doses were significantly different from lower radiation doses except for A549 cells pretreated with DMEM followed by radiation of 4 Gy vs. 8 Gy, A549 cells pretreated with 5 mM MβCD followed by radiation of 0 Gy vs. 4 Gy, A549 cells pretreated with 10 mM MβCD followed by radiation of 0 Gy vs. 4 Gy, and H1993 cells pretreated with 5 mM MβCD followed by radiation of 0 Gy vs. 4 Gy. As shown in Additional file 1: Table S1 and Additional file 2: Table S2 and Fig. 2, the PEs of A549 and H1993 cells decreased in a radiation dose-dependent way. The PEs of A549 and H1993 cells in each group pretreated with the same concentration of MβCD irradiated with 8 Gy or 12 Gy X-ray compared with control group were significantly different. But this trend was not shown in each group irradiated with 4 Gy compared with control group. The

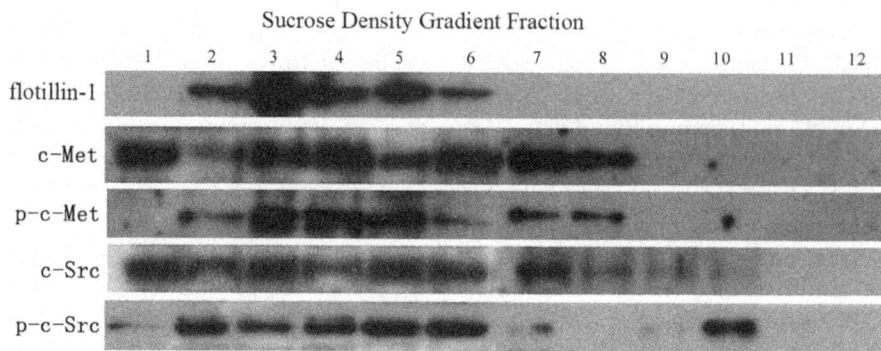

Fig. 1 Lipid rafts were separated by a sucrose density gradient centrifugation procedure, and immunoblotting was performed for c-Met, p-c-Met, c-Src, p-c-Src and flotillin-1. Blots are representative of at least three independent experiments. Fractions 2–6 were determined to be lipid raft fractions due to the presence of the lipid raft-specific protein flotillin-1. c-Met was mainly distributed in fractions 1 and 3–8; p-c-Met was mainly distributed in fractions 2–8; c-Src was mainly distributed in fractions 1–8; and p-c-Src was mainly distributed in fractions 2–6 and 10

PEs of A549 and H1993 cells pretreated with either DMEM or MβCD and irradiated with 12 Gy were too low to continue the remaining experiments; therefore, we chose 8 Gy as the proper radiation dose in our further experiments. Our results showed that the PEs of A549 cells in each group pretreated with 10 mM MβCD compared with DMEM followed by the same radiation dose (0, 4, 8 and 12 Gy, respectively) were significantly different, but the PEs were not significantly different in each radiation group pretreated with 5 mM MβCD vs. DMEM or 5 mM MβCD vs. 10 mM MβCD (Additional file 1: Table S1 and Fig. 2). This trend was also shown in H1993 cells (Additional file 2: Table S2 and Fig. 2). Therefore, we chose 10 mM as the proper concentration of MβCD for our further experiments. These results showed that MβCD suppressed the proliferation of A549 and H1993 cells whether followed by X-ray irradiation or not.

The combined treatment of MβCD and radiation resulted in additive increases in apoptosis of A549 and H1993 cells

In this study, we aimed to ascertain whether the combination of MβCD and radiation had an additive or supra-additive effect on the apoptosis of A549 and H1993 cells. Notably, pretreatment with 5 mM MβCD alone produced little apoptosis in both A549 and H1993 cells (Fig. 3). Increasing the concentration of MβCD to 10 mM greatly increased the apoptosis rate in both cell lines (Fig. 3). The combined treatment of 5 mM MβCD and X-ray irradiation (8 Gy) did not significantly differ from that of X-ray irradiation alone at 4, 8, or 24 h in A549 cells or at 4 h in H1993 cells with respect to an additive effect on apoptosis (at 4, 8 and 24 h in A549 cells: $P = 0.1124$, $P = 0.0650$, $P = 0.1110$; at 4 h in H1993 cells: $P = 0.7438$; respectively; Fig. 3); however, the combined treatment of 5 mM MβCD and X-ray irradiation (8 Gy) significantly increased apoptosis at 8 and 24 h in H1993 cells (at 8 h and 24 h: $P = 0.0071$, $P = 0.0010$,

respectively; Fig. 3). The combination of 10 mM MβCD and radiation (8 Gy) markedly increased the apoptosis rate when compared with that of radiation alone at 4, 8 and 24 h, and the differences were statistically significant (at 4, 8 and 24 h in A549 cells: $P = 0.0026$, $P = 0.0013$, and $P = 0.0016$; at 4, 8 and 24 h in H1993 cells: $P = 0.0038$, $P = 0.0020$, and $P = 0.0002$, respectively; Fig. 3). These results showed that the combination of MβCD and radiation resulted in additive increases in the apoptosis of A549 and H1993 cells.

X-ray irradiation induced the redistribution of c-met and c-Src in lipid rafts

To investigate the impact of X-ray irradiation on the redistribution of c-Met and c-Src in lipid rafts, A549 cells were treated with 10 mM MβCD or control (DMEM) for 1 h followed by X-ray irradiation to a dose of 0 or 8 Gy. Sixteen hours later, the distribution of c-Met and c-Src in lipid rafts was determined (Fig. 4). The results showed that X-ray irradiation alone induced the aggregation of lipid rafts and clustering of c-Met and c-Src to lipid rafts. Through destroying the integrity of lipid rafts, MβCD pretreatment blocked both the aggregation of lipid rafts and clustering of c-Met and c-Src to lipid rafts.

The activation of c-met and c-Src and the accumulation of c-met and c-Src to lipid rafts were restrained by MβCD

In agreement with the sucrose density gradient centrifugation procedure [10, 11], the original location of c-Met, p-c-Met, c-Src and p-c-Src in A549 cells with no MβCD treatment and no X-ray irradiation was revealed (Fig. 1): c-Met was mainly distributed in fractions 1 and 3–8; p-c-Met was mainly distributed in fractions 2–8; c-Src was mainly distributed in fractions 1–8; and p-c-Src was mainly distributed in fractions 2–6 and 10. As we mentioned before, fractions 2–6 were determined to be the lipid raft fractions.

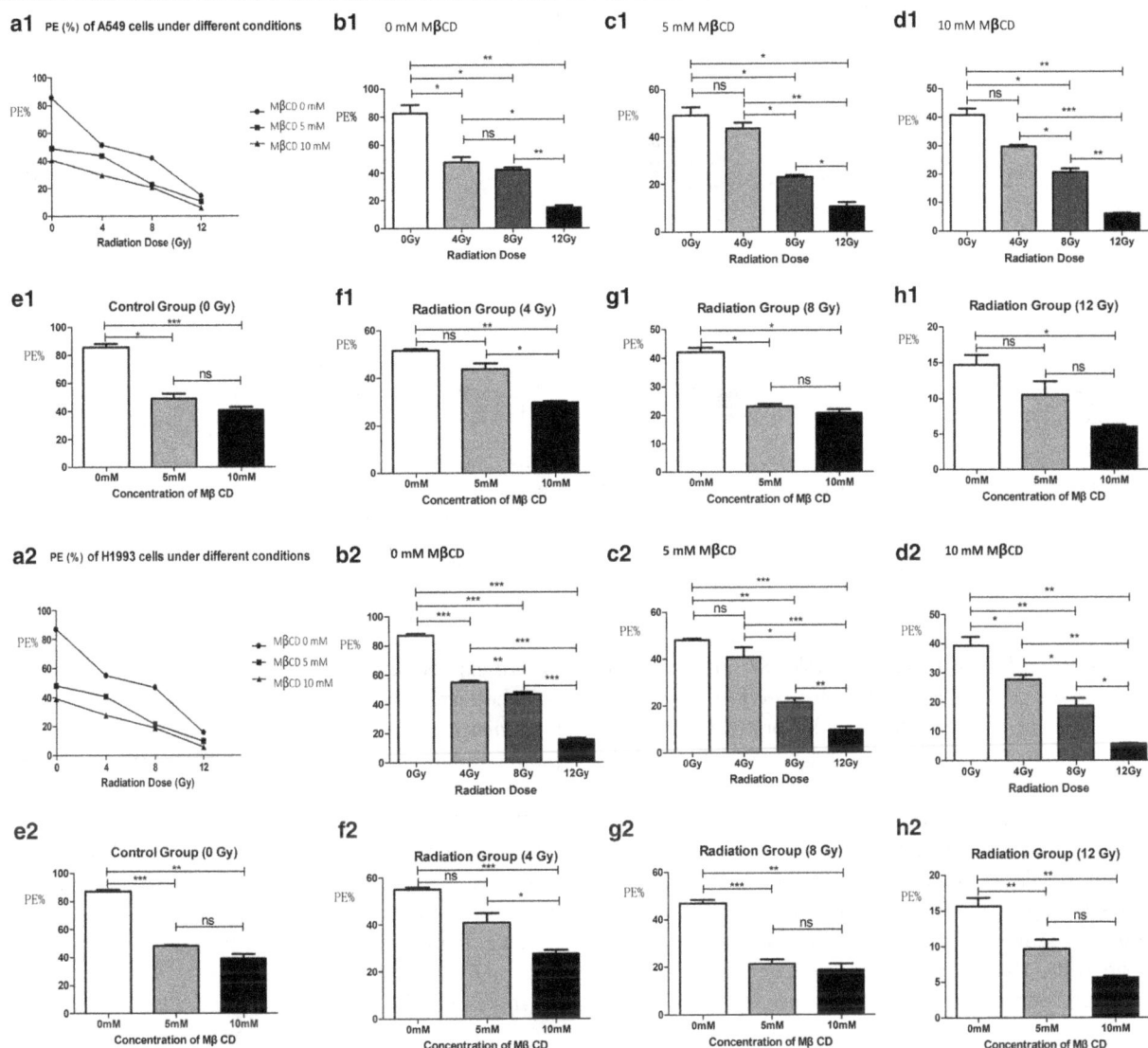

Fig. 2 MβCD suppressed proliferation of A549 and H1993 cells whether followed by X-ray irradiation or not. Cells were pretreated with either control (DMEM) or MβCD (5 or 10 mM) for 1 h followed by X-ray irradiation to a discontinuous rising dose of 0, 4, 8 and 12 Gy. Then, cells were incubated for 30 days to allow macroscopic colony formation. The results showed that exposing A549 and H1993 cells to a rising dose of radiation either pretreated with DMEM or 5 or 10 mM MβCD inhibited cell proliferation in a radiation dose-dependent manner (**a1** represents PE(%) of A549 cells under different conditions. **b1-d1** represents PE(%) of A549 cells pretreated with the same concentration of MβCD (0, 5 or 10 mM, respectively) followed by different doses of X-ray(0, 4, 8 and 12 Gy). **e1-h1** represents PE(%) of A549 cells pretreated with different concentration of MβCD (0, 5 or 10 mM) followed by the same doses of X-ray(0, 4, 8 and 12 Gy, respectively). **a2** represents PE(%) of H1993 cells under different conditions. **b2-d2** represents PE(%) of H1993 cells pretreated with the same concentration of MβCD (0, 5 or 10 mM, respectively) followed by different doses of X-ray(0, 4, 8 and 12 Gy). **e2-h2** represents PE(%) of H1993 cells pretreated with different concentration of MβCD (0, 5 or 10 mM) followed by the same doses of X-ray(0, 4, 8 and 12 Gy, respectively). "no statistical significance" is shown as "ns", "$P < 0.05$" is shown as "*", "$P < 0.01$" is shown as "**", and "$P < 0.001$" is shown as "***")

The expression levels of c-Met, p-c-Met (activated c-Met), c-Src and p-c-Src (activated c-Src) in the whole-cell samples were significantly increased after X-ray irradiation (c-Met, p-c-Met, c-Src, and p-c-Src: $P = 0.0406$, $P = 0.0012$, $P = 0.0085$, and $P = 0.0045$, respectively; Additional file 3: Table S3 and Fig. 5) when compared with those of the control group. However, this up-regulation of c-Met, p-c-Met, c-Src and p-c-Src in the whole-cell samples was blocked by

pretreatment with MβCD (c-Met, p-c-Met, c-Src, and p-c-Src: $P = 0.0033$, $P = 0.0005$, $P = 0.0012$, and $P = 0.0024$, respectively; Additional file 3: Table S3 and Fig. 5). The sucrose density gradient centrifugation results showed that the accumulation of c-Met, p-c-Met, c-Src and p-c-Src to lipid rafts was significantly induced by X-ray irradiation (c-Met, p-c-Met, c-Src, and p-c-Src: $P < 0.0001$, $P < 0.0001$, $P = 0.0030$, and $P = 0.0051$,

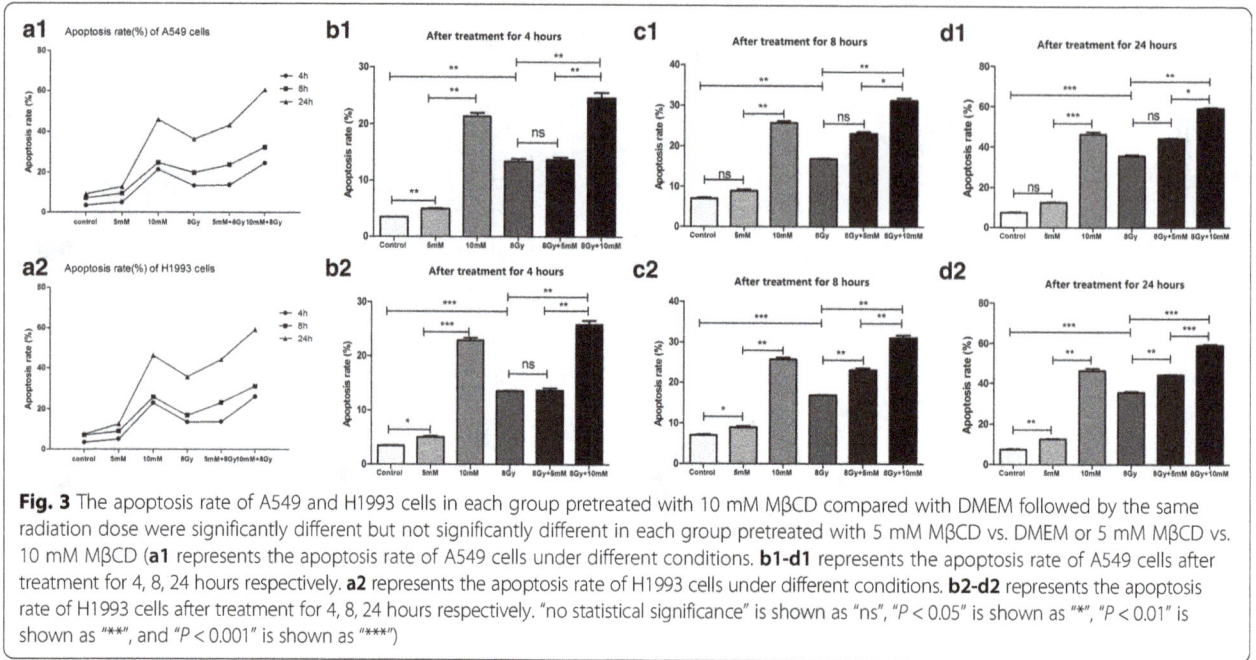

Fig. 3 The apoptosis rate of A549 and H1993 cells in each group pretreated with 10 mM MβCD compared with DMEM followed by the same radiation dose were significantly different but not significantly different in each group pretreated with 5 mM MβCD vs. DMEM or 5 mM MβCD vs. 10 mM MβCD (**a1** represents the apoptosis rate of A549 cells under different conditions. **b1-d1** represents the apoptosis rate of A549 cells after treatment for 4, 8, 24 hours respectively. **a2** represents the apoptosis rate of H1993 cells under different conditions. **b2-d2** represents the apoptosis rate of H1993 cells after treatment for 4, 8, 24 hours respectively. "no statistical significance" is shown as "ns", "P < 0.05" is shown as "*", "P < 0.01" is shown as "**", and "P < 0.001" is shown as "***")

respectively; Additional file 4: Table S4 and Fig. 6). Moreover, this accumulation of c-Met, p-c-Met, c-Src and p-c-Src to lipid rafts was blocked by pretreatment with MβCD (c-Met, p-c-Met, c-Src, and p-c-Src: $P < 0.0001$, $P < 0.0001$, $P = 0.0028$, and $P = 0.0082$, respectively; Additional file 4: Table S4 and Fig. 6).

Interestingly, compared with the MβCD alone group, the combined treatment group showed significantly increased expression of p-c-Met and p-c-Src in the whole-cell samples. However, there was no significant change in the accumulation of p-c-Met or p-c-Src to lipid rafts. More importantly, the percentages of p-c-Met and

p-c-Src expressed in lipid rafts out of those expressed in the whole-cell samples were obviously decreased in the combined group when compared with the MβCD alone group (Additional file 5: Table S5 and Fig. 7).

Discussion

Lung cancer is the leading cause of cancer death worldwide, and NSCLC accounts for approximately 85% of the total number of lung cancer diagnoses. Although significant progress in diagnosis and treatment has been made over the past several years, it is still too late for most NSCLC patients to have radical surgery at

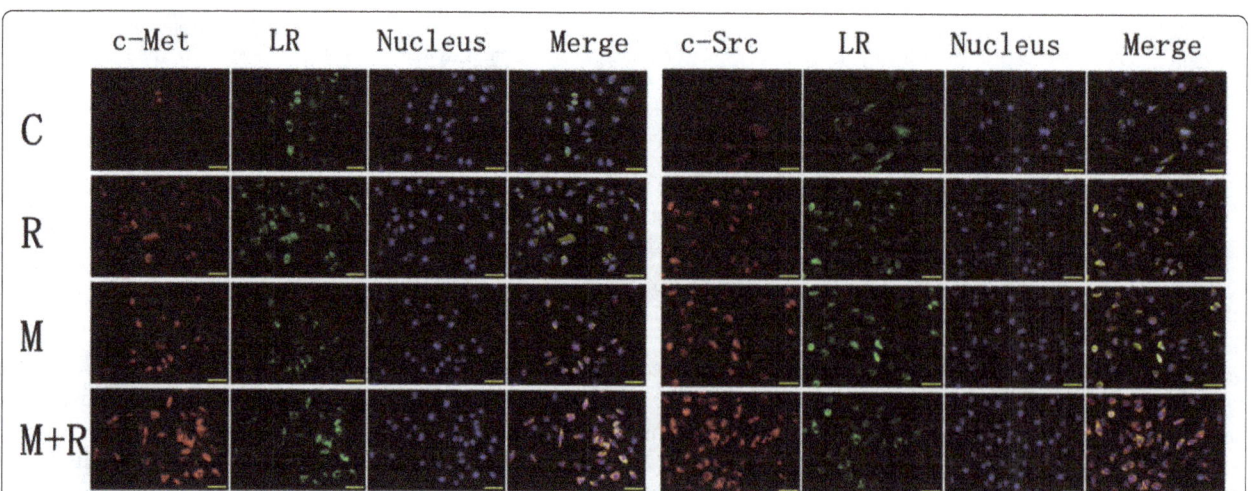

Fig. 4 X-ray irradiation induced the aggregation of lipid rafts and clustering of c-Met and c-Src to lipid rafts in A549 cells. MβCD blocked both the aggregation of lipid rafts and clustering of c-Met and c-Src to lipid rafts(C: control group, R: radiation only group, M: MβCD only group, M + R: MβCD and radiation combined group, LR: lipid raft marker)

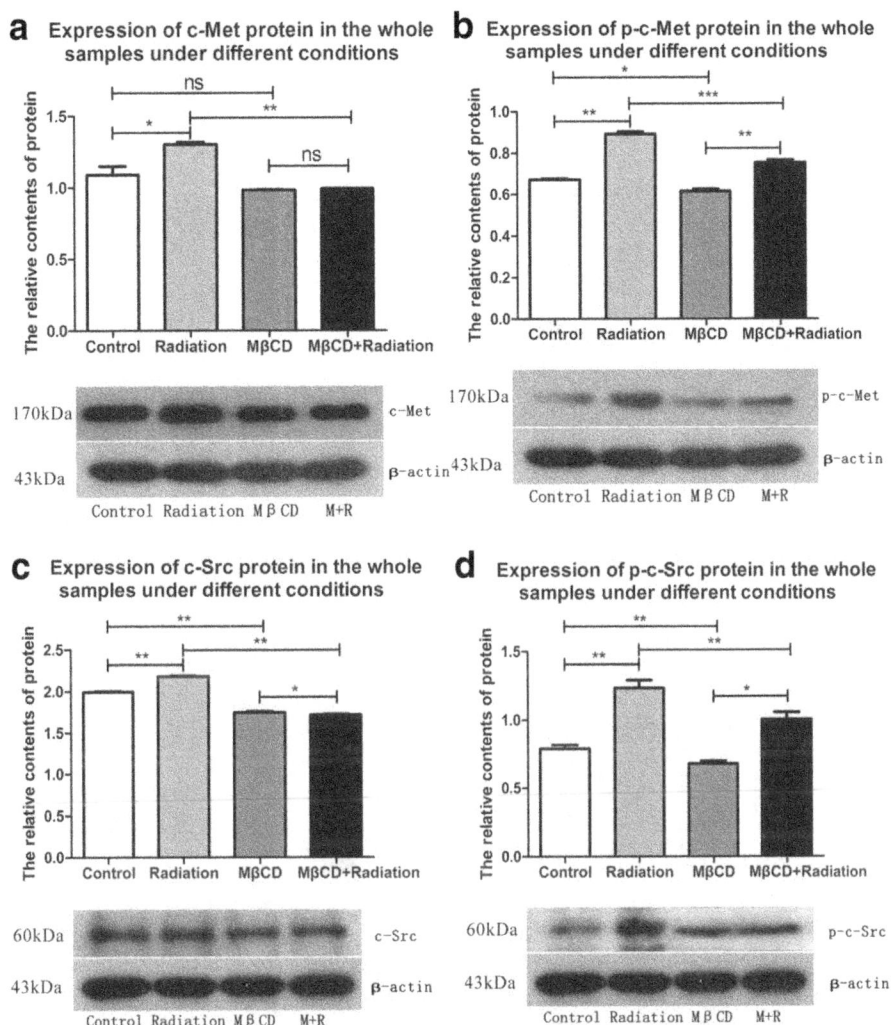

a Expression of c-Met protein in the whole samples under different conditions

b Expression of p-c-Met protein in the whole samples under different conditions

c Expression of c-Src protein in the whole samples under different conditions

d Expression of p-c-Src protein in the whole samples under different conditions

Fig. 5 Expression of c-Met, p-c-Met, c-Src and p-c-Src in the whole-cell samples was significantly increased by X-ray irradiation in A549 cells. However, this up-regulation was blocked by pretreatment with MβCD (**a-d** presents the expression of c-Met, p-c-Met, c-Src and p-c-Src in the whole-cell samples under different conditions respectively. "no statistical significance" is shown as "ns", "$P < 0.05$" is shown as "*", "$P < 0.01$" is shown as "**", and "$P < 0.001$" is shown as "***")

their first diagnosis. Radiotherapy is one of the basic treatments for unresectable NSCLC, but the resistance to radiation greatly limits the curative effect of radiotherapy. Currently, cellular survival pathways that regulate DNA damage repair after radiotherapy have been heavily researched to reveal the mechanism of NSCLC radiation resistance [13]. Many clinical studies have shown that the radiotherapy resistance of various solid tumors is associated with the overexpression of c-Met [14–16]. c-Met is a 170-kDa transmembrane protein that can be activated by binding hepatocyte growth factor (HGF) to its extracellular region [17]. De Bacco et al. demonstrated that irradiation directly induced the overexpression and activity of the Met oncogene and activated c-Met signaling through the ATM-NF-κB signaling pathway. In turn, the activated c-Met signaling triggered the activation of downstream signaling, mainly through the PI3K/Akt, MAPK, and

STAT pathways [18]. The activation of c-Met and its downstream signaling pathways has been shown to induce invasion and migration of cancer cells [19]. Fan et al. showed that the activation of c-Met protected tumor cells from DNA damage caused by radiation and led to radiation resistance [20]. Overexpression of c-Met has been noted in various tumors, and c-Met activation appears to be associated with increased tumor differentiation, shorter survival times and an overall worse prognosis in patients with NSCLC [21, 22]. c-Src, a non-receptor tyrosine kinase, is localized to intracellular membranes. c-Src is overexpressed or highly activated in a number of human malignancies, including carcinomas of the breast, lung, colon, esophagus, skin, parotid, cervix, and gastric tissues, as well as in the development of cancer and progression to distant metastases [23]. Recent studies have shown that c-Src enhances DNA damage repair and induces NSCLC

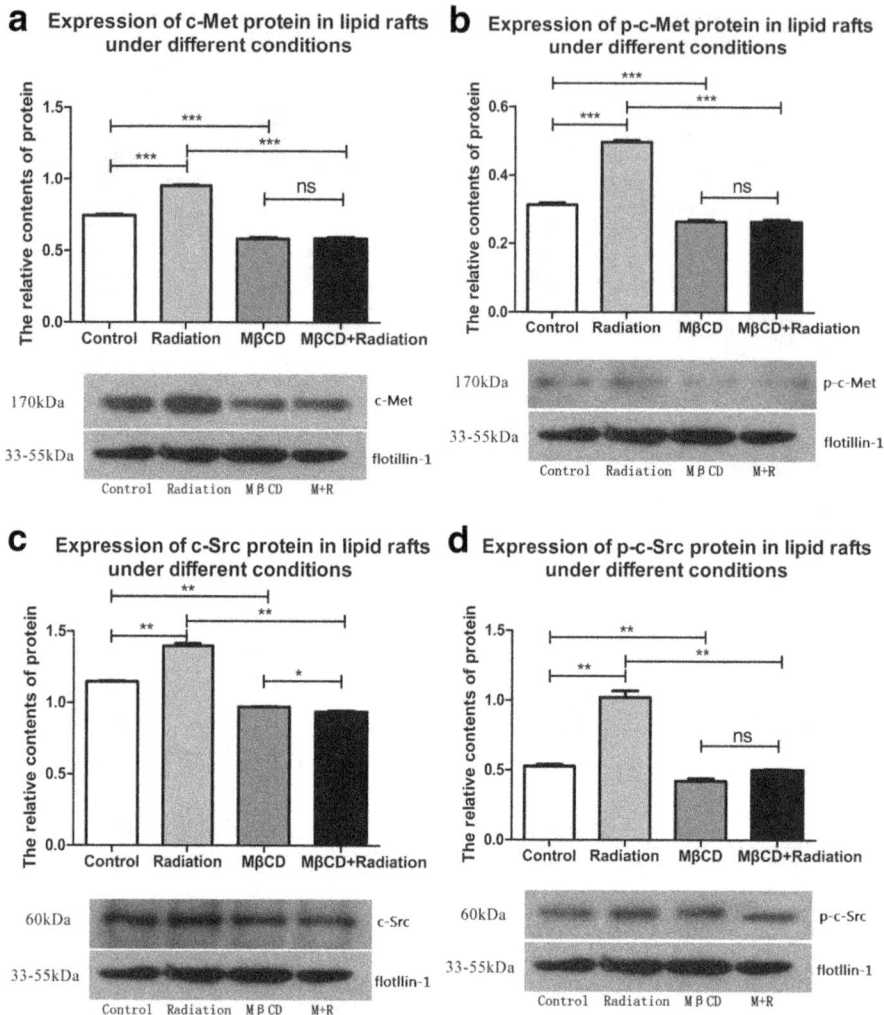

Fig. 6 Expression of c-Met, p-c-Met, c-Src and p-c-Src in lipid rafts was significantly increased by X-ray irradiation in A549 cells. However, this up-regulation was blocked by pretreatment with MβCD (**a-d** presents the expression of c-Met, p-c-Met, c-Src and p-c-Src in lipid rafts under different conditions respectively. "no statistical significance" is shown as "ns", "$P < 0.05$" is shown as "*", "$P < 0.01$" is shown as "**", and "$P < 0.001$" is shown as "***")

radiation resistance through ERK, AKT, and NF-κB pathways [13]. c-Met activates the PI3K/Akt, ERK, and NF-κB pathways via c-Src in cervical cancer cells [24–26]. c-Src might be the bridge by which the c-Met signaling pathway induces radiation resistance.

The plasma membrane is the structural basis for signal transduction. Lipid rafts are small (10–200 nm), heterogeneous, highly dynamic, sterol- and sphingolipid-enriched domains that compartmentalize cellular processes. Smaller lipid rafts can stabilize their structure and form a larger platform through protein-protein and protein-lipid interactions [27]. As a "highly dynamic platform", the lipid raft environment plays an important role in cell proliferation, apoptosis, and functional activities through regulating various cell signal transduction mechanisms. Hanahan et al. summarized that the occurrence and development of tumors is closely connected with uncontrolled cell

proliferation, resisting apoptosis, evading growth suppressors, enabling replicative immortality, inducing angiogenesis, activating invasion and metastasis, reprogramming of energy metabolism and evading immune destruction [28]. A growing body of evidence has shown that lipid raft microdomains provide signaling platforms that regulate a variety of cellular signaling pathways through which tumors can be initiated and developed [29–31]. Recent studies have shown that the activated residual of c-Met located in lipid rafts, which serve as a huge signaling platform for the activation of c-Met and its downstream pathways [3]. Localization of c-Src to lipid rafts has been demonstrated in a variety of cancer cell lines [32]. We hypothesized that disturbing the integrity of lipid rafts would block the activation of the c-Met signaling pathway and reverse the radiation resistance of NSCLC cells in some way.

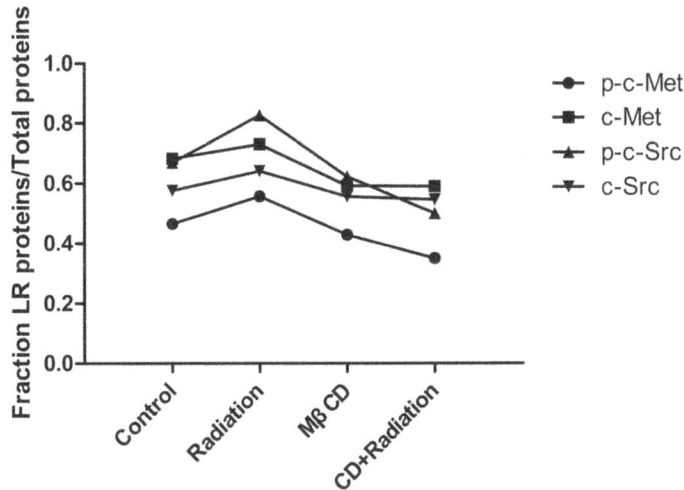

Fig. 7 The percentages of c-Met, p-c-Met, c-Src and p-c-Src expressed in lipid rafts out of the whole samples in A549 cells

In this study, the clonogenic survival assays showed that X-ray irradiation inhibited the proliferation of A549 and H1993 cells in a radiation dose-dependent manner regardless of MβCD pretreatment. Our results further confirmed that inhibiting the integrity of lipid rafts suppressed the proliferation of A549 and H1993 cells whether followed by X-ray irradiation or not. Furthermore, we found the proper concentration of MβCD (10 mM) and the proper radiation dose (8 Gy) for our remaining experiments.

Next, we found that pretreating A549 and H1993 cells with 10 mM MβCD alone obviously increased the apoptosis rate in both control (0 Gy) and irradiated cells (8 Gy) but not for 5 mM MβCD alone. Our results also showed that the combined treatment of MβCD and radiation significantly increased the apoptosis rates of A549 and H1993 cells when compared with those of radiation alone at 4, 8 and 24 h, but this effect was not significant for the combination of 5 mM MβCD and radiation (8 Gy) compared with radiation alone. These results suggest that disturbing the integrity of lipid rafts by MβCD sensitized A549 and H1993 cells to radiotherapy in both time-dependent and concentration-dependent manners. Our findings also indicate that lipid rafts play an important role in increasing the radiation sensitivity of NSCLC cells, and the combination of MβCD and radiation may provide a new effective therapeutic strategy for the treatment of radiation-resistant NSCLC.

To investigate the impact of X-ray irradiation on the redistribution of c-Met and c-Src in lipid rafts, A549 cells were treated with 10 mM MβCD or DMEM for 1 h followed by X-ray irradiation to a dose of 0 or 8 Gy, and the distribution of c-Met and c-Src in lipid rafts was determined 16 h later. The results showed that X-ray

irradiation induced the aggregation of lipid rafts and the clustering of c-Met and c-Src to lipid rafts. The results also demonstrated that destroying the integrity of lipid rafts restrained both the aggregation of lipid rafts and the clustering of c-Met and c-Src to lipid rafts. These results indicate that X-ray irradiation-induced redistribution of c-Met and c-Src in lipid rafts might result in radiation resistance in NSCLC cells.

Western blotting results showed that X-ray irradiation significantly increased the expression of c-Met, p-c-Met, c-Src and p-c-Src in the whole-cell samples, but this up-regulation was blocked by pretreatment with MβCD. The sucrose density gradient centrifugation analysis showed that X-ray irradiation significantly induced the accumulation of c-Met, p-c-Met, c-Src and p-c-Src to lipid rafts. Furthermore, the accumulation of these four proteins to lipid rafts was blocked by pretreatment with MβCD. Interestingly, we also found that the expression levels of p-c-Met and p-c-Src in the whole-cell samples were significantly increased in the combined group compared with those in the MβCD alone group. However, there was no significant change in the accumulation of these two proteins to lipid rafts. The percentages of p-c-Met and p-c-Src expressed in lipid rafts out of the whole-cell samples was obviously decreased in the combined treatment group when compared with those in the MβCD alone group. Collectively, these results show that X-ray irradiation might activate c-Met and c-Src through both lipid raft-dependent and lipid raft-independent mechanisms.

By analyzing the percentages of c-Met, p-c-Met, c-Src, and p-c-Src proteins expressed in lipid rafts out of the whole-cell samples, we found that in A549 cells, the expression of p-c-Met and p-c-Src in lipid rafts induced by X-ray irradiation was significantly higher than that of c-Met and c-Src. Furthermore, the inhibition of p-c-Met and p-c-Src expressed in lipid rafts was more obvious than that of c-Met and c-Src by the destruction of lipid rafts.

In summary, this study confirmed that MβCD suppressed the proliferation of human NSCLC cell lines A549 and H1993 with or without X-ray irradiation, and the combination of MβCD and radiation resulted in additive increases in the apoptosis of A549 and H1993 cells. X-ray irradiation induced the aggregation of lipid rafts and the clustering of c-Met and c-Src to lipid rafts through both lipid raft-dependent and lipid raft-independent mechanisms. Our results also demonstrated that destroying the integrity of lipid rafts significantly inhibited the aggregation of c-Met and c-Src to lipid rafts. More importantly, the expression of p-c-Met and p-c-Src in lipid rafts induced by X-ray irradiation was notably higher than that of c-Met and c-Src. Furthermore, the inhibition of p-c-Met and p-c-Src expressed in lipid rafts was more obvious than that of c-Met and c-Src by destruction of lipid rafts.

Conclusions

Taken together, we draw a conclusion that lipid rafts serve as the signaling platforms for the lipid raft-dependent activation of c-Met and c-Src induced by X-ray irradiation. The lipid raft-dependent activation of c-Met and its downstream pathways play an important role in radiation resistance of NSCLC cells mediated by c-Met. Destroying the integrity of lipid rafts can reverse these signaling pathways and improve the radiosensitivity of NSCLC cells, which can provide a new strategy for developing radiation sensitizing agents and for improving the therapeutic effect of radiotherapy. Further studies are still required to explore the molecular mechanisms of the activation of c-Met and c-Src in lipid rafts induced by radiation.

Additional files

Additional file 1: Table S1. Colony-plating efficiency (PE) of A549 cells treated with either control or MβCD followed by irradiation. (DOC 28 kb)

Additional file 2: Table S2. Colony-plating efficiency (PE) of H1993 cells treated with either control or MβCD followed by irradiation. (DOC 29 kb)

Additional file 3: Table S3. Expression of proteins in the whole-cell samples under different conditions in A549 cells. (DOC 28 kb)

Additional file 4: Table S4. Expression of proteins in lipid rafts under different conditions in A549 cells. (DOC 28 kb)

Additional file 5: Table S5. The percentage of protein expressed in lipid rafts out of the whole-cell samples in A549 cells. (DOC 28 kb)

Abbreviations
c-Met: Mesenchymal-epithelial transition factor; DAPI: 4′,6-Diamidine-2′-phenylindole dihydrochloride; HGF: Hepatocyte growth factor; MβCD: Methyl-β-cyclodextrin; NSCLC: Non-small cell lung cancer; PE: Colony-plating efficiency; PI: Propidium iodide; PMSF: Phenylmethanesulfonyl fluoride; RIPA: Radioimmunoprecipitation assay; SF: Survival fraction

Acknowledgements
The following individuals and institutions participated in this study: Juan Zeng, Heying Zhang, Yonggang Tan, Cheng Sun, Yusi Liang, Jinyang Yu, Huawei Zou, Shengjing Hospital affiliated with China Medical University, Shenyang, China. We are grateful to all the library staff of Shengjing Hospital affiliated with China Medical University for helping us with data collection, sorting, verification and analysis.

Funding
This study has received a major funding from national natural science foundation of China, and the award number is 81472806. This foundation does not affect the study design, analysis and interpretation of data, and the writing the manuscript.

Authors' contributions
JZ drafted the manuscript. JZ, HYZ, YGT, CS, YSL, JYY, HWZ planned, coordinated, and conducted the study. YGT contributed to data management. HYZ, CS and YSL conducted the statistical analysis. JZ, YGT and HWZ participated in revising the manuscript. All authors read and approved the final manuscript.

Competing interests
The authors declare that they have no competing interests.

References
1. Patra SK, Bettuzzi S. Epigenetic DNA methylation regulation of genes coding for lipid raft-associated components: a role for raft proteins in cell transformation and cancer progression. Oncol Rep. 2007;17:1279–90.
2. Brown DA, London E. Structure and function of sphingolipids- and cholesterol-rich membrane rafts. J Biol Chem. 2000;275:17221–4.
3. Duhon D, Bigelow RLH, Coleman DT, Steffan JJ, Yu C, Langston W, et al. The polyphenol epigallocatechin-3-gallate affects lipid rafts to block activation of the c-Metreceptor inprostate cancer cells. Mol Carcinog. 2010;49:739–49.
4. Coleman DT, Bigelow R, Cardelli JA. Inhibition of fatty acid synthase by luteolin post-transcriptionally down-regulates c-met expression independent of proteosomal/lysosomal degradation. Mol Cancer Ther. 2009; 8(1):214–24.
5. Aleshin A, Finn RS. SRC: a century of science brought to the clinic. Neoplasia. 2010;12:599–607.
6. Shimm DS, Miller PR, Lin T. Effects of v-src oncogene activation on radiation sensitivity in drug-sensitive and in multidrug-resistant rat fibroblasts. Radiat Res. 1992;129(2):149–56.
7. Radhakrishnan A, Anderson TG, McConnell HM. Condensed complexes, rafts, and the chemical activity of cholesterol in membranes. Proc Natl Acad Sci U S A. 2000;97:12422–7.
8. Franken NA, Rodermond HM, Stap J, Haveman J, van BC. Clonogenic assay of cells in vitro. Nat Protoc. 2006;1(5):2315–9.
9. Bigelow RLH, Cardelli JA. The green tea catechins, (−)-Epigallocatechin-3-gallate (EGCG) and (−)-Epicatechin-3-gallate (ECG), inhibit HGF/met signaling in immortalized and tumorigenic breast epithelial cells. Oncogene. 2006;25:1922–30.
10. Macdonald JL, Pike LJ. A simplified method for the preparation of detergent-free lipid rafts. J Lipid Res. 2005;46:1061–7.
11. Song KS, Li S, Okamoto T, Quilliam LA, Sargiacomo M, Lisanti MP. Co-purification and direct interaction of Ras with caveolin, an integral membrane protein of caveolae microdomains. Detergent-free purification of caveolae microdomains. J Biol Chem. 1996;271:9690–7.
12. Yancey PG, Rodrigueza WV, Kilsdonk EP, Stoudt GW, Johnson WJ, Phillips MC, et al. Cellular cholesterol efflux mediated by cyclodextrins. Demonstration of kinetic pools and mechanism of efflux. J Biol Chem. 1996; 271:16026–34.
13. Begg AC, Stewart FA, Vens C. Strategies to improve radiotherapy with targeted drugs. Nat Rev Cancer. 2011;11(4):239–53.
14. Yu H, Li X, Sun S, Gao X, Zhou D. C-met inhibitor SU11274 enhances the response of the prostate cancer cell line DU145 to ionizing radiation. Biochem Biophys Res Commun. 2012;427:659–65.
15. Li B, Torossian A, Sun Y, Du R, Dicker AP, Lu B. A novel selective c-met inhibitor with radiosensitizing effects. Int J Radiat Oncol Biol Phys. 2012;84: e525–e31.

16. Buchanan IM, Scott T, Tandle AT, Burgan WE, Burgess TL, Tofilon PJ, et al. Radiosensitization of glioma cells by modulation of met signalling with the hepatocyte growth factor neutralizing antibody. AMG102. J Cell Mol Med. 2011;15:1999–2006.

17. Birchmeier C, Birchmeier W, Gherardi E, Vande Woude GF. Met, metastasis, motility and more. Nat Rev Mol Cell Biol. 2003;4(12):915–25.

18. De Bacco F, Luraghi P, Medico E, Reato G, Girolami F, Perera T, et al. Induction of MET by ionizing radiation and its role in radioresistance and invasive growth of cancer. J Natl Cancer Inst. 2011;103:645–61.

19. Qian LW, Mizumoto K, Inadome N, Nagai E, Sato N, Matsumoto K, et al. Radiation stimulates HGF receptor/c-met expression that leads to amplifying cellular response to HGF stimulation via upregulated receptor tyrosine phosphorylation and MAP kinase activity in pancreatic cancer cells. Int J Cancer. 2003;104:542–9.

20. Fan S, Wang JA, Yuan RQ, Rockwell S, Andres J, Zlatapolskiy A, et al. Scatter factor protects epithelial and carcinoma cells against apoptosis induced by DNA-damaging agents. Oncogene. 1998;17:131–41.

21. Nakamura Y, Niki T, Goto A, Morikawa T, Miyazawa K, Nakajima J, et al. C-met activation in lung adenocarcinoma tissues: an immunohistochemical analysis. Cancer Sci. 2007;98:1006–13.

22. Masuya D, Huang C, Liu D, Nakashima T, Kameyama K, Haba R, et al. The tumour-stromal interaction between intratumoral c-met and stromal hepatocyte growth factor associated with tumour growth and prognosis in non-small-cell lung cancer patients. Br J Cancer. 2004;90:1555–62.

23. Yeatman TJ. A renaissance for SRC. Nat Rev Cancer. 2004;4:470–80.

24. Kim MJ, Byun JY, Yun CH, Park IC, Lee KH, Lee SJ. C-Src-p38 mitogen-activated protein kinase signaling is required for Akt activation in response to ionizing radiation. Mol Cancer Res. 2008;6(12):1872–80.

25. Ishizawar R, Parsons SJ. C-Src and cooperating partners in human cancer. Cancer Cell. 2004;6(3):209–14.

26. Funakoshi-Tago M, Tago K, Andoh K, Sonoda Y, Tominaga S, Kasahara T. Functional role of c-Src in IL-1-induced NF-kappa B activation: c-Src is a component of the IKK complex. J Biochem. 2005;137(2):189–97.

27. Pike LJ. Rafts defined: a report on the keystone symposium on lipid rafts and cell function. J Lipid Res. 2006;47:1597–8.

28. Hanahan D, Weinberg RA. Hallmarks of cancer: the next generation. Cell. 2011;144(5):646–74.

29. Algeciras-Schimnich A, Shen L, Barnhart BC, Murmann AE, Burkhardt JK, Peter ME. Molecular ordering of the initial signaling events of CD95. Mol Cell Biol. 2002;22:207–20.

30. Bang B, Gniadecki R, Gajkowska B. Disruption of lipid rafts causes apoptotic cell death in HaCaT keratinocytes. Exp Dermatol. 2005;14:266–72.

31. Li HY, Appelbaum FR, Willman CL, Zager RA, Banker DE. Cholesterol-modulating agents kill acute myeloid leukemia cells and sensitize them to therapeutics by blocking adaptive cholesterol responses. Blood. 2003;101:3628–34.

32. Arcaro A, Aubert M, Espinosa del Hierro ME, Khanzada UK, Angelidou S, Tetley TD, et al. Critical role for lipid raft-associated Src kinases in activation of PI3K-Akt signalling. Cell Signal. 2007;19:1081–92.

13

A study on volatile organic compounds emitted by in-vitro lung cancer cultured cells using gas sensor array and SPME-GCMS

Reena Thriumani[1][*] (iD), Ammar Zakaria[1][*], Yumi Zuhanis Has-Yun Hashim[2,3], Amanina Iymia Jeffree[1], Khaled Mohamed Helmy[4], Latifah Munirah Kamarudin[1], Mohammad Iqbal Omar[1], Ali Yeon Md Shakaff[1], Abdul Hamid Adom[1] and Krishna C. Persaud[5]

Abstract

Background: Volatile organic compounds (VOCs) emitted from exhaled breath from human bodies have been proven to be a useful source of information for early lung cancer diagnosis. To date, there are still arguable information on the production and origin of significant VOCs of cancer cells. Thus, this study aims to conduct in-vitro experiments involving related cell lines to verify the capability of VOCs in providing information of the cells.

Method: The performances of e-nose technology with different statistical methods to determine the best classifier were conducted and discussed. The gas sensor study has been complemented using solid phase micro-extraction-gas chromatography mass spectrometry. For this purpose, the lung cancer cells (A549 and Calu-3) and control cell lines, breast cancer cell (MCF7) and non-cancerous lung cell (WI38VA13) were cultured in growth medium.

Results: This study successfully provided a list of possible volatile organic compounds that can be specific biomarkers for lung cancer, even at the 24th hour of cell growth. Also, the Linear Discriminant Analysis-based One versus All-Support Vector Machine classifier, is able to produce high performance in distinguishing lung cancer from breast cancer cells and normal lung cells.

Conclusion: The findings in this work conclude that the specific VOC released from the cancer cells can act as the odour signature and potentially to be used as non-invasive screening of lung cancer using gas array sensor devices.

Keywords: E-nose, In-vitro, GCMS-SPME, Lung cancer, VOCs

Background

Cancer is one of the leading causes of mortality among humans worldwide. These phenomena are mainly because cancer commonly detected at a very late stage. The American Cancer Society [1], estimated about 1,685,210 new cases of cancer to be diagnosed and 595,690 cancer related deaths to be reported in the United States in the year 2016. It is also reported that lung cancer (LC) is the second most common cancer affecting men (14%) and women (13%) behind only prostate cancer (21%) and breast cancer (29%) respectively [1]. In Malaysia, LC has been reported to be the second most common cancer affecting men and the third most common cancer affecting females with 2,100 Malaysians diagnosed each year [2].The diagnosis of lung cancer at an early stage, particularly when the tumour is discovered at its local site, has been shown to improve the survival rate of patients [3, 4]. Hence it is critical that high risk patients are screened. However, the established and widely used screening techniques, such as chest radiography and cytological examination, often give poor results in detecting small and resectable cancers [5].

* Correspondence: thriumanireena@yahoo.com; ammarzakaria@unimap.edu.my
[1]Centre of Excellence for Advanced Sensor Technology, Universiti Malaysia Perlis, Arau, Perlis, Malaysia
Full list of author information is available at the end of the article

Currently, the application of low dose computed tomography (LDCT) as an early stage lung cancer screening technique shows reduction in the number of lung cancer-based deaths [6]. Yet, this method exposed patients to great risk as the high amount of radiation used can lead to several complications [4, 7]. Generally, conventional methods are invasive and might delay the therapy if the cancer is found [8, 9]. In addition, only selected hospital with the right expertise and facilities can perform such screening tests. Thus, a new screening approach based on the cell biology theory [4] using the analysis of volatile organic compounds (VOCs) linked to lung cancer has been receiving considerable attention from researchers. This new screening technique is non-invasive, reliable and inexpensive [10, 11].

The change in metabolic pathways (gene or protein changes) in cancerous cells during tumour growth may lead to peroxidation of the cell membrane and production of certain VOCs [12, 13]. These VOCs can be detected directly on the headspace of the cancer cells [8, 14], or exhaled breath of cancer patients [10, 15, 16]. In the case of exhaled breath air, VOCs generated by the cancer cells are released by blood and exchanged through the alveolus in the lung [17]. The potential of detection of VOCs in the breath of lung cancer patients to be used as diagnostic or screening tools have been extensively analysed and studied for several years [18]. However, in order to provide cellular and biochemical origin information of VOCs to clinicians for the decision on the specific treatment for the cancer, the analysis should also be compared with cancer cells (0either in-vivo or in-vitro) [19, 20].

Many studies of in-vitro cultured cells as a model system to demonstrate the discrimination between tumour and normal cells using spectrometric technique have been reported [21–32]. However, the results are somewhat equivocal and more studies are essential to identify VOC biomarkers of lung cancer [32]. There are only few studies conducted using an array of sensors to distinguish types of lung cancer cells based on in-vitro cultured cell lines samples [8, 33, 34] as shown in Table 1. These reports show substantial results in term of performance of the sensors. However, the use of the right

classification algorithms for e-nose performance with the aid of SPME-GCMS analysis is crucial to strengthen the findings and progress the aim of non-invasively cancer diagnosis [35, 36].

In this study, the VOCs signature of the two types of lung cancer cell lines which are A549 and Calu3 will be investigated. The normal lung cell line and the breast cancer cell line are used as control samples to differentiate the lung cancer-related VOCs. As to date, no known reported work investigating VOC patterns released by both lung and breast cancer cultured cell lines under the same conditions, environment and at different growth stages.

This paper presents new results distinguishing the VOCs generated by two types of cancer cell lines, namely lung cancer (A549 and Calu-3) and breast cancer (MCF7), as well as normal lung (WI38VA13) cell lines at different proliferation stages using the Cyranose320 e-nose device. Also presented are results of five different classifiers for the e-nose to perform the VOCs classification. To the best of author knowledge, this paper also presents a novel work by investigating the use of Naïve Bayes (NB) and One versus All-Support Vector Machine (OVA-SVM) to classify the VOCs emitted by the in-vitro cell lines using e-nose. Table 2 shows the parameters used in this study.

The Cyranose320 is an array of 32 conducting polymer coated carbon black sensor-based e-nose and the pattern of change in the resistance of the sensor array is used to identify smells [37]. This feature can assist to detect even the slightest difference in headspace or complex volatile organic compounds (VOCs) emitted by the exhaled breath [38] or in vitro cultured cells [34, 39–41]. The Cyranose320 was used to detect and discriminate the volatiles collected from the different cell lines with the aid of pattern recognition methods.

The VOCs collected were classified using different multiclass classifiers that best utilise the effectiveness of Cyranose 320 in distinguishing the lung cancer cells from control samples. GCMS-SPME analysis also performed for each sample. This pre-concentrated volatile compound extraction method was able to determine the

Table 1 List of sensor array used, cell lines, cell growth time considered for measurement (incubated period) and type of matrix used in in-vitro studies aiming to distinguish type of lung cancer by previous studies

Sensor Type	Cell lines	Control	Incubation (hours)	Matrix Type	Statistical Approach	Reference
GNP	NSCLC: A549, Calu-3, H1650, H4006, H1435, H820 and H1975	Pure medium	-	Culture medium with cells	PCA	[8]
GNP	NSCLC: A549, Calu-3, H1650, H4006, H1435, H820, H1975, H2009, HCC95, HCC15, H226 and NE18 SCLC: H774, H69, H187, and H526	IBE, pure medium	68	Culture medium with cells	Linear nu-SVC-SVM; cross validation	[33]
C320	NSCLC: L55, L65, A549, H460, M51 and REN	NHDF and HASM	-	Cells in saline solution	MD	[34]

Table 2 List of sensor array used, cancer cell lines, cell growth time considered for measurement (incubated period) and type of matrix used in this work

Sensor Type	Cell lines	Control	Incubations (hours)	Matrix Type	Statistical Approach
C320	NSCLC: A459 and Calu-3	WI38VA13, MCF7 and pure medium	24, 48, 72	Culture medium with cells	*Savitsky Golay filtering;* LDA,PCA, PNN, KNN, OVA-SVM, NB; 10-k-fold cross validation

specific compound emitted by each type of cells. The compounds were identified using NIST library and compared with e-nose data. Thus, the significance of this preliminary results and its support in the application in lung cancer clinical screening are discussed.

Methods

Cell culture preparation

Cancerous lung cell lines A549 (ATCC ® CCL-185™) and Calu-3(ATCC® HTB-55™), normal lung cell line WI38VA13 (ATCC® CCL75.1™) and breast cancer cell line MCF7 (ATCC® HTB-22™) were obtained from the American Type Culture Collection and being maintained at the Cell and Tissue Culture Engineering Lab (CTEL), Department of Biotechnology Engineering, IIUM. Table 3 shows the characteristics of the cell lines used in this project. Based on the Table 3, the A549 and Calu3 are representing same histology which is adenocarcinoma but claimed to be from different origin. Thus, the VOCs signature of both A549 and Calu3 will be also covered in this work.

The A549, WI38VA13 and MCF7 cells were revived and cultivated in DMEM (Dulbecco's Modified Eagles Medium) supplemented with 10% (v/v) FBS (Fetal Bovine Serum). Meanwhile, the Calu-3 cell line was grown in Eagle's Minimum Essential Medium (EMEM) with 10% (v/v) FBS. The cells were grown in 25cm^2 T-flasks and incubated in a carbon dioxide (CO_2) incubator at 37°C/5% CO_2 [22, 23, 36].

Upon reaching 70-90% confluence, the cells were harvested and then seeded into new flasks with an initial density of 1×10^5 cells/ml in 5ml media for each cell line respectively. The culture condition was as reported in our previous work [39]. The blank mediums, DMEM (without cells) and EMEM (without cells) samples were also triplicates respectively as control samples and incubated together with A549, Calu-3, MCF7 and

WI38VA13. Same cell culture preparation and environmental conditions were maintained for both e-nose and SPME-GCMS measurement. The odour samplings were taken after 24 h of incubation using SPME fiber (Divinylbenzene/Carbonexen/Polydimethylsiloxane), while for Cyranose320, the measurement commenced at 24th, 48th and 72nd hours of incubation.

E-nose headspace sampling

The prepared samples in fully sealed T-flasks were placed in the biosafety cabinet. Then the flasks were connected to the inlet of Cyranose 320 for data collection. The sampling setup using e-nose is shown in Fig. 1. Table 4 shows the configuration of the data collection process using Cyranose 320. The baseline purge was set to be at 10 s before data collection. The odour samples were drawn for 180 s to allow it to cover all the 32 sensors. This duration will enable all the sensors inside the Cyranose320 to detect the VOCs in the odour. The sniffing process was set to be repeated for 5 times.

Data analysis

The collected data were then analysed using SPSS 17.0 and MATLAB R2012a to evaluate the e-nose performance. Each individual sample was described by a unique set of measurement known as features. The Cyranose 320 used in the work contains 32 conducting polymer sensors, and hence creates 32 features for each odour sample. Each feature forms a dimension in a space known as feature space. For each sample including the blank mediums, the experiments were replicated 3 times and each sniffing was repeated for 5 times at 24th, 48th and 72th hours respectively. For the e-nose analysis, each sample including blank mediums were replicated into three flasks, with datasets of two flasks used for training and the final one for testing. The sample datasets were divided into two parts and assigned as training and testing sets with a 2:1 ratio

Table 3 Characteristic of the cell lines

Cell Lines	Oncogene	Histology	Patient Type	Tissue Type	Growth Medium
A549	K-Ras mutation	Adeno-carcinoma	Male, 58 years Caucasian	Lung (epithelial cell)	DMEM
Calu-3	EGFR, K-Ras, TP53 and CDKNA genes mutation	Adeno-carcinoma	Male, 25 years, Caucasian	Lung (epithelial cell) from pleural effusion	EMEM
MCF-7	WNT7B mutation	Adeno-carcinoma	Female, 68 years	Mammary gland (epithelial cell) from pleural effusion	DMEM
WI38VA13	-	Normal cell	Female,Caucasian,3 months	Lung (Fibroblast)	DMEM

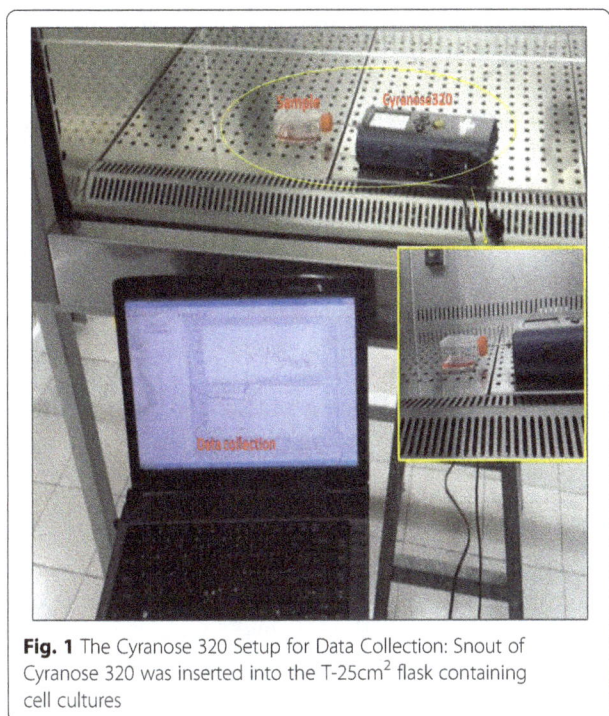

Fig. 1 The Cyranose 320 Setup for Data Collection: Snout of Cyranose 320 was inserted into the T-25cm² flask containing cell cultures

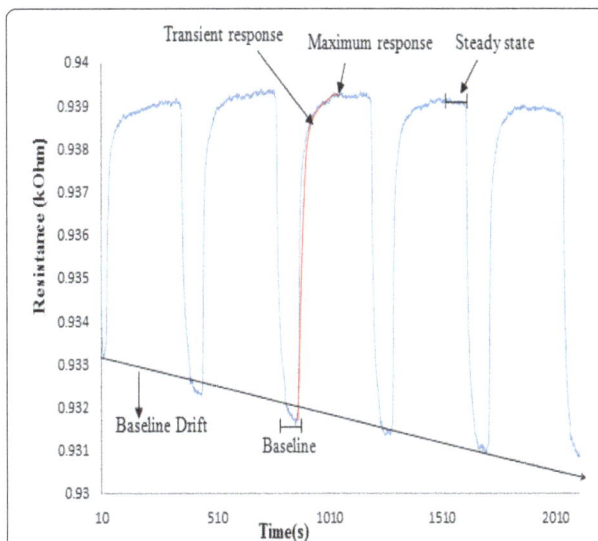

Fig. 2 Example of five complete cycles of the feature space extracted from sensor 12 of the e -nose using A549 sample at 24th hour

respectively. This study uses 18 different classes for classification purposes (total of six (6) classes multiplied by three varying incubation times).

Figure 2 shows an example of five complete cycles of feature space from sensor 12 of the Cyranose 320. Figure 3 shows the block diagram of the summary of data analysis conducted in this study.

Signal pre-processing

The Savitzky-Golay filter was selected to remove noise from the gas sensor signal while preserving the height, width, amplitude and overall profile of the response [37, 39]. The datasets were normalized using fractional difference method as in Eq. (1) [42]:

$$dR = (R{-}Ro)/R \qquad (1)$$

Where Ro is the baseline and the R is the steady state of the sensor response to the gas sample of the

system. This fractional method helps to reduce the signal drift problem [43]. All data were further normalized using sensor auto scaling global method, scaled to zero mean and standard deviation of one [42, 44].

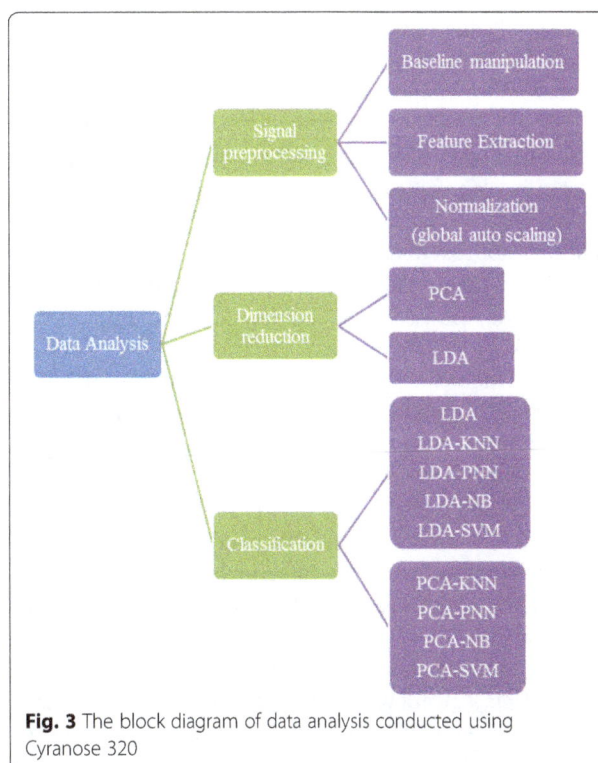

Fig. 3 The block diagram of data analysis conducted using Cyranose 320

Table 4 Parameter settings of the Cyranose 320 for data collection procedure [85]

Parameters	Time (s)	Pump Speed (cc/min)
Baseline Purge	10	160
Sample Draw	180	120
Snout Removal	3	-
1st Air Intake Purge	40	180
Filter: ON	-	-

The e-nose was set to be at 37°C (optimum temperature for culture growth)

Feature extraction

The consideration of features extraction is essential to point out the discriminating information that would aid the improvement of classification performance [38].

Principal component analysis (PCA) and linear discriminant analysis (LDA) are two commonly used feature extraction techniques [45, 46]. In this present study, both techniques were conducted to evaluate the best method for reducing dimensionality by preserving the minimum information about the dataset. Hence the component and discriminants from PCA and LDA respectively were used for class separability visualisation. The PCA provides unbiased projection, which gives better information on the clustering behaviour of each class, while LDA maximizes the intergroup variance and minimizes within group variance. Further, the LDA data was considered as the input for different classifiers. This LDA data able to provide the highest possible discrimination between different classes of data and help to classify the data accurately [47–50].

Proposed classification algorithms

To date, various classification algorithms are proposed for cancer detection particularly those related to e-nose. In this study, the effectiveness and robustness of e-nose in distinguishing lung cancer cell lines were tested using several classification algorithms namely LDA with fisher criterion, K-Neighbour Neural Network (KNN), Probabilistic Neural Network (PNN), Naïve Bayes (NB) and Multi-class Support Vector Machine (SVM). The statistical significance of all 32 independent sensors was evaluated by comparing the mean score of 18 different groups using the Wilk's Lamda method. A multi-class odour classification model (LDA-based classifier) was later proposed to evaluate the robustness of an e-nose system in classifying cancerous cell samples.

The LDA classification was conducted using leave-one-out approach for the error estimation. The fisher criteria was reported to be able to overcome the non-normally distributed data [51], hence being employed in this work.

PNN, which is defined as an implementation of Kernel discriminant analysis contains operations, which are organized into multi-layered feed forward network with four layers [52]. Although PNN algorithm required a large memory for training, it requires less training time [52, 53]. The spread value (σ) was determined using 10-fold cross validation and a value of 0.1 were obtained as appropriate for the dataset with acceptable classification accuracy [54].

On the other hand, KNN classification is known as the simplest classification which uses neighbour characteristics to determine the class of the data samples. This classifier is able to rapidly evaluate the unknown inputs by

calculating the distance between a new sample and mean of training data samples in each class weight by their covariance matrices [23]. By considering the theoretical method the best k-value (one; 1) and the distance metric of Euclidean were selected as maximum accuracy obtained using these parameters [24].

Meanwhile, naïve Bayesian (NB) is a simple probabilistic classifier which applies Bayes's theorem with naïve independence assumption. It is known as an efficient and effective classification technique to create models with predictive capabilities [55]as the algorithm does not have several free parameter settings, does not require large amounts of data for training and computationally fast in decision making [56, 57]. In this study, the NB classification with normal (Gaussian) was chosen and the prior probabilities for the classes specified to empirical.

Finally, SVM analysis is a linear classifier which is able to find the best separating line between two classes in higher dimensions [58]. However, the SVM can be directly used for binary classes only. For cases with more than two classes, the multi-class SVM can be implemented by dividing the single multiclass problem into multiple binary classification problems. There are three type of multi-class SVM, namely one versus all (OVA), one versus one (OVO) and Direct Acyclic Graph (DAG)-SVM [59]. The OVA based SVM was used in this work to classify the 18 classes. This classification was trained with RBF kernel functions which were obtained from optimization method [60]. Various pairs of box constraint (C) and sigma (σ) were tested for each dataset and the final obtained values were: C: 2^{10} and σ: 2^{-3} for this dataset.

Performance evaluation

The performance of each of the classifiers are presented using the accuracy (ACC) achieved. This is defined as the percentage (%) of correct classification over the total cases presented. However, since the accuracy alone might not give the best classification performance; sensitivity (SEN), specificity (SPE), precision (PREC) and Matthews Correlation Coefficient (MCC) measurements for each class were calculated to provide more relevant and interpretable information about the results [61, 62]. There are a few terms that are commonly used to measure the performance rate, namely, true positive (TP), true negative (TN), false positive (FP) and false positive (FP) [63].

The application of MCC in the multiclass case was originally reported in [64] which was used to measure the classification correlation. The value of MCC varies between -1 and 1 (where 1 is perfect prediction quality, while -1 is in the extreme misclassification of a confusion matrix and 0 specify random correlation) [62, 65]. This paper will report the accuracy, sensitivity, specificity, precision and MCC measures as well for all 18 classes for the best results.

Gas chromatography mass spectrometry- solid phase micro extraction (GCMS-SPME)
GCMS-SPME headspace sampling
The SPME-GCMS was used to identify the headspace VOCs that were released by each type of cultured cell lines (A549, Calu-3, WI38VA13 and MCF7) and blank mediums. Preheated solid phase micro extraction (SPME) was used to collect the VOCs released from the cells. The inner needle, which is the fiber of SPME or known as Divinylbenzene/Carbonexen/Polydimethylsiloxane (DVB/CAR/PDMS), was used in this work. The DVB/CAR/PDMS coated fiber was chosen as it has been optimized to extract a wide range of molecular range of molecular weight of both volatile and semi volatile molecules [66]. The needle was exposed to headspaces of cell cultured in the 25cm² T-flask for 15 min as shown in Fig. 4. At the end of the VOCs extraction time, the fiber was immediately inserted into GCMS Agilent 7890 sample point.

The DB-WAX capillary column (30 m x 250 μm x 0. 25 μm) was used with the injector temperature of 250 ° C to allow desorption of VOCs thermally. The oven temperature was initially set to be 50°C and held for 0.5 min, then ramped 10°C/minutes up to 180°C for 1 min and then again ramped 15°C per minute until it reached 250°C and held for 5 min. The carrier gas Helium flow rate was 1ml/min. The total analysis took 24.17 min to obtain the results. The MS analyses were done in full scan mode (TIC mode) with the scan range between 40 to 200 a.m.u and the electron impact ionization was done at 70eV to separate the compounds [30].

Identification of VOCs
The potential VOCs were only identified by using the spectral match in this study [29, 64]. The identity of each compound was determined using the Agilent Chem Station Software by searching on the "NIST" Mass Spectral Library 11 which provides the use of retention time and m/z of VOCs of interest. Each chromatograph was integrated and the peaks were matched and aligned in order to obtain a matrix that contains all peaks found in the whole set of measurements. The peaks or compounds that are missing in other replicate samples were eliminated. In this analysis, peaks less than 80% of the matching percentage to the NIST library (Qualitative) and peak area less than 3000 were excluded [27]. Those peaks identified as arising from column, empty flask and fiber (siloxanes) were excluded in this study [19, 29]. The significant differences on the relative abundances of identified VOCS were conducted using the t-test and considered significant at $P < 0.05$.

Results
E-nose performance
Table 5 shows a representative result of Wilk's Lambda test of day 1 dataset to show the contribution of variation in the discriminant function (df). The functions with p-value less than 0.05 ($p < 0.05$) were chosen, as this corresponds to the ability of the function to discriminate the groups.

Figures 5 and 6 show 3D scatter plots to visualize the variability between VOCs of cell lines detected by e-nose using LDA and PCA analysis respectively.

Based on Fig. 5, the result shows that the samples of A549, Calu-3, MCF7, WI38VA13 and blank mediums were well separated with 100% discriminant function. The test data samples were matched closely with the distribution of different groups of cell lines in the training data. A significant clustering between lung cancer cell, breast cancer and the control samples was observed. This indicates that the different cell lines are emitting different profile of VOCs and that the e-nose is able to

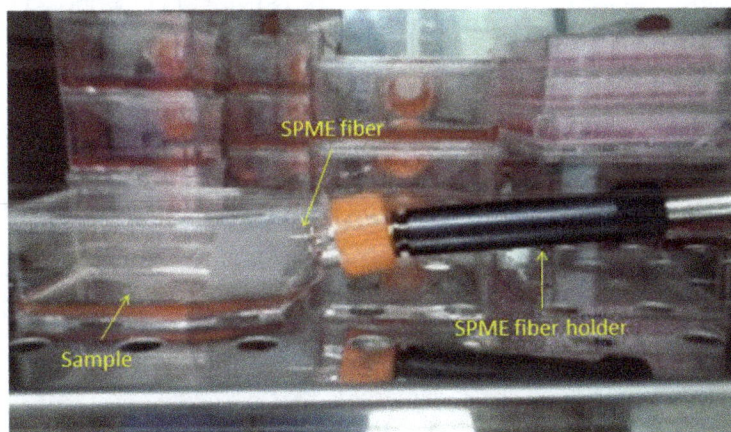

Fig. 4 The GCMS-SPME odour sampling procedure. SPME coated needle was exposed to the headspace of cultured cell. The experiment was conducted in an incubator (37°C/5% CO_2)

Table 5 The Significant test using Wilk's Lambda for LDA

Test of Function(s)	Wilks' Lambda	Chi-square	df	Sig.
1 through 5	.000	8432.165	75	.000
2 through 5	.000	3116.215	56	.000
3 through 5	.033	1214.302	39	.000
4 through 5	.246	496.519	24	.000
5	.911	32.974	11	.001

Df different function, Sig significant value

detect these variations. Both of the non-small lung cancer cells, A549 and Calu-3 ,were observed to be very close together but with a distinct separation. The scores of other samples were well distributed within each group, respectively with visible separation for the combination of all days.

PCA was performed on the data and the eigenvectors and eigenvalues were calculated using correlation matrix. The eigenvectors of eigenvalue higher than 1.0 can be selected as principal components (PC) and value lower than 1.0 can be considered to be excluded, in this study, the first three PCs with eigenvalue higher than 1. 0, were selected for dataset at 24th, 48th and 72nd hours. Based on Fig. 6a, the samples were observed to

be well separated. The total percentage of principal components (PC1, PC2, and PC3) in the PCA analysis as shown in Fig. 6a is 93.56%, which indicates that the each of the cell lines are separable. In order to emphasise the ability of sensors to distinguish the different lung cancer type, the PCA plot for Calu-3 and A549 were enlarged in Fig. 6b. The sensors managed to distinguish the 2 types of lung cancer each other might be due to the specific VOCs emitted from the cell lines since the origin of the A549 and Calu-3 cells are from epithelium and pleural effusion, respectively.

However, based on the PCA grouping behavior, it is observed that the features within the group were separated spatially compared to the LDA. The clustering of A459 and Calu-3 (lung cancer cells) observed to be significantly separated from the MCF7 (breast cancer cell) and WI38VA13 (normal cell) clusters. Overall, the extracted feature by LDA indicates good separability of different samples. Thus the LDA-based features were used to test the four different classifiers.

Classification results

The LDA-based features were used to test the four classifiers (LDA, PNN, KNN, NB and OVA-SVM) using 10-

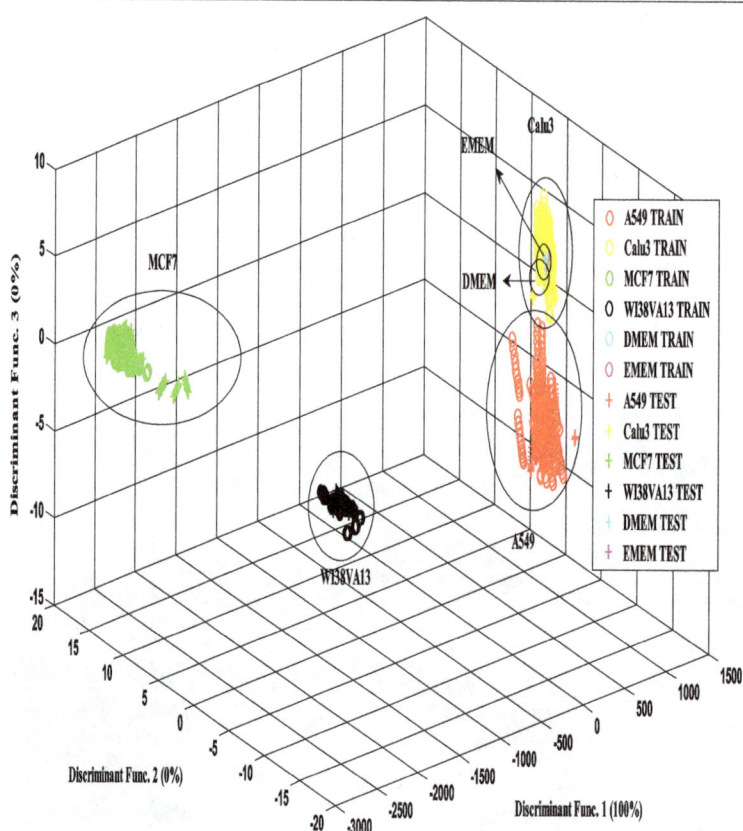

Fig. 5 LDA plot of volatile compounds from cultured cells (combination of all 3 days). The separability of 4 types of cell lines and two different blank medium shows the effectiveness of the e-nose

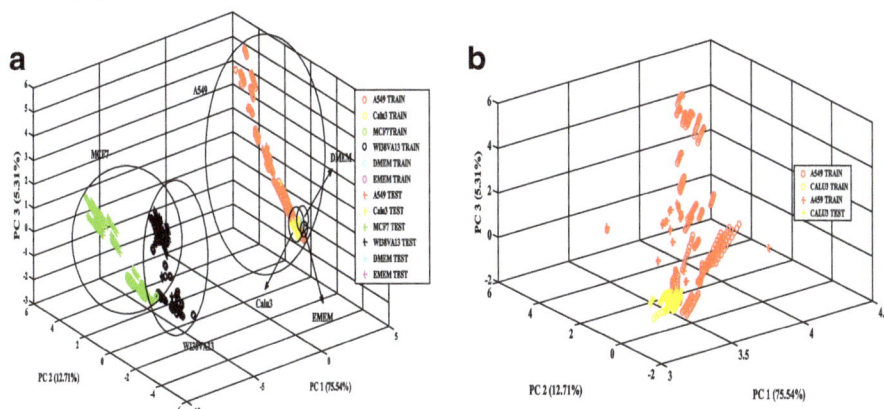

Fig. 6 a PCA plot of volatile compounds of cultured cells (combination of all 3 days). The separability of 4 types of cell lines and two different blank medium shows the effectiveness of the e-nose. **b** PCA plot of volatile compounds of lung cancer cultured cells (combination of all 3 days). The separability of 2 types of lung cancer cell lines shows the effectiveness of the e-nose

fold cross validation. The performance of these classifiers was measured by their accuracy, sensitivity, specificity, precision and MCC of training and testing data. The performances of the e-nose and the classifiers on differentiating the VOCs emitted by lung cancer from the control samples were evaluated by comparing of the performance each classifier.

Tables 6, 7, 8, 9, 10 show the of the classification results of five different classifiers performance in detecting

each type of cell lines samples at three different times of incubation.

Tables 6, 7, 8, 9, 10 shows that three out of five LDA-based classifiers (SVM, PNN, KNN and NB) were able to achieve accuracy, sensitivity, specificity and precision of 90% while MCC has the value of 1 (high prediction quality). However, the OVA-SVM classifier gives the best results as compared to the other classifiers for classifying lung cancer cell lines volatile data. This algorithm shows

Table 6 Performance rate of Fisher-Linear Discriminant Analysis

Time (h)	Classes	Performance rate of LDA (%)									
		Train and Validate					Test				
		ACC	SEN	SPEC	PREC	MCC	ACC	SEN	SPEC	PREC	MCC
24	A549	90.86	98.41	98.93	98.41	0.91	96.89	98.61	98.88	98.44	0.94
	Calu3	94.84	94.38	95.50	98.52	0.75	95.15	95.26	96.18	97.52	0.74
	MCF7	94.32	94.92	95.50	88.89	0.80	95.01	94.72	96.30	90.32	0.82
	WI38VA13	94.73	93.20	95.72	92.86	0.89	95.56	94.50	94.53	92.99	0.89
	DMEM	93.25	93.33	95.18	87.69	0.75	92.96	92.63	95.75	93.17	0.78
	EMEM	90.22	92.25	91.33	84.39	0.70	90.96	89.84	95.65	83.01	0.67
48	A549	94.89	98.45	98.94	98.50	0.98	96.90	99.47	99.87	98.51	0.98
	Calu3	92.99	98.21	95.81	98.64	0.78	96.75	94.18	98.17	97.88	0.82
	MCF7	95.32	96.86	95.78	90.38	0.85	96.51	91.30	97.64	95.45	0.90
	WI38VA13	95.32	96.30	96.07	94.11	0.88	95.90	96.51	95.20	94.14	0.92
	DMEM	93.65	80.00	55.58	92.86	0.50	93.89	50.00	93.00	97.13	0.53
	EMEM	94.11	91.38	92.38	89.74	0.45	94.09	93.10	97.36	90.19	0.86
72	A549	94.91	98.62	98.97	98.50	0.98	96.92	99.54	99.89	98.63	0.96
	Calu3	94.04	98.67	94.52	98.34	0.86	97.41	95.33	98.04	97.71	0.85
	MCF7	95.95	96.98	96.00	92.32	0.92	97.12	92.91	97.76	95.71	0.95
	WI38VA13	95.59	97.05	96.57	94.23	0.93	96.34	96.54	97.30	94.70	0.88
	DMEM	93.52	83.08	96.00	94.30	0.65	93.68	52.31	93.21	97.25	0.71
	EMEM	94.44	88.89	94.80	73.85	0.52	91.85	88.89	95.21	90.75	0.37

Table 7 Performance rate of Naïve Bayes classifier

Time (h)	Classes	Performance rate of NB (%)									
		Train and Validate					Test				
		ACC	SEN	SPEC	PREC	MCC	ACC	SEN	SPEC	PREC	MCC
24	A549	96.87	97.00	99.32	99.45	0.97	99.39	99.27	99.68	99.47	0.95
	Calu3	97.56	96.13	98.41	99.35	0.95	99.34	96.25	99.54	99.49	0.94
	MCF7	98.70	97.44	97.68	95.79	0.93	99.23	98.31	99.29	90.63	0.84
	WI38VA13	98.83	94.91	95.67	99.22	0.96	99.34	94.23	99.65	94.23	0.88
	DMEM	92.86	61.52	98.09	70.59	0.38	97.10	73.68	98.63	77.78	0.53
	EMEM	91.71	60.22	96.77	56.12	0.33	92.81	73.02	94.18	46.46	0.87
48	A549	99.93	97.00	99.92	98.80	0.98	99.96	97.35	99.94	99.93	0.94
	Calu3	96.72	97.48	99.54	83.00	0.47	96.27	97.18	98.74	79.63	0.52
	MCF7	99.50	95.06	99.89	99.87	0.97	99.23	91.30	99.88	98.44	0.93
	WI38VA13	99.33	95.81	99.61	93.59	0.87	99.12	94.52	99.52	94.52	0.89
	DMEM	93.72	84.80	97.11	64.29	0.74	93.58	85.52	98.57	60.91	0.77
	EMEM	98.60	83.96	99.45	91.95	0.81	99.01	88.28	99.06	87.69	0.79
72	A549	99.93	97.00	99.92	98.99	0.98	100.00	100.00	100.00	100.00	1.00
	Calu3	96.41	95.90	96.24	64.75	0.36	96.78	90.00	97.25	69.23	0.43
	MCF7	99.75	97.00	100.00	100.00	1.00	100.00	100.00	100.00	100.00	1.00
	WI38VA13	99.70	97.00	99.68	96.19	0.94	99.78	97.96	99.88	97.96	0.96
	DMEM	92.56	87.53	96.85	91.75	0.66	93.19	80.00	97.01	91.23	0.67
	EMEM	97.25	90.75	97.51	73.77	0.59	98.47	94.44	98.73	82.26	0.69

Table 8 Performance rate of K-Nearest Neighbour classifier

Time (h)	Classes	Performance rate of KNN (%)									
		Train and Validate					Test				
		ACC	SEN	SPEC	PREC	MCC	ACC	SEN	SPEC	PREC	MCC
24	A549	99.08	97.67	99.17	99.50	0.91	99.47	97.97	99.20	99.60	0.91
	Calu3	99.87	99.98	99.86	97.75	0.96	92.70	99.84	99.07	99.57	0.98
	MCF7	99.01	99.77	99.54	99.65	0.97	99.04	99.87	99.92	99.80	0.97
	WI38VA13	99.41	99.48	99.37	99.33	0.95	98.80	99.40	98.80	92.30	0.89
	DMEM	99.54	92.47	97.32	96.35	0.92	93.80	87.50	97.38	96.45	0.94
	EMEM	99.93	98.85	96.37	91.02	0.88	87.10	71.40	98.40	85.20	0.92
48	A549	99.89	99.01	99.78	96.39	0.94	99.00	99.23	99.81	96.85	0.95
	Calu3	99.60	98.81	99.65	94.32	0.91	99.71	99.05	99.50	94.29	0.93
	MCF7	99.87	98.02	100.00	100.00	0.99	100.00	100.00	100.00	100.00	1.00
	WI38VA13	99.86	97.47	100.00	95.62	0.95	99.37	99.59	99.60	95.36	0.94
	DMEM	94.73	58.67	96.51	45.36	0.32	92.20	50.80	96.10	54.10	0.39
	EMEM	94.53	89.02	97.86	80.98	0.79	93.70	97.20	97.00	89.00	0.72
72	A549	99.94	98.98	99.93	98.98	0.93	99.90	99.89	99.83	99.93	0.96
	Calu3	99.60	96.41	98.98	98.79	0.96	99.75	99.58	99.55	95.20	0.95
	MCF7	100.00	100.00	100.00	100.00	1.00	100.00	100.00	100.00	100.00	1.00
	WI38VA13	100.00	100.00	100.00	100.00	1.00	99.80	99.67	100.00	100.00	0.97
	DMEM	96.46	78.04	95.72	86.34	0.63	86.80	100.00	85.80	86.36	0.66
	EMEM	99.60	100.00	99.58	94.12	0.91	94.20	18.50	100.00	100.00	0.40

Table 9 Performance rate of Probabilistic Neural Network classifier

Time (h)	Classes	Performance rate of PNN (%)									
		Train and Validate					Test				
		ACC	SEN	SPEC	PREC	MCC	ACC	SEN	SPEC	PREC	MCC
24	A549	99.62	98.77	99.22	99.59	0.92	99.65	99.08	99.39	99.69	0.94
	Calu3	99.89	99.98	99.89	98.05	0.97	99.87	99.89	98.70	98.91	0.96
	MCF7	99.11	99.80	99.58	99.69	0.98	99.04	99.87	99.92	99.80	0.97
	WI38VA13	99.50	99.57	99.43	99.44	0.94	99.61	99.62	99.47	99.49	0.96
	DMEM	99.57	95.97	99.31	97.33	0.93	99.80	95.99	99.48	97.75	0.95
	EMEM	99.90	98.93	96.47	91.02	0.89	99.93	97.14	95.14	91.22	0.89
48	A549	99.91	99.75	99.93	98.80	0.97	99.90	98.51	97.02	98.87	0.96
	Calu3	99.93	98.93	99.75	99.86	0.98	99.94	98.51	100.00	100.00	0.99
	MCF7	99.90	96.43	99.86	97.59	0.94	99.95	97.00	99.92	98.57	0.95
	WI38VA13	99.90	98.00	100.00	100.00	1.00	100.00	100.00	100.00	100.00	1.00
	DMEM	95.24	94.43	94.93	96.67	0.92	91.57	81.03	95.05	62.47	0.79
	EMEM	96.93	98.22	98.66	90.87	0.82	96.97	98.36	98.78	92.39	0.84
72	A549	99.93	100.00	99.93	98.99	0.97	100.00	100.00	100.00	100.00	1.00
	Calu3	99.94	98.90	100.00	100.00	0.99	99.69	100.00	99.67	95.24	0.93
	MCF7	99.92	97.00	99.91	97.73	0.93	99.97	97.54	99.68	94.23	0.92
	WI38VA13	100.00	100.00	100.00	100.00	1.00	100.00	100.00	100.00	100.00	1.00
	DMEM	91.24	94.41	95.80	88.11	0.70	91.66	94.62	96.01	88.57	0.68
	EMEM	97.73	58.53	98.90	94.82	0.67	97.99	58.99	98.97	95.63	0.69

Table 10 Performance rate of Support Vector Machine classifier

Time (h)	Classes	Performance rate of SVM (%)									
		Train and Validate					Test				
		ACC	SEN	SPEC	PREC	MCC	ACC	SEN	SPEC	PREC	MCC
24	A549	99.69	99.24	99.93	99.67	0.98	99.86	99.65	99.96	99.82	0.98
	Calu3	99.93	99.81	99.92	99.89	0.98	99.84	99.87	99.72	99.76	0.98
	MCF7	99.98	99.87	99.97	99.92	0.96	99.94	99.95	99.98	99.89	0.98
	WI38VA13	99.72	99.80	99.72	99.84	0.97	99.71	99.82	99.83	99.87	0.97
	DMEM	99.46	96.77	99.65	98.32	0.94	99.85	96.99	99.69	98.75	0.96
	EMEM	99.86	100.00	99.85	97.75	0.97	96.38	96.19	97.83	91.64	0.87
48	A549	99.82	99.72	99.94	99.30	0.97	99.97	99.79	99.97	99.76	0.97
	Calu3	99.79	99.70	100.00	100.00	0.98	99.47	99.64	99.88	99.89	0.98
	MCF7	99.99	99.45	100.00	100.00	0.99	100.00	100.00	100.00	100.00	1.00
	WI38VA13	99.86	99.89	100.00	100.00	0.99	100.00	100.00	100.00	100.00	1.00
	DMEM	97.52	97.83	97.49	92.00	0.81	92.62	76.07	94.55	41.86	0.78
	EMEM	100.00	100.00	100.00	100.00	1.00	99.12	100.00	99.06	87.88	0.80
72	A549	99.98	99.71	99.93	99.82	0.90	100.00	100.00	100.00	100.00	1.00
	Calu3	100.00	100.00	100.00	100.00	1.00	99.96	99.93	99.88	99.83	0.98
	MCF7	100.00	100.00	100.00	100.00	1.00	100.00	100.00	100.00	100.00	1.00
	WI38VA13	99.64	80.20	100.00	100.00	0.89	100.00	100.00	100.00	100.00	1.00
	DMEM	97.52	88.82	99.86	96.15	0.71	95.36	82.31	100.00	100.00	0.85
	EMEM	97.84	100.00	91.31	82.67	0.81	95.76	81.85	98.43	86.67	0.84

high accuracy, sensitivity, specificity, precision and MCC in the testing phase. On the contrary, the LDA classifier has the least performance achieved and many samples were wrongly classified.

Although LDA-based OVA-SVM showed the best performance, the percentage of accuracy, sensitivity, specificity, precision and MCC values using PNN algorithm shows consistently high for every class. The prediction quality value (MCC) of DMEM using LDA-based PNN algorithm shows only 0.3 lesser than the SVM. To support this fact, a study conducted by F.Moderasi (2014), suggested that the PNN algorithm can be used as an appropriate alternative for SVM as the training process of the PNN algorithm is easier than SVM algorithm [67].

The performance of NB was observed to be less than SVM, KNN and PNN classifier because it is a generative classifier, and generally this classifier is not as accurate as the discriminative classifiers [68]. However, the NB is still preferred to be used for the medical diagnosis application because of it is simple to build, easy to train and able to deal with the missing information [56, 57]. According to K. Huang (2005), the NB performance can be improved by training the NB classifier in a discriminative way [68] .Thus, this method can be considered in future work to obtain excellent results from NB classifier.

When the LDA-based OVA-SVM performance rate was investigated according to samples at different incubation time, it was found that the classification accuracy rate improved significantly, achieving approximately 99% for the growth features of 24th-hour incubation period. The performance rate was observed to also improve for samples at 48th and 72nd-hour of cell growth. These may indicate that the VOCs of each sample increased with prolonged incubation periods.

The low performance of OVA-SVM for the 24th-hour compared to the 2nd day data may due to the insufficient time for the metabolites or compounds to be released by the cells to into the headspace. This may also happen due to relatively low cell numbers which cause the lower production of VOCs compared to the 48th and 72nd-hour of incubations. This corresponds to a previous study on in-vitro lung cancer cells by Smith. D (2003), where a number of compounds in the headspace are directly proportional to number of cells. This problem can be overcome using more concentrated cell seeding that might also help the differentiation between the other cell lines at an early stage of growth [69].

Identification of the VOCs of lung cancer cell lines and normal cell lines by SPME-GCMS analysis

The VOCs related to lung cancer cell metabolism were investigated using SPME-GCMS analysis. The headspaces of cultured lung cells have been compared to the headspace of medium with breast cancer cells, the normal lung cells and without cells, respectively. The complete list of identified VOCs, based on the average peak of total chromatograms of three replicates of each sample is tabulated in Table 11. These 32 selected compounds are supposed to emitted from the both background culture media and the metabolic activity of the cells.

Statistical significance of the relative abundances of the VOCs released from the lung cancer cell lines and the blank mediums have been evaluated using the t-test by considering p value less than 0.05 as statistically significant. This analysis conducted to eliminate confounding VOCs which are due to the different substrates rather than to the cell metabolism. The results were shown in Table 12. The same analysis also has been conducted on the VOCs released by the different cancer cell (MCF7) and the normal lung cancer (WI38VA13). The compounds and their significant differences have been tabulated in Table 13.

Among the 32 VOC compounds detected, 20 are related to the lung cancer cell lines. Out of these, 18 are observed to be significantly more in the headspace of lung cancer samples compared to the blank medium (Table 12). Out of those 18, nine were observed to be absent from the blank samples. This indicates that these nine VOC compounds have specific association with the lung cancer cell metabolism.

In order to eliminate the influence of VOCs of culture media on the VOCs of lung cancer, the VOCs that found exclusively in the blank medium (statistically not significant) have been removed in the further analysis aimed at studying the properties of cancer cell lines. Furthermore, the aromatic compounds such as styrene, dimethyl silanediol, benzene and ethylbenzene are more linked to the contaminants [19, 50, 70, 71], thus these compounds are also eliminated for further analysis.

Overall, the 11 VOCs identified as statistically significant in previous analysis for the discrimination between normal lung cell and breast cancer cell line. The abundances of each VOC related to lung cancer cells was compared to both lung cells and breast cancer samples and tabulated in Table 13.

As seen in Table 13, four VOCs, namely dodecane, decanal 2-ethyldodecanol and heneicosane, are specific to lung cancer cells. They are absent from the control samples. The VOC whose abundance significantly decreases in the lung cancer cells are propylbenzene, nonanal, 3, 4-dimethylheptane, 2, 4-dimethylundecane and 2-ethylhexanol. The decane was observed to be increases significantly in the cancer related cell samples compared to normal lung cell line, indicating this compound more related to cancerous volatile. These results indicated that the headspaces of lung cancer cell lines are characterized by a specific VOCs signature.

Table 11 Compounds detected from the headspace of in vitro cultured cell lines (>80% of the NIST matching percentage)

Retention Time (min)	Library/ID	Summary of All Substances Identified by Spectral Match						CAS number
		A549	Calu-3	MCF7	WI38VA13	DMEM	EMEM	
3.33	Amphetamine	-	-	-	+	-	-	300-62-9
3.44	Decane	+	+	+	-	-	-	124-18-5
4.25	Ethylbenzene	+	+	+	+	+	-	100-41-4
4.95	O-Xylene	-	-	-	+	-	-	95-47-6
5.30	Propylbenzene	+	+	+	+	+	-	103-65-1
5.51	1-Ethyl-2-methylbenzene	+	+	+	+	-	-	611-14-3
5.74	Styrene	+	++	++	++	++	-	100-42-5
6.18	Dodecane	-	+	+	-	-	-	112-40-3
6.28	1,2,4-Trimethyl-benzene	-	-	-	+	-	-	95-63-6
6.57	Trimethyl[4(trimethylsilyl)butoxy]silane	+	+	+	+	+	-	7140-91-2
7.52	Cyclohexanol	+	+	+	+	+	-	108-93-097
7.64	Decanal	+	-	-	-	-	-	112-31-2
7.68	Nonanal	+	-	-	+	-	-	124-19-6
7.69	3,4-Dimethylheptane	-	-	+	-	-	-	922-28-1
8.02	2,4-DimethylUndecane	-	-	-	+	-	-	17312-80-0
8.33	1,3-Bis(1,1-dimethylethyl)benzene	+	+	+	+	+	-	1014-60-4
8.67	Tetradecane	+	-	+	+	+	-	629-59-4
8.74	2-Ethyldodecanol	-	+	-	-	-	-	19780-33-7
8.75	2-Ethylhexanol	-	+	-	+	-	-	104-76-7
9.00	Benzaldehyde	+	-	+	+	+	-	100-52-7
10.25	Dimethylsilanediol	+	+	+	+	+	+	1066-42-8
10.55	Acetophenone	+	-	+	+	+	-	98-86-2
10.60	Ethanedioic acid, bis(trimethylsilyl)ester	+	+	+	+	+	-	18294-04-7
10.88	2-Ethyl-1,3-dimethyl-benzene	-	+	+	-	-	-	2870-04-4
10.92	1-Methyl-2-Pyrrolidinone	+	-	+	-	+	-	872-50-4
11.30	Heptadecane	-	-	-	+	-	-	629-78-7
11.22	Heneicosane	+	+	-	-	-	-	629-94-7
11.30	Hexadecane	-	-	+	-	-	-	544-76-3
11.37	2-(Aminooxy)-Propanoic acid	-	-	-	-	-	+	2786-22-3
11.48	3-Methyl-3-Hexanol	-	-	-	-	-	+	597-96-6
11.55	Methoxyphenyl_Oxime	+	+	+	+	+	+	1000222-86-6
12.96	2-Phenyl-2-Butanone	-	-	+	-	-	-	2550-26-7-97

++: Percentage of peak area more than 50%; +: percentage of peak area less than 50%; - : not detected (peak area < 1%)

Discussion

The VOCs analysis in the medical field offered a great alternative approach to cancer diagnosis. However, till date the use of VOCs analysis in the clinical approach is still limited due to the lack of validation of cancer related metabolites and sensing performance of VOCs sensors. In this work, the VOCs emitted by the 2 different lung cancer cell lines and the controlled cell lines, both breast cancer cell and normal lung cell lines were analyzed using the commercialized CP gas sensors (Cyranose 320) and GSMS-SPME. This work is highlighting the potential of these analysis techniques in providing meaningful information in the clinical application of lung cancer diagnosis. The Cyranose 320 e-nose used to analyze the headspace of conditioned culture cell lines (in-vitro) in the proliferative conditions for 3 days to discriminate the VOCs patterns released in the headspace of the cell lines during normal and proliferation stage. Results from the e-nose analysis highlighted that the cancer cell lines are able to classified with high accuracy using the VOCs patterns even at the early stage of cell proliferation (24th hours of incubation time).

Table 12 VOCs discriminating the headspace of lung cancer cell lines and blank mediums. Analysis of abundances of VOCS in the headspace of lung cancer cell lines using GCMS-SPME. VOCs increased (emitted) and or decreases (consumed) by lung cancer are reported with respect to blank medium. A p-value < 0.05 has been considered statistically significant

Trend	Library/ID	P-value
Increase	Decane	1.50E-5
	Ethylbenzene	0.052
	Propylbenzene	0.011
	1-Ethyl-2-methylbenzene	0.037
	Styrene	0.135
	Dodecane	0.033
	Cyclohexanol	0.102
	Decanal	0.001
	Nonanal	0.002
	1,3-Bis(1,1-dimethylethyl)benzene	0.084
	Tetradecane	0.506
	2-Ethyldodecanol	3.88E-5
	2-Ethylhexanol	3.52E-5
	Benzaldehyde	0.590
	Acetophenone	0.750
	2-Ethyl-1,3-dimethyl-benzene	0.036
	1-Methyl-2-Pyrrolidinone	0.319
	Heneicosane	3.35E-6
Decrease	Trimethyl[4(trimethylsilyl)butoxy]silane	0.101
	Ethanedioic acid, bis(trimethylsilyl)ester	0.107

The ability for the Cyranose320 to be able to discriminate the VOCs of the cell samples with high accuracy even at the 24th hour of incubation provides a motivation to perform GCMS-SPME analysis. This allows the identification of the specific VOCs that are associated with the cancer cell growth. This was achieved by comparing the VOCs from lung and breast cancer cells to those of the blank mediums. Comparison of the chromatograms indicated that there were significant differences between the cell culture samples based on several compounds. There are total four specific VOCs identified as lung cancer related volatile, namely, heneicosane, dodecane, 2-ethyldodecanol and decanal.

The GCMS result also shows that higher alkanes group; heneicosane was found in both lung cancer cell lines, A549 and Calu-3, statistically significant from the controlled samples. This indicates that the heneicosane has high potential to be the lung cancer related biomarker. There are studies claimed the heneicosane as a candidate of the biomarker from lung cancer patients breath [28, 72, 73]. However, the origin of heneicosane in lung cancer cell remains unclear.

Another compound with a higher alkane group known as dodecane was observed to increases significantly in Calu-3 during the incubation period. There are few studies on lung cancer biomarker suggested n-dodecane to be associated with lung cancer in adenocarcinoma tissues [29], patient's breath, especially in EGRF mutated adenocarcinoma patient's breath [74]. Dodecane also found to be related to breast cancer [75].

Among the detected VOCs, one specific compound, namely decane, which is also from the high alkanes group, was observed to be emitted by all of the three cancer cells. Similar results were obtained by Yishan. W and B G.Hyun. the decane is found in the lung cancer

Table 13 VOCs discriminating the headspace of lung cancer cell lines and control cell lines. Analysis of abundances of VOCS in the headspace of lung cancer, breast cancer and normal lung cell lines using GCMS-SPME. A p-value < 0.05 has been considered statistically significant

Compounds	P-values				
	A549/Calu3	A549/MCF7	A549/WI38VA13	Calu3/MCF7	Calu3/WI38VA13
Decane	0.326 (↑)	0.154 (↑)	1.04E-4 (↑)	0.127 (↓)	0.016 (↑)
Propylbenzene	0.507 (↑)	0.533 (↑)	0.104 (↓)	0.988 (↓)	0.071 (↓)
Dodecane	1.67E-6 (↓)	2.23E-5 (↓)	-	0.011 (↑)	1.67E-6 (↑)
Decanal	0.001 (↑)	0.001 (↑)	0.001 (↑)	-	-
Nonanal	0.002 (↑)	0.002 (↑)	1.17E-4 (↓)	-	2.21E-4 (↓)
3, 4-Dimethylheptane	-	2.75E-4 (↓)	-	2.75E-4 (↓)	-
2, 4-DimethylUndecane	-	-	0.017 (↓)	0.017 (↓)	-
2-Ethyldodecanol	3.88E-5 (↓)	-	-	3.88E-5 (↑)	3.88E-5 (↑)
2-Ethylhexanol	3.53E-5 (↓)	-	2.47E-7 (↓)	3.53E-5 (↑)	9.40E-5 (↑)
Heneicosane	0.334 (↓)	0.002 (↑)	0.002 (↑)	3.40E-4 (↑)	3.40E-4 (↑)

The (↑) and (↓) shows the trend of abundances increases and decreases in lung cancer cell line samples respectively

tissue of patients [29, 72]. Another study by Chen. X, using different lung cancer cells also found that decane to be one of the 11 compounds with higher concentrations compared to those of normal cells [76]. Decane also considered as a lung cancer biomarker in a patient's breath [77, 78]. A significant difference found in the concentrations of decane in the patient's breath before and after surgery [79]. Still, the origin of decane in breast cancer cell has never been reported in any previous studies.

According to a study by Meggie. H (2010), representative of hydrocarbon is reported as potential biomarker of lung cancer and suggested that these compounds are probably the outcome of oxidative stress [80]. The alkanes are mostly produced from lipid peroxidation by reactive oxygen species (ROS) supported by few studies stating that alkanes and methylated alkanes are found in lung cancer [50, 70, 71, 80] and breast cancer [31, 34, 81].

A specific VOC released by A549 cell lines distinguished this cell line from other cell lines and blank medium which is decanal. A study in 2011 reported that decanal was used as a biomarker to detect non-small lung cancer using electronic nose with 95% sensitivity and 70% specificity [82]. Decanal was used as one of the primary contributors to separate non-small cell lung cancer and small cell lung cancer as well, with 100% sensitivity and 75% specificity by Barash. O in a study conducted in 2012 [33]. Whereas, there is only one specific VOC, 2-ethyldodecanol has been emitted by Calu-3.

The obvious VOCs emitted by MCF7 cell in this study were 3, 4-dimethylheptane, hexadecane and 2-phenyl-2-butanone. This finding is in line with one study which found hexadecane in the breath of a breast cancer patient [31]. However, no previous published studies on volatiles from breast cancer have reported the existence of 3, 4-dimethylheptane and 2-phenyl-2-butanone. The

normal cell WI38VA13 emitted four different VOCs which were Amphetamine, Xylene, 2, 4-dimethylundecane and heptadecane. The 2-ethydodecanal, 3, 4-dimethylheptane, 2-phenyl-2-butanone, Amphetamine, Xylene, 2-4-dimethylundecane and heptadecane have not reported to date as biomarker in any in-vitro studies. Thus, the significance of these compounds remains unclear. Besides, the measurement time for VOCs collection used was in contrast with previous studies, where the VOCs collected after 24 h of cell growth. This is to ensure the compounds were collected at proliferation stage.

Nonanal and 2-ethylhexanol from WI38VA13 cells were found to be significantly more than that from A549 and Calu-3. In contrast to results observed in this study, it has been reported that the detection of nonanal is significant [83, 84] and used to separate adenocarcinoma and squamous cell carcinoma [74]. As for 2-ethylhexanol, the results here corresponds to other previous studies on lung cancer detection, and was never found to be one of the biomarkers. This indicates that these compounds might have a specific association related to cell metabolism. The WI38VA13 cells also share aromatic compounds with DMEM, which might be the reason for the overlapping of DMEM group in the WI38VA13 in the PCA and LDA analysis as shown in Figs. 5 and 6a.

In summary, the VOCs that exist in lung cancer cell lines but not in the control samples and those which exists in higher concentrations in the former may be considered as possible biomarkers as shown in Table 14. Decanal, dodecane, 2-ethyldodecanal and heneicosane may potentially be used to discriminate lung cancer cells from other type of cancer or normal cell lines. Decane on the other hand can potentially be used as a specific biomarker for cancer. These findings suggested that the identified VOCs are able to offer more information regarding in-vitro cultured cell line metabolism and aid

Table 14 The potential lung cancer biomarkers detected in this study were compared to the in-vitro and in vivo results of previous studies which were found in Scopus database

Class Specific compounds (In this study)		Origin	Comparison with Literature			
			Cell lines	[a]Tissues	Breath	References
Alkanes Straight chain	Dodecane Heneicosane	Endogenous- lipid peroxidation by reactive oxygen species (ROS) s	✓	✓	✓✓	[28, 29, 72, 76, 78–80]
			-	✓	✓	[29, 74, 80]
			-	-	✓	[28, 72, 73]
Aldehydes	Decanal Nonanal	Endogenous- peroxidation of omega3 and omega6 fatty acids (PUFAs), components of cell membrane phospholipids	✓	✓	-	[33, 80, 82, 86]
Alcohol	2-Ethyldodecanol	Endogenous- Hydroxylation of the lipid peroxidation biomarkers via cytochrome p450 enzymes	-	-	-	[80]

[a]Patient's tissue
✓Compounds that were detected as lung cancer biomarkers in previous studies
- Compounds that have not been detected in the previous study

the determination of lung cancer using the electronic nose technology. In order to reduce the possibility of false positive results, it is crucial to creating libraries of biomarkers for each of cancer cells and normal cells. This can be achieved by performing various chemometric or multivariate analysis to validate the biomarkers of the cancerous and normal cells of interest.

Conclusion

This study presents the possibility of using VOCs as biomarkers for cancer cells. Specific VOCs are verified to be specific to cancer cells compared to of the normal samples. The headspace of in-vitro cultured cell lines were analyzed using a Cyranose320 e-nose consisting of an array of sensors and GCMS coupled with SPME. Several classifiers were used to validate the ability of the e-nose to discriminate the cancer cells to that of the normal samples and blank mediums, namely the LDA, NB, KNN, PNN and OVA-SVM. The investigation was carried out to identify cell lines VOCs at three different proliferation stages under a normal laboratory condition.

The results from this study shows that the Cyranose320 was able to discriminate the VOCs released by the various cancer and healthy cells as well as the blank mediums. The classifiers tested were able to perform high levels of accuracy. The LDA based OVA-SVM records the best performance with 100% successful classification, even at the early stage of cell growth (24th hours of incubation) and managed to maintain this performance at 48th and 72nd hours.

The VOCs pattern collected from e-nose results were validated by the GCMS-SPME. The results show that particular cell lines produced specific VOCs. This study provides a list of possible VOCs, which is believed, can be specific biomarkers for lung cancer, even at the 24th hour of cell growth. The potential list of VOCs obtained from this study was compared with the previous studies as shown in Table 14. This also concludes that the e-nose in conjunction with GCMS-SPME is able to be a non-invasive screening tool at an early stage. This is particularly useful for the clinician to understand in the event any occurrences of overlapping groups in the e-nose results.

Besides, this study also shows that the use of existing tools such as GCMS-SPME and e-nose-based gas sensor array system promises the potentials to improve the cancerous VOCs detection system by optimizing the sensor selections. The sensors with higher selectivity and sensitivity are essential in order to capture the specific biomarkers. Therefore, further studies on optimizing the sensor system and using in-vivo studies (e.g. using breath samples) are underway with the ultimate goal to develop a complementary tool for clinical testing.

Abbreviation

A549: Lung cancer cell line; ACC: Accuracy; ANN: Artificial neural networks; Calu3: Lung cancer cell line; DMEM: Dulbecco's modification of Eagle medium; EMEM: Eagle's minimum essential medium; E-Nose: Electronic nose; FN: False negative; FP: False positive; GCMS: Gas chromatography mass spectrometry; GNP: Gold nanoparticles; HASM: Human airway smooth muscle; IBE: Immortal bronchial epithelium; KNN: K-Neural network; LDA: Linear discriminant analysis; LDCT: Low dose computed tomography; MCC: Matthews correlation coefficient; MCF7: Breast cancer cell line; MD: Mahalanobis distances; NB: Naïve bayes; NHDF: Normal human diploid fibroblast; NSCLC: Non-small cell lung cancer; OVA: One versus all; OVO: One versus one; PC: Principal component; PCA: Principal component analysis; PDMS: Polydimethylsiloxane; PNN: Probabilistic neural network; PREC: Precision; Rmax: Maximum value of response; Rms: Root mean square roughness; Rs: Steady state of response; SCLC: Small cell lung cancer; SEN: Sensitivity; SGF: Savitzky-Golay smoothing filter; SPE: Specificity; SPME: Solid phase micro extraction; SVM: Support vector machine; TIC: Total ion chromatogram; TN: True negative; TP: True positive; VOCs: Volatile organic compounds; WI38VA13: Normal lung cell line

Acknowledgements

The author would like to thank School of Chemical Engineering and Analytical Science, University of Manchester, United Kingdom for their support and funding for this project. The authors also would like to thank Hospital Tuanku Fauziah (HTF), Kangar, Perlis for their collaboration in this project. Special thanks to Cell and Tissue Engineering Lab, Kulliyyah of Engineering, International Islamic University Malaysia for their guidance in cell culture technique and funding for the project.

Funding

This work is supported by the Centre of Excellence for Advanced Sensor Technology Research Board. The funder had no role in study design, data collection and analysis, decision to publish, or preparation of the manuscript.

Authors' contributions

The research problem was defined by: RT, AZ, MIO, AHA and AYMS. Designed the methods: AZ, RT, MIO, YZHYH, KMH, AHA and KCP. Design the algorithm and statistical analysis: RT, AZ, LMK, AYMS and KCP. The experimental design was carried out by: RT, AZ, YZHYH, AIJ, MIO and KMH. Methods mostly implemented by RT with help from YZHYH, AIJ, AZ, KCP and MIO. Experiment and analysed the data: RT and AZ. RT wrote the paper with help from the other authors. All authors read and approved the final manuscript.

Competing interest

The authors declare that they have no competing interests.

Author details

[1]Centre of Excellence for Advanced Sensor Technology, Universiti Malaysia Perlis, Arau, Perlis, Malaysia. [2]Cell and Tissue Engineering Lab (CTEL), Department of Biotechnology Engineering, Kulliyyah of Engineering, International Islamic University Malaysia (IIUM), Kuala Lumpur, Malaysia. [3]International Institute for Halal Research and Training (INHART), International Islamic University Malaysia (IIUM), Kuala Lumpur, Malaysia. [4]Department of Respiratory, Hospital Tuanku Fauziah, Jalan Kolam, Kangar, Perlis, Malaysia. [5]School of Chemical Engineering and Analytical Science, University of Manchester, Oxford Road, Manchester, United Kingdom.

References

1. American Cancer Society. Cancer Facts & Figures 2017. Alanta: American Cancer Society; 2017.
2. Types of Cancer. Natl. Cancer Soc. Malaysia. 2016. Retrieved from "www.cancer.org.my/national-cancer-society-malaysia-and-ibm-team-up-to-use-data-to-combat-cancer/" at 23rd March 2016
3. Hirsch FR, Franklin WA, Af G, PAJ B. Early detection of lung cancer: clinical perspectives of recent advances in biology and radiology. Clin Cancer Res. 2001;7:5–22.

4. Peng G, Hakim M, Broza YY, Billan S, Abdah-Bortnyak R, Kuten a, et al. Detection of lung, breast, colorectal, and prostate cancers from exhaled breath using a single array of nanosensors. Br. J. Cancer. 103:542–51.

5. Fossella FV, Komaki MR, Putnam MJB M Jr. Lung cancer. Texas: Springer-Verlag New York; 2002.

6. The National Lung Screening Trial Research Team. Reduced lung cancer mortality with low-dose computed tomographic screening. N. Engl.J.Med. 2011;365:395–409.

7. Culter DM. Are we finally winning the war on cancer? J Eco Perspec. 2008; 22:3–26.

8. Barash O, Peled N, Hirsch FR, Haick H. Sniffing the unique "odor print" of non-small-cell lung cancer with gold nanoparticles. Small. 2009;5:2618–24.

9. Mazzone PJ. Exhaled breath volatile organic compound biomarkers in lung cancer. J. Breath Res. 2012;6:027106.

10. Amann A, Spanel P, Smith D. Breath analysis: the approach towards clinical applications. Mini Rev Med Chem. 2007;7:115–29.

11. Mazzone PJ. Analysis of volatile organic compounds in the exhaled breath for the diagnosis of lung cancer. J Thorac Oncol. 2008;3:774–80.

12. Singer SJ, Nicolson GL. The fluid mosaic model of the structure of cell membranes. Science. 1972;175:720–31.

13. Alberts B, Johnson A, Lewis J. Molecular biology of the cell. New York: Garl. Publ; 2002.

14. Bajaj A, Miranda OR, Kim I-B, Phillips RL, Jerry DJ, Bunz UHF, et al. Detection and differentiation of normal, cancerous, and metastatic cells using nanoparticle-polymer sensor arrays. Proc. Natl. Acad. Sci. U. S. A. 2009;106: 10912–6.

15. Montuschi P, Barnes PJ. Analysis of exhaled breath condensate for monitoring airway inflammation. Thrends Phamacol. 2002;23:232–7.

16. Bajtarevic A, Ager C, Pienz M, Klieber M, Schwarz K, Ligor M, et al. Noninvasive detection of lung cancer by analysis of exhaled breath. BMC Cancer. 2009;9:348.

17. Horváth I, Lázár Z, Gyulai N, Kollai M, Losonczy G. Exhaled biomarkers in lung cancer. Eur. Respir. J. 2009;34:261–75.

18. Gordon SM, Szldon JP, Krotoszynski BK, Gibbons RD, Neill JO. Volatile organic compounds in exhaled air from patients with lung cancer. Clin. Chem. 1985;31:1278–82.

19. Lavra L, Catini A, Ulivieri A, Capuano R, Salehi LB, Sciacchitano S, et al. Investigation of VOCs associated with different characteristics of breast cancer cells. Sci. Rep. 2015;5:1–12.

20. Boots AW, Bos LD, Van Der SMP, Van SF, Sterk PJ. Exhaled molecular fingerprinting in diagnosis and monitoring: validating volatile promises. Trends Mol. Med. 2015;21:633–44.

21. Smith D, Wang T, Sulé-Suso J, Spanel P, Haj A E. Quantification of acetaldehyde released by lung cancer cells in vitro using selected ion flow tube mass spectrometry. Rapid Commun. Mass Spectrom. 2003;17:845–50.

22. Filipiak W, Sponring A, Mikoviny T, Ager C, Schubert J, Miekisch W, et al. Release of volatile organic compounds (VOCs) from the lung cancer cell line CALU-1 in vitro. Cancer Cell Int. 2008;8:17.

23. Sponring A, Filipiak W, Mikoviny T, Ager C, Schubert J, Miekisch W, et al. Release of volatile organic compounds from the lung cancer cell line NCI-H2087 in vitro. Anticancer Res. 2009;29:419–26.

24. Filipiak W, Sponring A, Filipiak A, Ager C, Schubert J, Miekisch W, et al. TD-GC-MS analysis of volatile metabolites of human lung cancer and normal cells in vitro. Cancer Epidemiol Biomarkers Prev. 2010;19:182–95.

25. Baranska A, Smolinska A, Boots AW, Dallinga JW, van Schooten FJ. Dynamic collection and analysis of volatile organic compounds from the headspace of cell cultures. J. Breath Res. 2015;9:047102.

26. Sponring A, Filipiak W, Ager C, Schubert J. Analysis of volatile organic compounds (VOCs) in the headspace of NCI-H1666 lung cancer cells. Cancer Biomarkers. 2010;7:3233.

27. Hanai Y, Shimono K, Oka H, Baba Y, Yamazaki K, Beauchamp GK. Analysis of volatile organic compounds released from human lung cancer cells and from the urine of tumor-bearing mice. Cancer Cell Int. 2012;12:7.

28. Yu J, Wang D, Wang L, Wang P, Hu Y, Ying K. Detection of lung cancer with volatile organic biomarkers in exhaled breath and lung cancer cells. AIP Conf. Proc. 2009:198–201.

29. Yishan W, Hub Y, Wanga D, Kai Y, Ling W, Yingchang Z, et al. The analysis of volatile organic compounds biomarkers for lung cancer in exhaled breath, tissues and cell lines. Cancer Biomarkers. 2012;11:129–0270.

30. Nozoe T, Goda S, Selyanchyn R, Wang T, Nakazawa K, Hirano T, et al. In vitro detection of small molecule metabolites excreted from cancer cells using a Tenax TA thin-film microextraction device. J. Chromatogr. B Anal. Technol. Biomed. Life Sci. 2015;991:99–107.

31. Wang C, Sun B, Guo L, Wang X, Ke C, Liu S, et al. Volatile organic metabolites identify patients with breast cancer, cyclomastopathy, and mammary gland fibroma. Sci. Rep. 2014;4:5383.

32. Calenic B, Filipiak W, Greabu M, Amann A. Volatile organic compounds expression in different cell types: an in vitro approach. Int. J. Clin. Toxicol. 2013;1:43–51.

33. Barash O, Peled N, Tisch U, Bunn P a, Hirsch FR, Haick H. Classification of lung cancer histology by gold nanoparticle sensors. Nanomedicine. Elsevier. 2012;8:580–9.

34. Gendron KB, Hockstein NG, Thaler ER, Vachani A, Hanson CW. In vitro discrimination of tumor cell lines with an electronic nose. Otolaryngol. Head. Neck Surg. 2007;137:269–73.

35. Broza YY, Haick H. Nanomaterial-based sensors for detection of disease by volatile organic compounds. Nanomedicine. 2013;8:785–806.

36. Marzluf BA, Krajc T, Mueller MR. Principles of lung cancer screening – exhaled breath analysis. Hamdan med. J. 2016;2016(9):17–38.

37. Bassey E, Whalley J, Sallis P. An evaluation of smoothing filters for gas sensor signal cleaning. Fourth. Int. Conf. Adv. Commun. Comput. 2014:19–23.

38. Pearce T, Schiffman S, Nagle H, Gardner J. Electronic nose technology. Hand B. Mach. Olfaction. Weinheim, Wiley-VCH; 2003.

39. Thriumani R, Jeffree AI, Zakaria A, Hasyim YZH-Y, Helmy KM, Omar MI, et al. A preliminary study on detection of lung cancer cells based on volatile organic compounds sensing using electronic nose. J. Teknol. 2015;77:67–71.

40. Thriumani R, Zakaria A, Jeffree AI, Hishamuddin NA, Omar MI, Adom AH, et al. A preliminary study on in-vitro lung cancer detection using E-nose technology. 2014. IEEE Int. Conf. Control Syst. Comput. Eng. 2014:601–5.

41. Thriumani R, Zakaria A, Jeffree AI, Hishamuddin NA, Omar MI, Adom AH, et al. Cancer detection using an electronic nose: a preliminary study on detection and discrimination of cancerous cells. Miri, Sarawak: IEEE Conf. Biomed. Eng. Sci; 2014. p. 752–6.

42. Dutta R, Hines EL, Gardner JW, Boilot P. Bacteria classification using Cyranose 320 electronic nose. Biomed. Eng. 2002;1:4.

43. Distante C, Siciliano PC, Persaud K. Dynamic cluster recognition with multiple self-Organising maps. Pattern Anal. Appl. 2002;5:306–15.

44. Scott SM, James D, Ali Z. Data analysis for electronic nose systems. Microchim. Acta. 2006;156:183–207.

45. Wei Z, Jin L, Jin Y. Independent component analysis. Statistics (Ber). New York: John Wiley & Sons; 2005. p. 504.

46. Stone JV. Independent component analysis: an introduction. Trends Cogn Sci. 2002;6:59.

47. Lu H, Plataniotis KN, Anastasios V. Multilinear Subspace Learning: Dimensionality Reduction of Multidimensional Data. illustrate. Herbrich R, Graepel T, editors. Boca Raton: CRC Press; 2013.

48. Xu Y, Lu G. Analysis on fisher discriminant criterion and linear separability of feature space. Int. Conf. Comput. Intell. Secur. ICCIAS. 2007;2006:1671–6.

49. Jin Z, Yang JY, Hu ZS, Lou Z. Face recognition based on the uncorrelated discriminant transformation. Pattern Recognit. 2001;34:1405–16.

50. Phillips M, Altorki N, Austin JHM, Cameron RB, Cataneo RN, Greenberg J, et al. Prediction of lung cancer using volatile biomarkers in breath. Cancer Biomark. 2007;3:95–109.

51. Li T, Zhu S, Ogihara M. Using discriminant analysis for multi-class classification: an experimental investigation. Knowl. Inf. Syst. 2006;10:453–72.

52. Mishra M, Jena AR, Das R. A probabilistic neural network approach for classification of vehicle. Int. J. Appl. or Innov. Eng. Manag. 2013;2:367–71.

53. Bhattacharyya N, Jana A. Incremental PNN Classifier for a Versatile Electronic Nose. 3rd Int. Conf. Sens. Technol; 2008. p. 242–7.

54. Antony R, Nandagopal MSG, Rangabhashiyam S, Selvaraju N. Probabilistic neural network prediction of liquid- liquid two phase flows in a circular microchannel. J. Sci. Ind. Res. 2014;73:525–9.

55. Al-Aidaroos K, Bakar A, Othman Z. Medical data classification with naive Bayes approach. Inf. Technol. J. 2012;11:1166–74.

56. Ashari A, Paryudi I, Tjoa AM. Performance comparison between Naïve Bayes, decision tree and k-nearest neighbor in searching alternative Design in an Energy Simulation Tool. Int. J. Adv. Comput. Sci. Appl. 2013;4:33–9.

57. Patil MRR. Heart disease prediction system using naive Bayes and Jelinek-mercer smoothing. Int. J. Adv. Res. Comput Commun. Eng. 2014;3:6787–9.

58. Seo N. A comparison of multi-class support vector machine methods for face recognition. 2007.

59. Naveen T. Word recognition in Indic scripts. International Institute of Information Technology; 2014.

60. Mishra A, Sankaran N, Ranjan V, Jawahar CV. Automatic localization and correction of line segmentation errors. Proceeding work. Doc. Anal. Recognit. - DAR '12; 2012. p. 1–8.

61. Shao X, Li H, Wang N, Zhang Q. Comparison of different classification methods for analyzing electronic nose data to characterize sesame oils and blends. Sensors. 2015;15:26726–42.

62. Dehzangi A, Paliwal K, Lyons J, Sharma A, Sattar A. Proposing a highly accurate protein structural class predictor using segmentation-based features. BMC Genomics. 2014;15:1–13.

63. Zhu W, Zeng N, Wang N. Sensitivity, specificity, accuracy, associated confidence interval and ROC analysis with practical SAS® implementations. Northeast SAS users gr. 2010 heal. Care. Life Sci. 2010:1–9.

64. Zhang Y, Gao G, Liu H, Fu H, Fan J, Wang K, et al. Identification of volatile biomarkers of gastric cancer cells and ultrasensitive electrochemical detection based on sensing interface of au-ag alloy coated MWCNTs. Theranostics. 2014;4:154–62.

65. Jurman G, Riccadonna S, Furlanello C. A comparison of MCC and CEN error measures in multi-class prediction. PLoS One. 2012;7:1–8.

66. Schmidt K, Podmore I. Solid phase microextraction (SPME) method development in analysis of volatile organic compounds (VOCS) as potential biomarkers of cancer. Mol. Biomark. Diagnosis. 2015;6:1–11.

67. Modaresi F, Araghinejad S. A comparative assessment of support vector machines, probabilistic neural networks, and K-nearest neighbor algorithms for water quality classification. Water Resour. Manag. 2014;28:4095–111.

68. Huang K, Zhou Z, King I, R Lyu M. Improving naive Bayesian classifier by discriminative training. Taipei, Taiwan: Proc. Int. Conf. Neural Inf. Process. (ICONIP 05); 2005.

69. Smith D, Wang T, Sulé-Suso J, Španěl P, Haj A. Quantification of acetaldehyde released by lung cancer cells in vitro using selected ion flow tube mass spectrometry. Rapid Commun. Mass Spectrom. 2003;17:845–50.

70. Silva CL, Passos M, Câmara JS. Investigation of urinary volatile organic metabolites as potential cancer biomarkers by solid-phase microextraction in combination with gas chromatography-mass spectrometry. Br. J. Cancer. 2011;105:1894–904.

71. D'Amico A, Pennazza G, Santonico M, Martinelli E, Roscioni C, Galluccio G, et al. An investigation on electronic nose diagnosis of lung cancer. Lung Cancer Elsevier. 2010;68:170–6.

72. Byun H, Yu J, Huh J, Lim J, Nose E, Diseases L. Exhaled breath analysis system based on electronic nose techniques applicable to lung diseases. Hanyang Med. Rev. 2014;34:125–9.

73. Yu J-B, Lim J-O, Byun H-G, Huh J-S. Exhaled breath analysis of lung cancer patients using metal oxide sensor. Journal of Sensor Science and Technology. 2011;20:281–4.

74. Handa H, Usuba A, Maddula S, Baumbach JI, Mineshita M, Miyazawa T. Exhaled breath analysis for lung cancer detection using ion mobility spectrometry. PLoS One. 2014;9:1–13.

75. Phillips M, Cataneo R, Saunders C, Hope P, Schmitt P, Wai J. Volatile biomarkers in the breath of women with breast cancer. J. Breath Res. 2010;4:1–8.

76. Chen X, Xu F, Wang Y, Pan Y, Lu D, Wang P, et al. A study of the volatile organic compounds exhaled by lung cancer cells in vitro for breath diagnosis. Cancer. 2007;110:835–44.

77. Phillips M, Herrera J, Krishnan S, Zain M, Greenberg J, Cataneo RN. Variation in volatile organic compounds in the breath of normal humans. J. Chromatogr. B. 1999;729:75–88.

78. Yu H, Xu L, Wang P. Solid phase microextraction for analysis of alkanes and aromatic hydrocarbons in human breath. J. Chromatogr. B Anal. Technol. Biomed. Life Sci. 2005;826:69–74.

79. Poli D, Carbognani P, Corradi M, Goldoni M, Acampa O, Balbi B, et al. Exhaled volatile organic compounds in patients with non-small cell lung cancer: cross sectional and nested short-term follow-up study. Respir. Res. 2005;6:71.

80. Meggie H, Yoav YB, Orna B, Nir P, Michael P, Anton A, et al. Volatile organic compounds of lung cancer and possible biochemical pathways. Chem. Rev. 2012;112:5949–66.

81. Phillips M, Cataneo R, Ditkoff B, Fisher P, Greenberg J, Gunawardena R, Kwon C, et al. Volatile markers of breast cancer in the breath. Breast J. 2003; 9:184–91.

82. Zheng Z, Lin X. Study on application of medical diagnosis by electronic nose. World Sci. Technol. World Science and Technology Press. 2012;14: 2115–9.

83. Mochalski P, Theurl M, Sponring A. Analysis of volatile organic compounds liberated and metabolized by human umbilical vein endothelial cells (HUVEC) in vitro. Cell Biochem Biophyd. 2015;71:323–9.

84. Fuchs P, Loeseken C, Schubert JK, Miekisch W. Breath gas aldehydes as biomarkers of lung cancer. Int. J. Cancer. 2010;126:2663–70.

85. Nurlisa Y, Ammar Z, Mohammad IO, Shakaff AYM, Masnan MJ, Kamarudin LM, et al. In-vitro diagnosis of single and poly microbial species targeted for diabetic foot infection using e-nose technology. J. Med. Imaging Heal. Informatics. 2015;5:1251–4.

86. Filipiak W, Filipiak A, Sponring A, Schmid T, Zelger B, Ager C, et al. Comparative analyses of volatile organic compounds (VOCs) from patients, tumors and transformed cell lines for the validation of lung cancer-derived breath markers. J. Breath Res. 2014;8:1–13.

14

Re-challenging immune checkpoint inhibitor in a patient with advanced non-small cell lung cancer

Taiki Hakozaki[1], Yusuke Okuma[1*] ⓘ and Jumpei Kashima[2]

Abstract

Background: Currently, immune checkpoint (ICP) inhibitors are essential drugs for the treatment of non-small cell lung cancer (NSCLC). However, in patients previously treated with ICP inhibitors, the efficacy and safety of re-challenging the same or another ICP inhibitor remain unclear.

Case presentation: We present the case of a patient treated with nivolumab for advanced NSCLC who was previously treated with an ICP inhibitor as the first-line chemotherapy along with heavy cytotoxic chemotherapy. After the failure of five lines of chemotherapy, 3 cycles of nivolumab, as the ICP inhibitor re-challenge, the patient achieved a partial response.

Conclusions: This case might suggest that re-challenging an ICP inhibitor could be clinically active in selected patients with advanced NSCLC who progress after achieving an initial clinical benefit with an ICP inhibitor.

Keywords: Nivolumab, Immune checkpoint inhibitor, Non-small cell lung cancer, Immune-related adverse events, Re-challenge

Background

Immune checkpoint (ICP) inhibitors, including nivolumab, pembrolizumab, and atezolizumab, are currently approved for advanced non-small cell lung cancer (NSCLC). The CheckMate-017 [1], CheckMate-057 [2], KEYNOTE-010 [3], and OAK [4] trials demonstrated the clinical benefit, as well as the long-tailed effect, of these agents over docetaxel, which was the standard of care (SoC) in the second-line therapy. The KEYNOTE-024 [5] demonstrated the prolonged progression-free survival (PFS) with pembrolizumab over platinum doublet chemotherapy in the first-line setting. Reportedly, immune-related adverse events (irAEs), which occur in approximately 20% of patients, are the leading adverse events related to ICP inhibitors [2]. Once high-grade irAEs occur during treatment with ICP inhibitors, clinicians are required to discontinue the use of the ICP inhibitors. In a majority of cases, the resolution is

achieved with corticosteroids. However, re-initiation of ICP inhibitors is often challenging because further anti-PD-1/PD-L1 are required to obtain the best durable disease control. To date, limited data are available about the efficacy and safety of re-challenging ICP inhibitors. Furthermore, the median PFS of patients with advanced NSCLC treated with ICP inhibitors is approximately 3–4 months [2], although some patients achieve a long-lasting response with ICP inhibitors. At present, cytotoxic chemotherapy is the SoC for patients after the disease progression with ICP inhibitors. Nonetheless, the efficacy and safety of re-challenging the same or another ICP inhibitor in such settings remain unclear.

Herein, we present the case of a patient with advanced NSCLC who was previously treated with the first-line ICP inhibitor and demonstrated the clinical response to nivolumab as the sixth-line treatment receiving cytotoxic chemotherapy.

Case presentation

A 72-year-old Japanese male presented with an abnormal chest opacity that was determined to be adenocarcinoma

* Correspondence: y-okuma@cick.jp
[1]Department of Thoracic Oncology and Respiratory Medicine, Tokyo Metropolitan Cancer and Infectious Diseases Center Komagome Hospital, 3-18-22 Honkomagome, Bunkyo, Tokyo 113-8677, Japan
Full list of author information is available at the end of the article

of the left upper lobe at cT2aN1M1b Stage IV, without epidermal growth factor receptor (EGFR) mutation and anaplastic lymphoma kinase (ALK) translocation (Fig. 1a). The patient was a never smoker with no specific medical history, except for duodenal ulcer, appendicitis, and hypertension. His Eastern Cooperative Oncology Group (ECOG) performance status was 0. He was enrolled in the clinical trial and was randomized to receive a PD-1 inhibitor (an investigational new drug) as the first-line treatment. After 3 weeks of his second cycle, he presented with a productive cough. A computed tomography (CT) scan revealed an infiltrative shadow and the ground glass opacity around the primary lesion in the left upper lobe (Fig. 1c). In addition, transbronchial lung biopsy suggested drug-induced alveolitis, which was considered as grade 2 irAE caused by the ICP inhibitor (Fig. 2). Accordingly, we administered and down-titrated oral prednisolone (25 mg/day), which reduced alveolitis to grade 1 after 2 weeks and normalized by 6 months. After remaining at a stable disease (SD) for 2 months (Fig. 1d), the restaging CT scan of the patient at 4 months revealed an enlarging primary tumor (Fig. 1b). He was subsequently treated with cytotoxic agents, such as cisplatin, pemetrexed, docetaxel, S-1, and nanoparticle albumin–bound paclitaxel, all of which ended with the disease progression (Fig. 1e). After that, the patient was treated with nivolumab (2 mg/kg, day 1, every 2 weeks) as the sixth-line therapy. After 6 weeks of initiating nivolumab treatment, a CT scan revealed a partial response in the primary lung lesion (Fig. 1f). After 6 cycles of nivolumab, the routine imaging surveillance of the patient revealed no disease progression and no irAEs, including recurrence of alveolitis.

Discussion and conclusions

Here, we reported the case of a patient who responded to nivolumab in the later line of treatment, which had previously failed with a PD-1 inhibitor and cytotoxic

chemotherapy. Although the patient experienced irAE with the PD-1 inhibitor treatment, the recurrence of irAE was not observed in nivolumab treatment. To date, limited published data is available about the efficacy and safety of re-challenging ICP inhibitors. To the best of our knowledge, no study to date has elucidated the clinical benefit of re-challenging an ICP inhibitor in patients with advanced NSCLC.

In patients with metastatic melanoma, some studies have reported the efficacy and safety profile of retreatment with ipilimumab, a fully monoclonal antibody against cytotoxic T-lymphocyte-associated antigen-4 (CTLA-4), or a combination of nivolumab and ipilimumab, after an initial period of disease control (Table 1) [6–8]. Regarding the efficacy, re-challenging ICP inhibitors achieved a relatively favorable response. For patients who were retreated with ipilimumab after the initial failure with ipilimumab, the overall response rate (ORR) and disease control rate (DCR) were 11.8–23.0% and 48.4–60.5%, respectively. In contrast, for patients who were only retreated with nivolumab after the initial failure with a combination of ipilimumab and nivolumab, the ORR and DCR were 70.0 and 88.8%, respectively [6, 7, 9, 10]. In these studies, the response of some patients to ipilimumab improved upon re-challenging compared with induction, implying that the re-challenge with ipilimumab induced renewed or even deeper antitumor activity, although the precise mechanism remains poorly understood. In this case, the patient's immunity against the tumor, which shifted to "escape" phase at the time of pembrolizumab therapy failure, might have been reactivated by any changes during subsequent treatments. Possible justifications for the transition in the responsiveness to ICP inhibitors include changes in the (1) tumor mutation and neoantigen load, (2) tumor-infiltrating T-cell repertoire, and (3) immunosuppressive tumor microenvironment. In our patient, such changes might have been induced by previous ICP inhibitor and

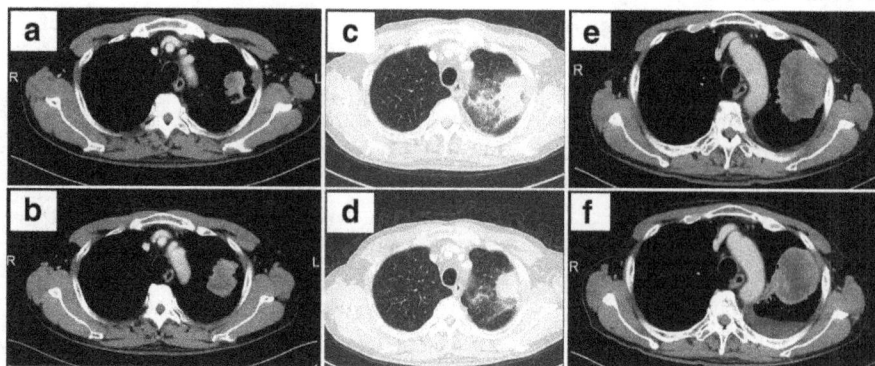

Fig. 1 Radiographic results before and after ICP inhibitors. The CT scan shows the primary lesion in the right upper lobe before the first-line ICP inhibitor (**a**), SD after 2 months accompanied by alveolitis (**c**, **d**), and enlarged after 4 months (**b**). After the failure of five lines of chemotherapy (**e**), the primary lesion responded to 3 cycles of nivolumab (**f**)

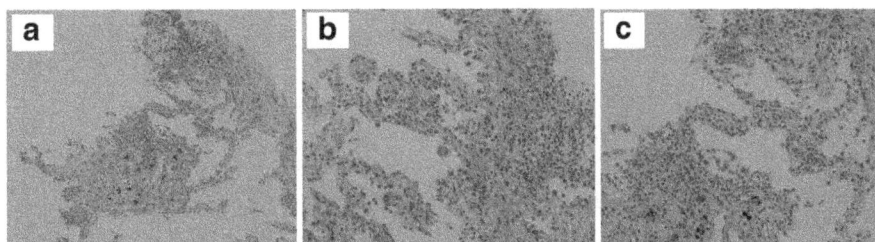

Fig. 2 Lung biopsy demonstrated mild fibrinolytic hyperplasia of alveolar septum and strong infiltration of lymphocytes, including small fraction of eosinophil. Alveolar cells were swollen and form cells were accumulated ((**a**): X100, (**b**, **c**): X200)

cytotoxic chemotherapy exposure or disease progression itself. Remarkably, a recent research of the T-cell repertoire demonstrated the association of responses to nivolumab with different patterns of the T-cell diversity dynamics according to previous ipilimumab exposure [11].

Regarding safety, ipilimumab retreatment was well tolerated [6–10], and any grade irAEs and grade 3 or 4 irAEs were observed in 21.6–60.4% and 5.9–30.0%, respectively (Table 1). In addition, the frequency of treatment-related irAEs during retreatment was similar to those observed during induction and was manageable with established algorithms used in induction immunotherapy. A study suggested that the type of toxicity in induction immunotherapy, the absence of steroids at re-challenge, and the interval before re-challenge could be potential predictors of recurrent or novel severe toxicities, whereas the severity of initial toxicity or the duration of immunosuppression demonstrated little correlation [7].

In a prior case series focusing on patients who developed pneumonitis associated with PD-1/PD-L1 inhibitors, three among twelve (25%) patients who underwent re-challenge with ICP inhibitors after an initial pneumonitis event experienced recurrent pneumonitis, which was resolved in all with corticosteroids or ICP inhibitor discontinuation [12]. Interestingly, some patients experienced recurrence of pneumonitis after initial clinical improvement without re-challenge of ICP inhibitors.

In addition, recent studies have highlighted the correlation of the development of irAEs with better clinical outcomes of ICP inhibitors treatment in NSCLC as well as melanoma [13–15]. The CheckMate-153 trial represented the prolonged PFS of patients with NSCLC receiving the continuous nivolumab treatment compared to those who discontinued within a year [16]. The increment in the incidence of irAE is proportional to the duration of ICP inhibitors treatment, raising the conflict about the efficacy of ICP inhibitors re-challenge for patients with NSCLC. Hence, further research is warranted to establish the optimal sequence of treatment, including the consideration for ICP inhibitors re-challenge based on these insights. At present, with little evidence on efficacy and safety of ICP inhibitors in patients with advanced NSCLC, ICP inhibitors require deliberation on the risk–benefit of re-challenging on the individual basis with adequate informed consent.

This case might suggest the potential efficacy of re-challenging ICP inhibitors in selected patients with advanced NSCLC who progress after achieving initial clinical benefit with ICP inhibitor treatment. Nevertheless, further investigation is warranted to validate the efficacy and safety of re-challenging ICP inhibitors in patients with NSCLC.

Abbreviations
CT: Computed tomography; irAEs: Immune-related adverse effects; NSCLC: Non-small cell lung cancer; PD-1: Programmed death receptor-1; PD-L1: Programmed death receptor ligand 1;; SoC: Standard of care

Acknowledgments
The authors would like to thank Enago (https://www.enago.jp) for English language editing.

Funding
No specific funding was received for this work.

Table 1 Retreatment with ICP inhibitors in metastatic melanoma

	Ipi → Ipi			Ipi + Nivo→ Nivo
	Robert et al. [5] (n = 38)	Chiarion-Sileni et al [7] (n = 51)	Lebbe et al [10] (n = 122)	Pollack et al [8] (n = 80)
ORR (%)	18.4	11.8	23.0	70.0
DCR (%)	60.5	54.9	48.4	88.8
All grade irAE (%)	57.9	21.6	64.0	50.0
Grade 3/4 irAE (%)	10.5	13.5	13.5	30.0

Ipi ipilimumab, *Nivo* nivolumab, *ORR* overall response rate, *DCR* disease control rate, *irAE* immune-related adverse event

Authors' contributions
TH, JK, and YO acquired the clinical data and drafted the manuscript, read and approved the final manuscript. JK was responsible for pathological diagnosis.

Competing interests

All authors declare that they have no competing interests.

Author details

[1]Department of Thoracic Oncology and Respiratory Medicine, Tokyo Metropolitan Cancer and Infectious Diseases Center Komagome Hospital, 3-18-22 Honkomagome, Bunkyo, Tokyo 113-8677, Japan. [2]Department of Pathology, Tokyo Metropolitan Cancer and Infectious Diseases Center Komagome Hospital, Tokyo 113-8677, Japan.

References

1. Brahmer J, Reckamp KL, Baas P, Crino L, Eberhardt WE, Poddubskaya E, Antonia S, Pluzanski A, Vokes EE, Holgado E, et al. Nivolumab versus docetaxel in advanced squamous-cell non-small-cell lung Cancer. N Engl J Med. 2015;373(2):123–35.
2. Borghaei H, Paz-Ares L, Horn L, Spigel DR, Steins M, Ready NE, Chow LQ, Vokes EE, Felip E, Holgado E, et al. Nivolumab versus docetaxel in advanced nonsquamous non-small-cell lung Cancer. N Engl J Med. 2015;373(17):1627–39.
3. Herbst RS, Baas P, Kim DW, Felip E, Perez-Gracia JL, Han JY, Molina J, Kim JH, Arvis CD, Ahn MJ, et al. Pembrolizumab versus docetaxel for previously treated, PD-L1-positive, advanced non-small-cell lung cancer (KEYNOTE-010): a randomised controlled trial. Lancet. 2016;387(10027):1540–50.
4. Rittmeyer A, Barlesi F, Waterkamp D, Park K, Ciardiello F, von Pawel J, Gadgeel SM, Hida T, Kowalski DM, Dols MC, et al. Atezolizumab versus docetaxel in patients with previously treated non-small-cell lung cancer (OAK): a phase 3, open-label, multicentre randomised controlled trial. Lancet. 2017;389(10066):255–65.
5. Reck M, Rodriguez-Abreu D, Robinson AG, Hui R, Csoszi T, Fulop A, Gottfried M, Peled N, Tafreshi A, Cuffe S, et al. Pembrolizumab versus chemotherapy for PD-L1-positive non-small-cell lung Cancer. N Engl J Med. 2016;375(19): 1823–33.
6. Robert C, Schadendorf D, Messina M, Hodi FS, O'Day S, investigators MDX. Efficacy and safety of retreatment with ipilimumab in patients with pretreated advanced melanoma who progressed after initially achieving disease control. Clin Cancer Res. 2013;19(8):2232–9.
7. Pollack MH, Betof A, Dearden H, Rapazzo K, Valentine I, Brohl AS, Ancell KK, Long GV, Menzies AM, Eroglu Z, et al. Safety of resuming anti-PD-1 in patients with immune-related adverse events (irAEs) during combined anti-CTLA-4 and anti-PD1 in metastatic melanoma. Ann Oncol. 2018;29(1):250–55.
8. Spain L, Walls G, Messiou C, Turajlic S, Gore M, Larkin J. Efficacy and toxicity of rechallenge with combination immune checkpoint blockade in metastatic melanoma: a case series. Cancer Immunol Immunother. 2017; 66(1):113–7.
9. Lebbe C, Weber JS, Maio M, Neyns B, Harmankaya K, Hamid O, O'Day SJ, Konto C, Cykowski L, McHenry MB, et al. Survival follow-up and ipilimumab retreatment of patients with advanced melanoma who received ipilimumab in prior phase II studies. Ann Oncol. 2014;25(11):2277–84.
10. Chiarion-Sileni V, Pigozzo J, Ascierto PA, Simeone E, Maio M, Calabro L, Marchetti P, De Galitiis F, Testori A, Ferrucci PF, et al. Ipilimumab retreatment in patients with pretreated advanced melanoma: the expanded access programme in Italy. Br J Cancer. 2014;110(7):1721–6.
11. Riaz N, Havel JJ, Makarov V, Desrichard A, Urba WJ, Sims JS, Hodi FS, Martin-Algarra S, Mandal R, Sharfman WH, et al. Tumor and microenvironment evolution during immunotherapy with Nivolumab. Cell. 2017;171(4):934–49. e915
12. Naidoo J, Wang X, Woo KM, Iyriboz T, Halpenny D, Cunningham J, Chaft JE, Segal NH, Callahan MK, Lesokhin AM, et al. Pneumonitis in patients treated with anti-programmed death-1/programmed death ligand 1 therapy. J Clin Oncol. 2017;35(7):709–17.
13. Haratani K, Hayashi H, Chiba Y, Kudo K, Yonesaka K, Kato R, Kaneda H, Hasegawa Y, Tanaka K, Takeda M, et al. Association of Immune-Related Adverse Events with Nivolumab Efficacy in non-small-cell lung Cancer. JAMA Oncol. 2017;
14. Postow MA, Chesney J, Pavlick AC, Robert C, Grossmann K, McDermott D, Linette GP, Meyer N, Giguere JK, Agarwala SS, et al. Nivolumab and ipilimumab versus ipilimumab in untreated melanoma. N Engl J Med. 2015; 372(21):2006–17.
15. Sankarapandian V, Rehman SM, David KV, Christopher P, Ganesh A, Pricilla RA. Sensitizing undergraduate medical students to consultation skills: a pilot study. Natl Med J India. 2014;27(5):276–9.
16. Spigel DR, McLeod M, Hussein MA, Waterhouse DM, AU-Einhorn L, Horn L, Creelan B, Babu S, Leighl NB, Couture F, et al. Randomized results of fixed-duration (1-yr) vs continuous nivolumab in patients (pts) with advanced non-small cell lung cancer (NSCLC). Ann Oncol. 2017;28(suppl_5). https://doi.org/10.1093/annonc/mdx380.002

15

Association of genetic polymorphisms *CYP2A6*2 rs1801272* and *CYP2A6*9 rs28399433* with tobacco-induced lung Cancer

Nada Ezzeldin[1], Dalia El-Lebedy[3], Amira Darwish[2,5]*, Ahmed El Bastawisy[2], Shereen Hamdy Abd Elaziz[3], Mirhane Mohamed Hassan[3] and Amal Saad-Hussein[4]

Abstract

Background: Several studies have reported the role of CYP2A6 genetic polymorphisms in smoking and lung cancer risk with some contradictory results in different populations. The purpose of the current study is to assess the contribution of the *CYP2A6*2 rs1801272* and *CYP2A6*9 rs28399433* gene polymorphisms and tobacco smoking in the risk of lung cancer in an Egyptian population.

Methods: A case-control study was conducted on 150 lung cancer cases and 150 controls. All subjects were subjected to blood sampling for Extraction of genomic DNA and Genotyping of the *CYP2A6* gene SNPs (*CYP2A6*2 (1799 T > A) rs1801272* and *CYP2A6*9 (− 48 T > G)* rs28399433 by Real time PCR.

Results: AC and CC genotypes were detected in *CYP2A6*9*; and AT genotype in *CYP2A6*2*. The frequency of *CYP2A6*2* and *CYP2A6*9* were 0.7% and 3.7% respectively in the studied Egyptian population. All cancer cases with slow metabolizer variants were NSCLC. Non-smokers represented 71.4% of the *CYP2A6* variants. There was no statistical significant association between risk of lung cancer, smoking habits, heaviness of smoking and the different polymorphisms of *CYP2A6* genotypes.

Conclusion: The frequency of slow metabolizers *CYP2A6*2* and *CYP2A6*9* are poor in the studied Egyptian population. Our findings did not suggest any association between *CYP2A6* genotypes and risk of lung cancer.

Keywords: Lung cancer, CYP2A6, CYP2A6*2, CYP2A6*9, Polymorphism, Tobacco smoking, Nicotine metabolism, Egyptian

Background

Lung Cancer is the most common cancer worldwide in term of new cases (1.8 million, 12.9%) & in term of death (1.6 million death, 19.4%) [1]. Cytochrome *P450 2A6 (CYP2A6)*, one of the forms of CYP expressed in the human respiratory tract, is the main enzyme involved in the metabolic activation of tobacco-specific nitrosamines to their carcinogenic forms [2]. CYP2A6

* Correspondence: amiradd@yahoo.com
[2]Medical Oncology, National Cancer Institute, Cairo University, Cairo, Egypt
[5]National Cancer Institute (NCI), Fom-Elkhalig Square, P.O.Box: 11796, Cairo, Egypt
Full list of author information is available at the end of the article

inactivates nicotine, the principle component in cigarette smoke, to cotinine [3]. Thus it is reasonable to hypothesize that CYP2A6 activity may be related to the susceptibility of developing lung cancer among smokers.

The existence of a *CYP2A6* genetic polymorphism was suggested by evidence that there was extensive inter individual difference in the capacity of coumarin 7-hydroxylation [4, 5]. Detecting the alleles of CYP2A6 can help us to describe different smoking behaviors and smoking-related diseases among individuals [6]. Numerous characterized alleles and some haplotypes that are uncharacterized have been identified & most of these are derived from single nucleotide polymorphisms (SNPS) in regulatory & coding regions [7]. The wild-type allele that is considered as a reference is CYP2A6*1A [8]. Currently CYP2A6*6, CYP2A6*7, CYP2A6*9, CYP2A6*10, CYP2A6*11, &, CYP2A6*13 are known to lead to reduced enzymatic activities while 5 variants (CYP2A6*2, CYP2A6*4, CYP2A6*5, CYP2A6*12, & CYP2A6*20) produce no functional enzyme [2, 9–12].

The CYP2A6*2 variant, appears to be one of the causal polymorphisms associated with decreased or virtually absent nicotine metabolism in Caucasians [13, 14]. In East and Southeast Asian populations such as Chinese, Korean, Japanese, Malaysian and Thai, CYP2A6*2 is non-existent [15–19]. CYP2A6*4C is the most widely studied allele in all populations. East Asian populations such as Japanese, Chinese, Korean & malysian showed the highest frequency among populations (4.9–25.6%) [2, 12, 17, 20]. Caucasians had a frequency lower than 3% while Middle East populations such as Turkish and Iranian showed a lower frequency [21].CYP2A6*7 has a higher frequency in East and Southeast Asian populations [6, 17, 19, 22]. On the other hand, in Indian, African, Canadian native this allele isn't found. It has also been reported in a lower frequency in Caucasian (≤0.3%) [21].

The CYP2A6*9 is present in all ethnic groups but its frequency varies from 6 to 8% in Europeans & Africans to 21% in Asian populations [23, 24]. Middle East population as Turkish [10] & Iranian [25] also showed a high frequency. CYP2A6*9 was reported as one of the most common variants of CYP2A6 in Caucasians that modifies the levels of enzyme expression [10].

Considerable studies have reported the role of CYP2A6 genetic polymorphisms in lung cancer risk with some contradictory results in different populations from ethnic variation [2, 26–30]. It seemed probable that genetic polymorphism in CYP2A6 causing a lack of or reduced activity might result in lowering tobacco-induced lung cancer risk, by decreased smoking. This is due to decreased activation of carcinogens such as nitrosamines present in tobacco smoke, or by lower nicotine catabolism or by both [2, 6].

Thus knowing that CYP2A6 activity affects genetic suscebility to tobacco- induced lung cancer, individuals possessing the CYP2A6*2 and/or CYP2A6*9, but not the CYP2A6*1A allele would be expected to be at lower risk for lung cancer.

We conducted a case-control study to assess the contribution of the CYP2A6*2 rs1801272 and CYP2A6*9 rs28399433 gene polymorphisms and tobacco smoking in the risk of lung cancer in an Egyptian population.

Methods
Subjects
This study was a collaboration between National Research Center and National Cancer Institute (NCI) Cairo University. A case-control study was conducted that included 150 unrelated adult patients with primary lung cancer and 150 unrelated controls. The case series consisted of patients presented to NCI details of which have been described elsewhere [31]. Almost half of the patients seen at NCI-Cairo came from the Cairo metropolitan area, whereas the rest of the patients were from other regions in South and North Egypt. Patients from the non-Cairo regions sought management at NCI-Cairo because it has the largest lung cancer services in Egypt for surgical and medical oncology & radiotherapy. All subjects included in the study were interviewed to fulfill questionnaire covering demographic information, data on smoking, occupational history and family history of malignancy. All subjects were aware of the study protocol and gave written informed consent. The study was approved by the ethical committee of the National Research Center.

DNA extraction
A peripheral blood sample is obtained from each subject through venipuncture. Blood was collected in tubes with EDETA. Extraction of genomic DNA was performed using a QIAamp DNA extraction kit according to the manufacturer's protocol.

Selecting SNPs
We searched relevant publications from 1990 to 2013 in the National Center for Biotechnology Information (NCBI) data base using the following keywords: "CYP2A6", "cigarette smoking", "lung cancer" and "genetics". Based on publication in Caucasian, African and Asian populations, we expect that: CYP2A6*2 and CYP2A6*9 would be interesting because the kinetics of nicotine metabolism are altered in individuals carrying any or both of these alleles.

Genotyping of CYP2A6 gene
CYP2A6*2 and CYP2A6*9 polymorphisms were genotyped using TaqMan® SNP Genotyping Assays. Primers and probes were designed by Applied Biosystems (Foster City, CA, USA) and analyses were performed on ABI 7500 Real Time PCR system (Applied Biosystems) according to the manufacturer's protocol.

For CYP2A6*2 (1799 T > A) [rs1801272; assay ID: C_27861808_60], the VIC/FAM sequence was as follows: CCCCTGCTCACCGCCAGTGCCCCGG[T/A]GGGCGTCGATGAGGAAGCCCGCCTC.

For CYP2A6*9 (– 48 T > G) [rs28399433; assay ID: C_30634332_10], the VIC/FAM sequence was as follows: GTGACGGCTGGGGTGGTTTGCCTTT[A/C]TACTGCCTGAAAAAGAGGGATGGAC.

For genotyping quality control, negative controls were included in all SNPs and 10% of samples were randomly selected and analyzed in duplicates and the concordance rate was 100%.

Statistical analysis

Data were analyzed using SPSS version 18.0 (Chicago, IL, USA). Data were expressed as number and percentages of total for categorical variables. The Chi-square test (χ^2) was used to compare the distribution of CYP2A6 genotypes between the groups. Likelihood ratio was used when the expected count was less than 5 in more than 20% of the cells. The associations between genotype and risk of lung cancer were estimated by odds ratio (OR) and 95% confidence interval (95% CI) using logistic regression models. The ORs were adjusted for age, smoking status, and pack-years. P-value < 0.05 was considered significant.

Results

Table 1 presents the baseline characteristics of 150 lung cancer cases and 150 controls. There were statistically significant differences between age & gender. The mean age of patients is (56.7 ± 9.79 years) and that of controls is (43.3 ± 11.1 years) ($p < 0.001$),

denoting that older age is associated with higher risk of lung cancer. A statistically significant gender difference was found between the 2 groups; 48.7% males and 51.3% females in controls and 76% males and 24% females in cancer cases, ($X^2 = 25.82$, $P < 0.0001$) with increased males risk to develop lung cancers than females.

Smoking was significantly higher among cancer cases (62% smokers) compared to control (20% smokers), $P < 0.0001$, and (OR = 2.78, CI: 2.0–3.86) denoting a higher risk to develop lung cancer in smokers by 2.78 times the non-smokers, independent of the heaviness of smoking.

Two genotypes were detected in CYP2A6*9; heterozygote AC and homozygote CC. AC genotype was found in 4 cases in control group; 3 males and 1 female, all cases were non-smokers and 6 cases in lung cancer group; 4 males and 2 females from which 2 males were smokers > 20 pack-year. All cases were diagnosed as NSCLC (2 adenocarcinoma, 1 squamous and 3 others). CC genotype was found in 1 control case, a male, smoking > 20 pack-year (Fig. 1). One heterozygous genotype was detected in CYP2A6*2; AT. It was found in one case of lung cancer; a non-smoker male diagnosed as adenocarcinoma (Fig. 2). The 2 polymorphisms CYP2A6*9 AC

Table 1 Characteristics of control and lung cancer cases and association between cigarette smoking and risk of lung cancer

	Control n = 150	Lung cancer n = 150	P value	
Age(years) Mean + SD	43.3 ± 11.1	56.7 ± 9.79	< 0.001	
Sex n(%)				
Male	73 (48.7%)	114 (76%)	< 0.0001	
Female	77 (51.3%)	36 (24%)		
Histological Types n (%)				
SCLC		20 (13.3%)		
NSCLC		130 (87.7%)		
Adenocarcinoma		73 (56.2%)		
Squamous cell carcinoma		18 (13.8%)		
Others[a]		39 (30%)		
	Control n (%)	Lung cancer n (%)	OR (95% C.I.)	P value
Smoking Status				
Smoker n (%)	30(20%)	93(62%)	2.78 (2.0–3.86)	0.0001
Non-smoker n (%)	120(80%)	57(38%)		
Pack-year				
< 20 n (%)	16(53.3%)	37(39.8%)	0.58 (0.25–1.32)	NS
> 20 n (%)	14(46.7%)	56(60.2%)		

SCLC small cell lung cancer, NSCLC non- small cell lung cancer
[a]Large cell carcinoma, undifferentiated, spindle, mucinous, Broncho alveolar carcinoma, carcinoid, sarcomatoid carcinoma, anaplastic

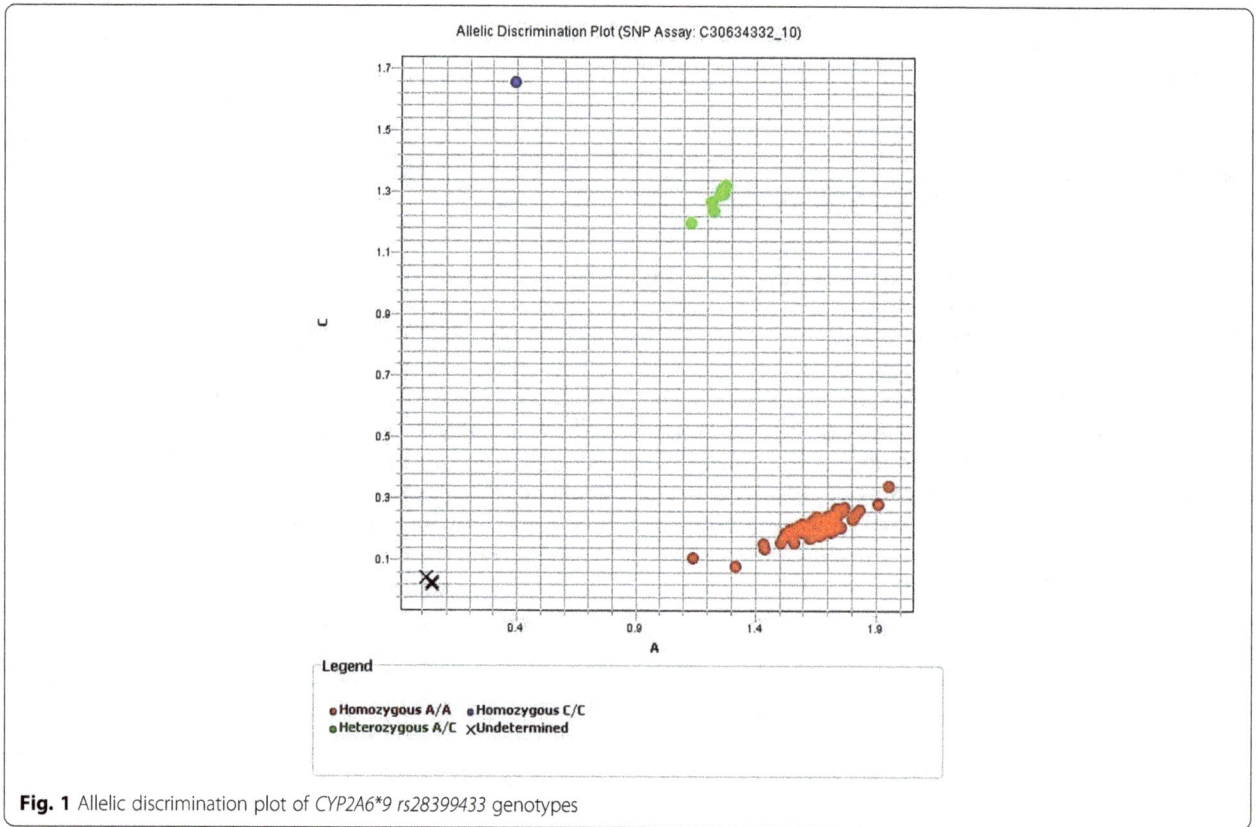

Fig. 1 Allelic discrimination plot of *CYP2A6*9 rs28399433* genotypes

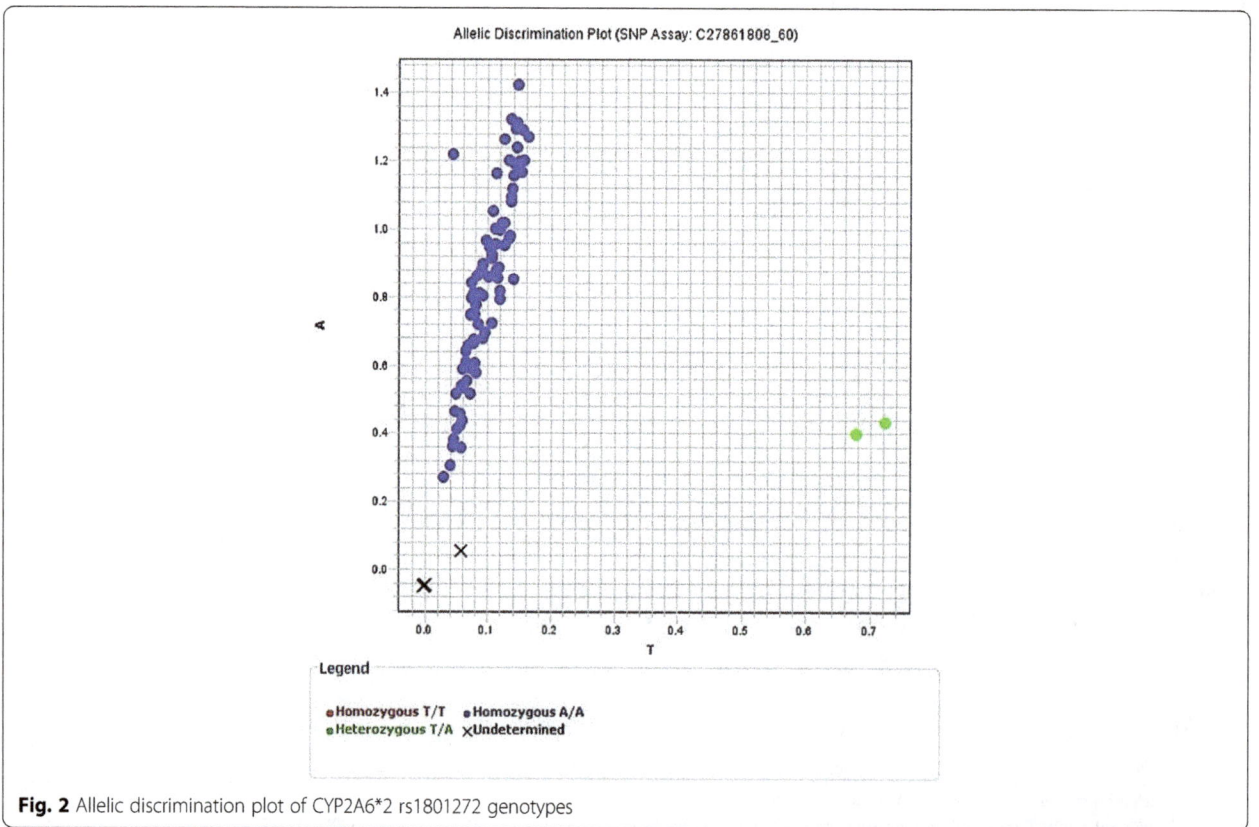

Fig. 2 Allelic discrimination plot of CYP2A6*2 rs1801272 genotypes

Table 2 Frequency of *CYP2A6* genotypes in the studied Egyptian population

Total n = 300	CYP2A6*1 AA n = 287 [a]	CYP2A6*9 n=12[a]	P-value	CYP2A6*2 n=2[a]	P-value
Age(years)					
Mean + SD	49.8 ± 12.3	51.6 ± 13.3	0.34	45.5 ± 6.4	0.62
Sex					
Male n (%)	178 (62%)	7 (63.6%)	0.74	1 (50%)	0.72
Female n (%)	109 (38%)	4 (36.4%)		1 (50%)	
Smoking Status					
Smoker n (%)	120 (41.8%)	3 (18.2%)	0.15	0 (0%)	0.15
Non-smoker n (%)	167 (58.2%)	9 (81.8%)		2 (100%)	
Pack-year					
< 20 n (%)	53 (44.2%)	0 (0%)	0.17	0 (0%)	
≥ 20 n (%)	67 (55.8%)	3 (100%)			

[a]One case had the 2 polymorphisms was added to both number of cases of CYP2A6*9 and CYP2A6*2

Table 3 *CYP2A6* genotypes, cigarette smoking and risk of lung cancer in the studied Egyptian population

	CYP2A6		
	CYP2A6*1 (AA)	CYP2A6*9 (AC)	CYP2A6*2 (AT)
Control/ cancer n	144/143	5/6	1/1
OR (95% C.I.)	1.2 (0.36–4.02)	0.8 (0.2–2.8)	0.99 (0.1–16)
P value	P = 0.77	P = 0.77	P = 0.99
Non-Smoker			
Control/ cancer n	114/52	5/4	1/1
OR (95% C.I.)	1.7 (0.4–6.7)	0.6 (0.1–2.2)	2.1 (0.1–34.6)
P value	P = 0.42	P = 0.42	P = 0.60
Smoker			
Control/ cancer n	30/91	0/2	(a)
OR (95% C.I.)	1.0 (0.99–1.1)	1.0 (1.0–1.1)	
P value	P = 0.30	P = 0.30	
Pack-year < 20			
Control/ cancer n	16/37		
OR (95% C.I.)	(a)	(a)	(a)
P value			
Pack-year ≥20			
Control/ cancer n	14/54	0/2	(a)
OR (95% C.I.)	1.0 (0.99–1.09)	1.0 (0.99–1.1)	
P value	P = 0.36	P = 0.36	

OR of the *CYP2A6*9 (CC)* cannot be calculated as it is one case only. (a): cannot be calculated there is no cases in one of the two groups

and *CYP2A6*2 AT* were detected in a non-smoker female control case.

There was no statistical difference between the Wild type *CYP2A6*1AA* and *CYP2A6*9, CYP2A6*2* polymorphisms regarding age, sex, smoking status, pack-year (Table 2). There was no statistical significant association between risk of lung cancer, smoking habits, heaviness of smoking and the different polymorphisms of *CYP2A6* genotypes (Table 3).

There was no statistical significant difference in the *CYP2A6* genotypes in different stages of lung cancer (Table 4).

Discussion

CYP2A6 has been proposed as a novel target for smoking cessation because of its major contribution to nicotine metabolism. To the best of our knowledge this is the first study to address the relationship between CYP2A6 status, smoking & lung cancer in an Egyptian population. Our data are valuable because cases that presented to NCI were from different governorates of Egypt. The CYP2A6*1A allele is considered the wild type, corresponding to normal enzymatic activity [16]. Based on reports in the literature, we expect that CYP2A6*2 & CYP2A6*9 would be intresting because they code for reduced activity. Many human nicotine pharmacokinetic & CYP2A6 studies have demonstrated the contribution of multiple decrease-, increase-, and loss-of-function polymorphisms in CYP2A6 to the variability in nicotine metabolism [23]. In our study the control group was sampled at random thus their age

Table 4 Effects of CYP2A6 genotypes on Stages of lung cancer in 150 lung cancer cases

Genotypes of CYP2A6 n = 150		Stage			Likelihood	P-value
		II n = 25	III n = 44	IV n = 81		
CYP2A6*1 AA	143 (95.3%)	23 (92%)	43 (97.7%)	77 (95.1%)	2.25	0.69
CYP2A6*9 AC	6 (4.0%)	2 (8%)	1 (2.3%)	3 (3.7%)		
CYP2A6*2 AT	1 (0.7%)	0 (0.0%)	0 (0.0%)	1 (1.2%)		

distribution was much younger than that of lung cancer cases. This explains the statistical significant difference in age between cases and control. Age isn't a confounder in our study and isn't intended to be examined in the analysis of CYP2A6 polymorphism. The tested polymorphisms are not affected by age and our aim was to to assess the contribution of the CYP2A6*2 and CYP2A6*9 gene polymorphisms and tobacco smoking in the risk of lung cancer.

Frequency and ethnic variation

Our results showed that the frequency of CYP2A6*2 and CYP2A6*9 were 0.7% and 3.7% respectively. There was no statististical significant difference in the frequency of the tested variants between control and lung cancer goups. Further statistical studies were difficult due to low frequency of variants. Neverthelss, these poor frequencies were reported in other studies. In African populations (Afro American & Ethiopian), the CYP2A6*2 frequency is less than 1% [16, 17, 19] while it was found to be one of the major variant alleles in Caucasians; with frequency 1–3% [17, 19]. The frequency of CYP2A6*2, and *9 detected in a Brazilian population was 1.7, and 5.7% respectively [32] while in Turkish population the CYP2A6* 2 is not existing [33]. Recent researches that had analysed different frequencies of CYP2A6 genetic variants in different ethnic groups; found that the frequency of CYP2A6*2, and *9 in Caucasian almost double our findings in the Egyptian population [23]. The frequencies of CYP2A6 *2 allele in different ethenic population were 1.1%, 0.0%, 2.2%, 0.0%, 0.0% and those of CYP2A6*9 were 7.1%, 15.5%, 7.1%, 15.6%, 20.3% in African American, Canadian, Caucasian, Chinese and Japanese respectively [9, 10, 12, 18, 19, 34–36].

Smoking

Many studies have concluded that CYP2A6 slow inactivator, or absent enzyme activity genotypes are associated with lower risk for smoking, altered smoking intensity, fewer cigarettes smoked, and increased quitting [2, 13, 19, 20, 37, 38]. Nevertheless, other studies are in disagreement with these conclusions [26, 39, 40].

Little is known about the genetic factors contributing to smoking in Egyptians. In the present study, although

no statistical difference were found between CYP2A6 variants and smoking status, most cases with CYP2A6 polymorphisms were non-smoker, 10 cases from 13; 100% and 81.8% non-smokers in CYP2A6*2 and CYP2A6*9 respectively compared to 58% in CYP2A6*1 indicating a role of CYP2A6 gene variants in affecting smoking status, with slow metabolizers smoking less than fast metabolizers. Verde & colleagues [41], found that CYP2A6*2 polymorphism was strongly linked to smoking status. Moreover, it was found that the amounts of cigarette consumed daily by individuals, who harbored CYP2A6*9, were significantly less than that consumed by those who carried CYP2A6*1 (P = 0.01) [6]. Slow metabolizers (as determined by CYP2A6*2, *4, *9 and *12 alleles), are very unlikely to be smokers, take smaller puff volumes and smoke fewer cigarettes per day. They also have lower levels of dependence, benefit more from nicotine patch replacement therapy and are more capable to quit compared to normal metabolizers [2, 16, 19, 38, 42–48].

Contrastingly two different meta-analyses failed to confirm any evidence of the association between the CYP2A6 diminished-activity polymorphisms and cigarette consumption. The investigators of both concluded that there is no association between the reduced-activity CYP2A6 alleles and the number of cigarettes smoked [49, 50].

Malaiyandi & colleagues [16] have postulated that the continued effect of slow metabolism on reducing the number of cigarette smoked, allthrough the smoking history of slow inactivators, may influence withdrawal mechanisms and consequently aids quitting among these individuals. The noticeable temporal effect of CYP2A6 on smoking behavior and nicotine dependence necessitates further research. The poor frequencies of the variant alleles of slow inactivators extend our understanding of the impact of CYP2A6 genotype on smoking risk and behavior in Egyptian, and have important implications for smoking aetiology. The number of smokers in Egypt is 13 million out of a population of 90 million according to statistics by the state-run Central Agency for Public Mobilization and Statistics. There is minimal change in the number of smokers inspite of 40% tax increments since 2010 or photos of damaged lungs placed on every pack of cigarettes as a warning from the hazardous health consequences of smoking [51] (Mansour, 2013).

According to the study by Loffredo & colleagues [52], the national prevalence of former cigarette smoking among males was 18.1%, and 27.5% reported current smoking.

Lung cancer

Sqamous cell carcinoma and Small cell lung cancer (SCLC) are major types of lung cancer caused by smoking, while adenocarcinoma isn't regarded as a common histological type in smokers [53, 54]. In the present study, all lung cancer cases (6), with *CYP2A6*2 and *9 polymorphisms* were diagnosed as NSCLC, 3 of them were adenocarcinoma. Statistical interpretations could not be done due to the low frequency of variants in the study. A former study [29], did not find a significant association between this CYP2A6 polymorphism and risk of adenocarcinoma or other histological types of lung cancer.

Studies of CYP2A6 inhibition demonstrated a role for the enzyme in the occurrence of lung cancer and hence have directed the interest in CYP2A6 as a target for cancer prevention [28, 55]. Investigating the role of CYP2A6 genotype in effective programs implemented for lung cancer screening may improve cancer risk prediction and assist selecting individuals who could benefit from preventative measures whether behavioural or pharmacological [56]. Ariyoshi & colleagues [2], demonstrated that individuals homozygous for the *CYP2A6*1A* allele (*1A/*1A) have the highest risk for tobacco-related lung cancer in Japanese male smokers. They also concluded that due to higher prevelence of the functionally active CYP2A6 gene in Caucasians compared to Asians, the genetic polymorphism of CYP2A6 may be a factor justifying the interindividual difference in predisposition to lung cancer among smokers. Consistent to the previous concept Benowitz et al. [57] concluded that the slower nicotine metabolism and therefore lower nicotine uptake per cigarette may explain lower incidence of lung cancer in Asians compared to Caucasians. In the present study we failed to find a significant association between CYP2A6 genotypes and risk of lung cancer. Our data is similar to the study by London & colleagues [39] who reported no significant relationship between the CYP2A6 inactive allele, mainly concentrating on the *CYP2A6*2*, and lung cancer risk.

Discordant results have been demonstrated on the association of CYP2A6 genetic polymorphisms and lung cancer risk [2, 26, 27, 29, 39, 58]. These contradictory results seem to be caused by the too small frequencies of the inactive alleles such as *CYP2A6*2* and *CYP2A6*4* in some studies to find a possible relationship with adequate statistical power [26, 29]. The protecting effect of CYP2A6 slow metabolism on lung cancer risk is more obvious in populations including subjects common to harbour CYP2A6 non-functional alleles as the Japanese compared to Caucasian & other populations who include individuals harbouring low frequency of CYP2A6 slow metabolizers. It is unclear whether the risk for lung cancer is mediated through the effect on smoking behavior or whether it also involves increased sensitivity to carcinogens present in cigarette smoke [59]. Liu & colleagues [60] suggested that decreasing or abolishing the activity of the CYP2A6 by means of specific inhibitors might prevent the frequency of occurrence of tobacco-induced lung cancer in smokers only. In this study, 5 out of 7 lung cancer cases (71.4%) with CYP2A6 slow metabolizer were non- smokers.

It is worth noting that our study has some limitations. First because the number of subjects is low, significant differences in smoking behaviors were not observed between those with and without *CYP2A6*2 & CYP2A6*9*. Further studies with larger population samples may present more detailed results. Second, we concentrated on only *CYP2A6*2 & CYP2A6*9* genetic polymorphisms. The effects of other polymorphisms of CYP2A6 on smoking habits should be examined; *CYP2A6*4 and *7* are also major functional polymorphisms.

Conclusions

Our study, in the setting of patients with lung cancer demonstrates that the frequency of slow metabolizer *CYP2A6*2* and *CYP2A6*9* are poor in the studied Egyptian population; who are non-smokers. Our findings did not suggest any association between CYP2A6 genotypes and risk of lung cancer.

Abbreviations
CI: Confidence interval; *CYP2A6*: Cytochrome *P450 2A6*; NCBI: National Center for Biotechnology Information; NCI: National Cancer Institute; NSCLC: Non small cell lung cancer; OR: Odds ratio; SCLC: Small cell lung cancer; SD: Standard deviation; SNPs: Single nucleotide polymorphisms

Acknowledgements
We would like to thank Science & Technology development Fund in Egypt (STDF) for the financial support of this study.

Funding
This study was supported financially by the Science and Technology Development Fund (STDF), Egypt, Grant No 5016. The funding body had no role in the design of the study and collection, analysis, and interpretation of data and in writing the manuscript.

Authors' contributions
All authors contributed to the present study. NE designed the study, AD & AE collected the samples & the clinicopathological data, DE, SA, and

MH performed the molecular analysis, AS analyzed the data, NE, DE & AD wrote the manuscript. All authors have read, revised & approved the final version of the manuscript.

Competing interests

The authors declare that they have no competing interests.

Author details
[1]Chest Diseases, National Research Center, Cairo, Egypt. [2]Medical Oncology, National Cancer Institute, Cairo University, Cairo, Egypt. [3]Clinical Pathology, National Research Center, Cairo, Egypt. [4]Environmental Health & Preventive Medicine, National Research Center, Cairo, Egypt. [5]National Cancer Institute (NCI), Fom-Elkhalig Square, P.O.Box: 11796, Cairo, Egypt.

References

1. Ferlay J, Soerjomataram I, Dikshit R, Eser S, Mathers C, Rebelo M, et al. Cancer incidence and mortality worldwide: sources, methods and major patterns in GLOBOCAN 2012. Int J Cancer. 2015;136:E359–86. https://doi.org/10.1002/ijc.29210.
2. Ariyoshi N, Miyamoto M, Umetsu Y, Kunitoh H, Dosaka-Akita H, Sawamura Y-I, et al. Genetic polymorphism of CYP2A6 gene and tobacco-induced lung cancer risk in male smokers. Cancer Epidemiol Biomark Prev. 2002;11:890–4.
3. Nakajima M, Yamamoto T, Nunoya K, Yokoi T, Nagashima K, Inoue K, et al. Role of human cytochrome P4502A6 in C-oxidation of nicotine. Drug Metab Dispos. 1996;24:1212–7.
4. Iscan M, Rostami H, Iscan M, Güray T, Pelkonen O, Rautio A. Interindividual variability of coumarin 7-hydroxylation in a Turkish population. Eur J Clin Pharmacol. 1994;47:315–8.
5. Rautio A, Kraul H, Kojo A, Salmela E, Pelkonen O. Interindividual variability of coumarin 7-hydroxylation in healthy volunteers. Pharmacogenetics. 1992;2:227–33.
6. Fujieda M, Yamazaki H, Saito T, Kiyotani K, Gyamfi MA, Sakurai M, et al. Evaluation of CYP2A6 genetic polymorphisms as determinants of smoking behavior and tobacco-related lung cancer risk in male Japanese smokers. Carcinogenesis. 2004;25:2451–8.
7. Kumondai M, Hosono H, Orikasa K, Arai Y, Arai T, Sugimura H, et al. Genetic polymorphisms of CYP2A6 in a case-control study on bladder Cancer in Japanese smokers. Biol Pharm Bull. 2016;39:84–9.
8. Yamano S, Tatsuno J, Gonzalez FJ. The CYP2A3 gene product catalyzes coumarin 7-hydroxylation in human liver microsomes. Biochemistry (Mosc). 1990;29:1322–9.
9. Kitagawa K, Kunugita N, Kitagawa M, Kawamoto T. CYP2A6*6, a novel polymorphism in cytochrome p450 2A6, has a single amino acid substitution (R128Q) that inactivates enzymatic activity. J Biol Chem. 2001;276:17830–5.
10. Pitarque M, von Richter O, Oke B, Berkkan H, Oscarson M, Ingelman-Sundberg M. Identification of a single nucleotide polymorphism in the TATA box of the CYP2A6 gene: impairment of its promoter activity. Biochem Biophys Res Commun. 2001;284:455–60.
11. Xu C, Rao YS, Xu B, Hoffmann E, Jones J, Sellers EM, et al. An in vivo pilot study characterizing the new CYP2A6*7, *8, and *10 alleles. Biochem Biophys Res Commun. 2002;290:318–24.
12. Yoshida R, Nakajima M, Watanabe Y, Kwon J-T, Yokoi T. Genetic polymorphisms in human CYP2A6 gene causing impaired nicotine metabolism. Br J Clin Pharmacol. 2002;54:511–7.
13. Minematsu N, Nakamura H, Iwata M, Tateno H, Nakajima T, Takahashi S, et al. Association of CYP2A6 deletion polymorphism with smoking habit and development of pulmonary emphysema. Thorax. 2003;58:623–8.
14. Oscarson M, Gullstén H, Rautio A, Bernal ML, Sinues B, Dahl ML, et al. Genotyping of human cytochrome P450 2A6 (CYP2A6), a nicotine C-oxidase. FEBS Lett. 1998;438:201–5.
15. Kitagawa K, Kunugita N, Katoh T, Yang M, Kawamoto T. The significance of the homozygous CYP2A6 deletion on nicotine metabolism: a new genotyping method of CYP2A6 using a single PCR–RFLP. Biochem Biophys Res Commun. 1999;262:146–51. https://doi.org/10.1006/bbrc.1999.1182.
16. Malaiyandi V, Sellers EM, Tyndale RF. Implications of CYP2A6 genetic variation for smoking behaviors and nicotine dependence. Clin Pharmacol Ther. 2005;77:145–58. https://doi.org/10.1016/j.clpt.2004.10.011.
17. Nakajima M, Fukami T, Yamanaka H, Higashi E, Sakai H, Yoshida R, et al. Comprehensive evaluation of variability in nicotine metabolism and CYP2A6

18. polymorphic alleles in four ethnic populations. Clin Pharmacol Ther. 2006; 80:282–97.
18. Oscarson M, McLellan RA, Gullstén H, Agúndez JA, Benítez J, Rautio A, et al. Identification and characterisation of novel polymorphisms in the CYP2A locus: implications for nicotine metabolism. FEBS Lett. 1999;460:321–7.
19. Schoedel KA, Hoffmann EB, Rao Y, Sellers EM, Tyndale RF. Ethnic variation in CYP2A6 and association of genetically slow nicotine metabolism and smoking in adult Caucasians. Pharmacogenetics. 2004;14:615–26.
20. Iwahashi K, Waga C, Takimoto T. Whole deletion of CYP2A6 gene (CYP2A6AST;4C) and smoking behavior. Neuropsychobiology. 2004;49:101–4.
21. López-Flores LA, Pérez-Rubio G, Falfán-Valencia R. Distribution of polymorphic variants of CYP2A6 and their involvement in nicotine addiction. EXCLI J. 2017;16:174–96. https://doi.org/10.17179/excli2016-847.
22. Minematsu N, Nakamura H, Furuuchi M, Nakajima T, Takahashi S, Tateno H, et al. Limitation of cigarette consumption by CYP2A6*4, *7 and *9 polymorphisms. Eur Respir J. 2006;27:289–92.
23. Mwenifumbo JC, Tyndale RF. Genetic variability in CYP2A6 and the pharmacokinetics of nicotine. Pharmacogenomics. 2007;8:1385–402.
24. Park SL, Tiirikainen MI, Patel YM, Wilkens LR, Stram DO, Le Marchand L, et al. Genetic determinants of CYP2A6 activity across racial/ethnic groups with different risks of lung cancer and effect on their smoking intensity. Carcinogenesis. 2016;37:269–79. https://doi.org/10.1093/carcin/bgw012.
25. Emamghoreishi M, Bokaee H-R, Keshavarz M, Ghaderi A, Tyndale RF. CYP2A6 allele frequencies in an Iranian population. Arch Iran Med. 2008;11:613–7.
26. Loriot MA, Rebuissou S, Oscarson M, Cenée S, Miyamoto M, Ariyoshi N, et al. Genetic polymorphisms of cytochrome P450 2A6 in a case-control study on lung cancer in a French population. Pharmacogenetics. 2001;11:39–44.
27. Miyamoto M, Umetsu Y, Dosaka-Akita H, Sawamura Y, Yokota J, Kunitoh H, et al. CYP2A6 gene deletion reduces susceptibility to lung cancer. Biochem Biophys Res Commun. 1999;261:658–60.
28. Takeuchi H, Saoo K, Yokohira M, Ikeda M, Maeta H, Miyazaki M, et al. Pretreatment with 8-methoxypsoralen, a potent human CYP2A6 inhibitor, strongly inhibits lung tumorigenesis induced by 4-(methylnitrosamino)-1-(3-pyridyl)-1-butanone in female a/J mice. Cancer Res. 2003;63:7581–3.
29. Tan W, Chen GF, Xing DY, Song CY, Kadlubar FF, Lin DX. Frequency of CYP2A6 gene deletion and its relation to risk of lung and esophageal cancer in the Chinese population. Int J Cancer. 2001;95:96–101.
30. Wang H, Tan W, Hao B, Miao X, Zhou G, He F, et al. Substantial reduction in risk of lung adenocarcinoma associated with genetic polymorphism in CYP2A13, the most active cytochrome P450 for the metabolic activation of tobacco-specific carcinogen NNK. Cancer Res. 2003;63:8057–61.
31. Ezzeldin N, El-Lebedy D, Darwish A, El-Bastawisy A, Hassan M, Abd El-Aziz S, et al. Genetic polymorphisms of human cytochrome P450 CYP1A1 in an Egyptian population and tobacco-induced lung cancer. Genes Environ. 2017;39:7. https://doi.org/10.1186/s41021-016-0066-4.
32. Vasconcelos GM, Struchiner CJ, Suarez-Kurtz G. CYP2A6 genetic polymorphisms and correlation with smoking status in Brazilians. Pharmacogenomics J. 2005;5:42–8.
33. Çok I, Kocabaş NA, Cholerton S, Karakayal AE, Şardaş S. Dtermination of coumarin metabolism in Turkish population. Hum Exp Toxicol. 2001;20: 179–84. https://doi.org/10.1191/096032701678766804.
34. Chen GF, Tang YM, Green B, Lin DX, Guengerich FP, Daly AK, et al. Low frequency of CYP2A6 gene polymorphism as revealed by a one-step polymerase chain reaction method. Pharmacogenetics. 1999;9:327–32.
35. Nakajima M, Kwon JT, Tanaka N, Zenta T, Yamamoto Y, Yamamoto H, et al. Relationship between interindividual differences in nicotine metabolism and CYP2A6 genetic polymorphism in humans. Clin Pharmacol Ther. 2001;69:72–8.
36. Paschke T, Riefler M, Schuler-Metz A, Wolz L, Scherer G, McBride CM, et al. Comparison of cytochrome P450 2A6 polymorphism frequencies in Caucasians and African-Americans using a new one-step PCR-RFLP genotyping method. Toxicology. 2001;168:259–68.
37. Ando M, Hamajima N, Ariyoshi N, Kamataki T, Matsuo K, Ohno Y. Association of CYP2A6 gene deletion with cigarette smoking status in Japanese adults. J Epidemiol. 2003;13:176–81.
38. Rao Y, Hoffmann E, Zia M, Bodin L, Zeman M, Sellers EM, et al. Duplications and defects in the CYP2A6 gene: identification, genotyping, and in vivo effects on smoking. Mol Pharmacol. 2000;58:747–55.
39. London SJ, Idle JR, Daly AK, Coetzee GA. Genetic variation of CYP2A6, smoking, and risk of cancer. Lancet. 1999;353:898–9.

Association of genetic polymorphisms CYP2A6*2 rs1801272 and CYP2A6*9 rs28399433...

151

40. Sabol SZ, Hamer DH. An improved assay shows no association between the CYP2A6 gene and Cigarette smoking behavior. Behav Genet. 1999; 29:257–61. https://doi.org/10.1023/A:1021642323602.

41. Verde Z, Santiago C, Rodríguez González-Moro JM, de Lucas RP, López Martín S, Bandrés F, et al. "Smoking genes": a genetic association study. PLoS One. 2011;6:e26668.

42. Gu DF, Hinks LJ, Morton NE, Day IN. The use of long PCR to confirm three common alleles at the CYP2A6 locus and the relationship between genotype and smoking habit. Ann Hum Genet. 2000;64(Pt 5):383–90.

43. Lerman C, Jepson C, Wileyto EP, Patterson F, Schnoll R, Mroziewicz M, et al. Genetic variation in nicotine metabolism predicts the efficacy of extended-duration transdermal nicotine therapy. Clin Pharmacol Ther. 2010;87:553–7.

44. Lerman C, Tyndale R, Patterson F, Wileyto EP, Shields PG, Pinto A, et al. Nicotine metabolite ratio predicts efficacy of transdermal nicotine for smoking cessation. Clin Pharmacol Ther. 2006;79:600–8.

45. Malaiyandi V, Lerman C, Benowitz NL, Jepson C, Patterson F, Tyndale RF. Impact of CYP2A6 genotype on pretreatment smoking behaviour and nicotine levels from and usage of nicotine replacement therapy. Mol Psychiatry. 2006;11:400–9.

46. Strasser AA, Benowitz NL, Pinto AG, Tang KZ, Hecht SS, Carmella SG, et al. Nicotine metabolite ratio predicts smoking topography and carcinogen biomarker level. Cancer Epidemiol Biomark Prev. 2011;20:234–8.

47. Styn MA, Nukui T, Romkes M, Perkins KA, Land SR, Weissfeld JL. CYP2A6 genotype and smoking behavior in current smokers screened for lung cancer. Subst Use Misuse. 2013;48:490–4.

48. Wassenaar CA, Dong Q, Wei Q, Amos CI, Spitz MR, Tyndale RF. Relationship between CYP2A6 and CHRNA5-CHRNA3-CHRNB4 variation and smoking behaviors and lung cancer risk. J Natl Cancer Inst. 2011;103:1342–6.

49. Carter B, Long T, Cinciripini P. A meta-analytic review of the CYP2A6 genotype and smoking behavior. Nicotine Tob Res. 2004;6:221–7.

50. Munafò M, Clark T, Johnstone E, Murphy M, Walton R. The genetic basis for smoking behavior: a systematic review and meta-analysis. Nicotine Tob Res. 2004;6:583–97.

51. Smoking in Egypt | Egypt Independent. http://www.egyptindependent.com/news/smoking-egypt. Accessed 18 Apr 2017.

52. Loffredo CA, Radwan GN, Eltahlawy EM, El-Setouhy M, Magder L, Hussein MH. Estimates of the prevalence of tobacco smoking in Egypt. Open J Epidemiol. 2015;05:129. https://doi.org/10.4236/ojepi.2015.52017.

53. Le Marchand L, Sivaraman L, Pierce L, Seifried A, Lum A, Wilkens LR, et al. Associations of CYP1A1, GSTM1, and CYP2E1 polymorphisms with lung cancer suggest cell type specificities to tobacco carcinogens. Cancer Res. 1998;58:4858–63.

54. Wynder EL, Hoffmann D. Smoking and lung cancer: scientific challenges and opportunities. Cancer Res. 1994;54:5284–95.

55. Strasser AA, Malaiyandi V, Hoffmann E, Tyndale RF, Lerman C. An association of CYP2A6 genotype and smoking topography. Nicotine Tob Res. 2007;9:511–8.

56. Wassenaar CA, Ye Y, Cai Q, Aldrich MC, Knight J, Spitz MR, et al. CYP2A6 reduced activity gene variants confer reduction in lung cancer risk in African American smokers–findings from two independent populations. Carcinogenesis. 2015;36:99–103.

57. Benowitz NL, Pérez-Stable EJ, Herrera B, Jacob P. Slower metabolism and reduced intake of nicotine from cigarette smoking in Chinese-Americans. J Natl Cancer Inst. 2002;94:108–15.

58. Wang D, Gaba RC, Jin B, Riaz A, Lewandowski RJ, Ryu RK, et al. Intraprocedural transcatheter intra-arterial perfusion MRI as a predictor of tumor response to chemoembolization for hepatocellular carcinoma. Acad Radiol. 2011;18:828–36.

59. Raunio H, Rahnasto Rilla M. CYP2A6: genetics, structure, regulation, and function. Drug Metabol Drug Interact. 2012;27:73–88.

60. Liu T, Xie C-B, Ma W-J, Chen W-Q. Association between CYP2A6 genetic polymorphisms and lung cancer: a meta-analysis of case-control studies. Environ Mol Mutagen. 2013;54:133–40.

16

Helicase-like transcription factor expression is associated with a poor prognosis in Non-Small-Cell Lung Cancer (NSCLC)

Ludovic Dhont[1,2,3], Melania Pintilie[4], Ethan Kaufman[2], Roya Navab[2], Shirley Tam[2], Arsène Burny[5], Frances Shepherd[6], Alexandra Belayew[1], Ming-Sound Tsao[2,6,7] and Céline Mascaux[8,9*]

Abstract

Background: The relapse rate in early stage non-small cell lung cancer (NSCLC) after surgical resection is high. Prognostic biomarkers may help identify patients who may benefit from additional therapy. The Helicase-like Transcription Factor (HLTF) is a tumor suppressor, altered in cancer either by gene hypermethylation or mRNA alternative splicing. This study assessed the expression and the clinical relevance of wild-type (WT) and variant forms of *HLTF* RNAs in NSCLC.

Methods: We analyzed online databases (TCGA, COSMIC) for *HLTF* alterations in NSCLC and assessed WT and spliced *HLTF* mRNAs expression by RT-ddPCR in 39 lung cancer cell lines and 171 patients with resected stage I-II NSCLC.

Results: In silico analyses identified *HLTF* gene alterations more frequently in lung squamous cell carcinoma than in adenocarcinoma. In cell lines and in patients, WT and I21R *HLTF* mRNAs were detected, but the latter at lower level. The subgroup of 25 patients presenting a combined low WT *HLTF* expression and a high I21R *HLTF* expression had a significantly worse disease-free survival than the other 146 patients in univariate (HR 1.96, CI 1.17–3.30; $p = 0.011$) and multivariate analyses (HR 1.98, CI 1.15–3.40; $p = 0.014$).

Conclusion: A low WT *HLTF* expression with a high I21R *HLTF* expression is associated with a poor DFS.

Keywords: Non-small cell lung cancer, HLTF, Prognosis, Alternative splicing

Background

Lung cancer is responsible for the highest cancer-associated mortality rate worldwide. Only 16% of patients affected with Non-small cell lung cancer (NSCLC), which is the most common subtype, are alive 5 years after diagnosis, and this number has hardly improved over several decades [1]. One reason for this poor prognosis is that only 15% of lung cancers are diagnosed at an early stage. Till recently the standard of care for NSCLC at stages I-IIIA was surgery, resulting in patient survival rates of 23% in stage IIIA, 33% in stage IIB, and up to 89% in stages IA [2]. Adjuvant chemotherapy after radical resection of localized NSCLC improves survival at 5 years by about 5% [3]. However, there is still a relatively high risk of relapse, and up to 40% of all stage IB and 60% of stage II patients die from their disease despite receiving adjuvant chemotherapy [4]. The integration of prognostic and predictive biomarkers has the potential of identifying patients who are at a low-risk of relapse following surgery and do not need further therapy, and conversely, patients who are at a high risk of relapse and who potentially may derive the greatest benefit from adjuvant treatment, including chemotherapy or personalized treatment based on individual tumor profiling. Therefore, an effort to identify more robust prognostic and predictive biomarkers is needed [5].

The Helicase-like Transcription Factor (HLTF) is a member of the yeast mating SWItch/Sucrose Non Fermenting (SWI/SNF) family of proteins involved in

* Correspondence: celinejmmascaux@gmail.com
[8]Department of Muldisciplinary Oncology and Therapeutic Innovations, Assistance Publique des Hôpitaux de Marseille (AP-HM), Aix-Marseille University, Chemin des Bourrely, 13195 Marseille, Cedex 20, France
[9]Centre de Recherche en Cancérologie de Marseille (CRCM, Cancer Research Center of Marseille), Inserm UMR1068, CNRS UMR7258 and Aix-Marseille University UM105, Marseille, France
Full list of author information is available at the end of the article

chromatin remodeling. Several studies demonstrated its function in gene transcription [6], cell cycle [7], DNA repair [8, 9], and genome stability maintenance [10], supporting its tumor suppressor role. In cancer, two different alterations in *HLTF* expression were reported: (i) an epigenetic silencing by hypermethylation of its promoter and (ii) an alternative splicing of its mRNA, leading to the production of several shorter forms of the protein lacking DNA repair domains. The hypermethylation of *HLTF* promoter was first identified in colon cancer [11] and was reported in other types of cancers, including gastric cancers [12–16]. It was shown in HeLa cells that *HLTF* mRNA was alternatively spliced in the exons 19 to 22 region, resulting in the expression of shorter truncated protein forms. The distinctive character of the *HLTF* spliced mRNA variants (I21R) is that they contain the intron 21 between exons 21 and 22. To date, the expression of HLTF protein forms was reported in head and neck, cervix and thyroid [17–20] cancers and associated with a poor prognosis [16].

In lung cancer, one study assessed the hypermethylation of *HLTF* in a cohort of 54 patients with NSCLC [21]. Promoter hypermethylation was found in 21 patients (39.6%), including 9/20 squamous cell carcinoma (SCC) and 12/33 adenocarinoma (ADC). Patients whose tumors harboured *HLTF* hypermethylation had shorter survival, in comparison with patients whose tumors had a hypomethylated *HLTF* promoter (log-rank, $p = 0.035$). So far, to our knowledge, there are no published data about the expression of HLTF (wild-type and its truncated forms) in lung cancer.

The purpose of this study is to assess the expression of wild-type (WT) and spliced variants (I21R) of *HLTF* mRNAs in NSCLC and evaluate their clinical relevance. We analyzed publicly available databases for *HLTF* in lung cancer and assessed its expression in NSCLC cell lines and in a clinically annotated cohort of 171 patients with resected stage I-II NSCLC.

Methods

In silico analyses

Available genomic profiling data (mutation, copy number, DNA methylation [correlation only], and mRNA expression) for *HLTF* were downloaded from cBioPortal, an online portal for accessing data from The Cancer Genome Atlas (TCGA) project and other cancer genome profiling initiatives (http://www.cbioportal.org/public-portal). Additional cancer genome profiling data were obtained from the Catalogue of Somatic Mutations in Cancer (http://cancer.sanger.ac.uk/cosmic; [22]).

To obtain gene expression estimates for individual mRNA forms, paired-end RNAseq raw read data from the TCGA project were downloaded from the Cancer Genomics Hub (https://cghub.ucsc.edu/). In brief, reads

were mapped to the latest human reference assembly, hg19, using TopHat, a splice-aware short-read aligner (http://ccb.jhu.edu/software/tophat). Alignment output was then supplied to Cufflinks (http://cufflinks.cbcb.umd.edu/), which was run in the reference-guided mode to quantify the abundance of known transcripts as well as predict and estimate expression of novel isoforms. Pre- and post-alignment quality control was performed with FastQC (http://www.bioinformatics.babraham.ac.uk/projects/fastqc/) and RSeQC (http://rseqc.sourceforge.net/), respectively.

Patient characteristics

A total of 171 patients with resected stage I-II NSCLC collected at University Health Network (Toronto, Canada) were included in this study. These patients had surgery between 1996 and 2005. The length of follow-up: median 5.4 years, range 0.1–12 years. As these patients all underwent surgery before 2005, none of them received adjuvant chemotherapy as it did only become standard after 2005. The clinical and demographic characteristics of the patient cohort are listed in Table 2.

Cell lines and cell culture

NSCLC cell lines were purchased from the American Type Cell Collection (ATCC, http://www.atcc.org), and cultured according to ATCC recommendation. Among these, there were 33 of the adenocarcinoma (ADC) subtype (H1693, H2122, H2228, H2279, H1573, H1395, H522, H1792, H838, H1819, H4011, H2291, H2073, H1568, H920, H1993, H4006, HCC827, H3255, H23, H4019, H2126, H1437, H1944, H2009, H2405, H1373, H1355, H1975, HCC2935, A549, H650, H1650), two large cell carcinoma (H661, H4017), one mixed adenosquamous carcinoma (H647) and two of undefined histology (DFC1032, DFC1024). MGH7 cells (squamous cell carcinoma, SCC) were cultured as described [23].

mRNA expression

Total RNA was extracted from cell lines with RNeasy Mini Kit (QIAGEN) according to the manufacturer's instructions. RNA purity and concentration were assessed with Nanodrop (Thermo Scientific). Total RNA (input 150 ng) extracted from cell lines and patient tumours were reverse transcribed into cDNA (SuperScript III, Invitrogen). Droplet Digital polymerase chain reaction (ddPCR) was performed based on the manufacturer's recommendations (QX200, Bio-Rad). ddPCR is a highly sensitive qPCR due to a step of sample fractioning (limiting dilutions) by generation of droplets (water:oil emulsion). It allows retrieving an absolute count of RNA copies for each sample, and is particularly indicated for low-expressed targets. Each ddPCR was performed with 22.5 ng cDNA in triplicates. Reaction conditions were as follow: ddPCR cycle was set up at 95 °C for 5 min, 40 cycles of [30 s at 95 °C and 1 min at 58 °C], 5 min at 4 °C, and finally 5 min at 90 °C. Results were analyzed with QuantaSoft (Bio-Rad), and the cut-off to define positive and negative droplets was set up at 10,000 arbitrary units of fluorescence amplitude. This signal is then used in the calculation of *HTLF* copy number by a Poisson regression (QuantaSoft, Bio-Rad).

Primers to detect either WT *HLTF* mRNA (F: 5′-GTT CAAAGATTAATGCGCT-3′ and R: 5′-AAAGACAGGA ATGTTGTAAACTGAGA-3′) or *HLTF* mRNA variants I21R (F: 5′-TCCAGTTTCAAAGGTAAAGTACTC-3′ and R: 5′-GCCAGTGGTCAACAACAGAA-3′) by ddPCR were designed with Primer3 and purchased from Eurogentec. Primers were tested for nonspecific amplicons and primer dimers by visualizing PCR products on 1% agarose gels and droplet distribution profile (QuantaSoft, Bio-Rad).

Statistical analyses

Expression levels of different variants of *HLTF* were measured in triplicates. The reliability was assessed by calculating the intra-class correlation coefficient (ICC) based on the within and between variances estimated using the variance component analysis. For the outcome analysis, the three replicates were averaged for each sample. Two outcome variables were assessed: overall survival (OS) and disease-free survival (DFS). Both were measured from surgery date. For OS, the time was calculated up to the date of death or last follow-up with death of any cause as an event; for DFS, the time was calculated up to the date of relapse, death or last follow-up with death or relapse as events. There were 71 deaths (number of events for OS) and 81 events for DFS in the cohort. The averages of the three replicates of WT and I21R *HLTF* expressions were tested for their associations with OS and DFS using the Cox proportional hazards regression. Both variants of *HLTF* were also dichotomized at their respective medians and were tested as categorical variables using the log-rank test. The percentages for OS and DFS for the high and low values of each of these covariates were calculated using the Kaplan-Meier method. A composite covariate was created by combining WT and I21R *HLTF* expression levels and a data-driven covariate was defined as "Low WT *HLTF* and High I21R *HLTF*" vs. the rest. This new covariate was also tested for its association with OS and DFS by employing the log-rank test. These covariates were tested for their association with outcome, adjusting the model for age (≤65, >65), sex, stage (I vs. II), and histology (ADC vs. the rest) using Cox regression. All *p*-values were based on the Wald test. *HLTF* expressions (continuous) were also tested for their associations with the clinical factors (age, sex, histology, and stage) using

the Mann-Whitney test. A cut-off of p ≤ 0.05 was used for statistical significance.

Results

In silico analysis of *HLTF* alterations in NSCLC

We collected available online data for *HLTF* alterations in NSCLC from TCGA (Lung ADC and SCC, TCGA Provisional 2015/02/04) and COSMIC, focusing on mutations, copy number alterations (CNAs), and methylation data. We analyzed these data in association with *HLTF* expression. The type and the frequency of the different *HLTF* alterations in ADC and SCC are reported in Table 1. When all types of molecular alteration were considered, *HLTF* was more frequently altered in SCC (438/504 cases, 83%) than ADC (266/578 cases, 46.0%; *p* < 0.0001). While a high expression of *HLTF* was more frequently reported in SCC than in ADC (28.6% vs 7.5%, *p* < 0.0001), a negative correlation between *HLTF* expression and its methylation status was found in both SCC (Pearson: −0.475 and Spearman: −0.484; Fig. 1) and ADC (Pearson: −0.473 and Spearman: −0.420; Fig. 1). *HLTF* copy number gain was more frequent in SCC (57% vs 23.3%, *p* < 0.0001) as well as high amplifications (26.1% s 2.1%, *p* < 0.0001). Conversely, loss of heterozygosity was more frequent in ADC than in SCC (22.3% vs 2.9%, respectively, *p* < 0.0001), along with diploidy (52% vs 13.5%, respectively, *p* < 0.0001). *HLTF* mutation is a rare event both in ADC and SCC, 2.2 and 1.5%, respectively (Table 1). The majority of the 13 mutations (12 missense and 1 splice site mutation) reported in ADC

Table 1 HLTF alterations in lung adenocarcinoma and squamous cell carcinoma

	Adenocarcinoma (*n* = 578) Number of cases, n (%)	Squamous cell carcinoma (*n* = 504) Number of cases, n (%)	*P*-value (Fisher test)
Mutation	13 (2.2%)	8 (1.5%)	0.5110
Copy number alterations			
Homozygous deletion	1 (0.1%)	1 (0.2%)	1.00
Heterozygosity loss	115 (22.3%)	15 (2.9%)	< 0.0001
Diploid	268 (52.0%)	68 (13.5%)	< 0.0001
Gain	120 (23.3%)	286 (57.0%)	< 0.0001
High level of amplification	11 (2.1%)	131 (26.1%)	< 0.0001
No data	63	3	
mRNA expression level			
High expression	43 (7.5%)	141 (28.6%)	< 0.0001
Low expression	0 (0.0%)	6 (1.2%)	0.0101
Total number of altered cases			
	266 (46.0%)	438 (83.0%)	< 0.0001

Data collected from TCGA database

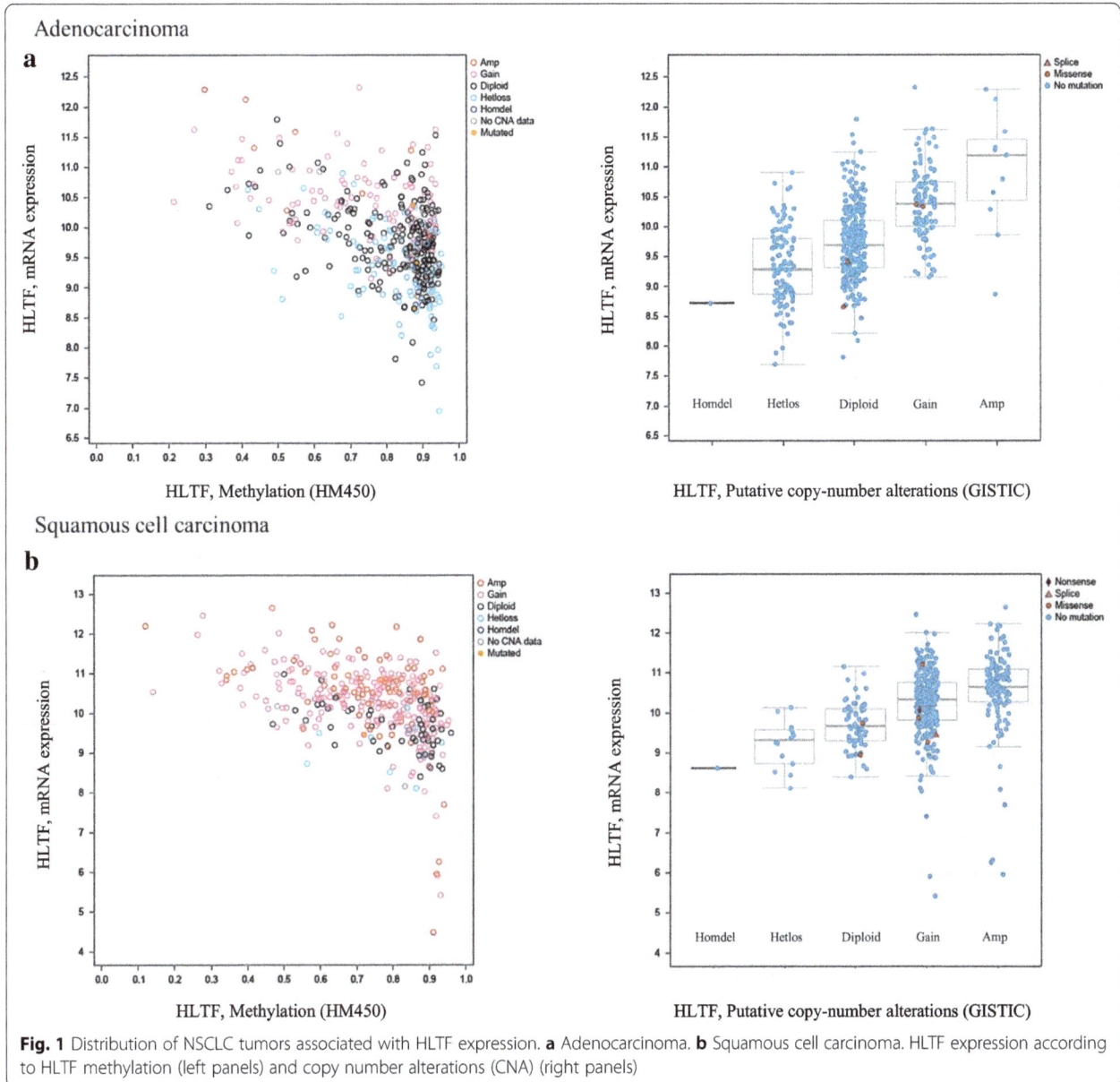

Fig. 1 Distribution of NSCLC tumors associated with HLTF expression. **a** Adenocarcinoma. **b** Squamous cell carcinoma. HLTF expression according to HLTF methylation (left panels) and copy number alterations (CNA) (right panels)

and 8 mutations (6 missense, 1 splice site and 1 non-sense mutations) in SCC are found in regions encoding functional domains involved in DNA binding (HIRAN domain), Sp1/Sp3 interaction (carboxyl-terminal domain), and DNA repair (SNF2_N/helicase-ATPase and RING finger domains) (Fig. 2).

In vitro screening of *HLTF* mRNA expression in a panel of NSCLC cell lines

We assessed *HLTF* mRNA expression in 39 NSCLC cell lines. Measurements for WT and I21R *HLTF* were considered reliable based on ICC values (0.878 and 0.933, respectively). Overall, the level of WT *HLTF* expression was significantly higher than the level of I21R *HLTF*

expression (Fig. 3) (median 71.5 vs. 18.3 respectively, Wilcoxon signed-rank test, $p = 4.5 \times 10^{-7}$).

Assessment of *HLTF* expression in a cohort of 171 patients with NSCLC

HLTF expression was assessed by RT-ddPCR in 171 tumours from patients with surgically resected stage I-II NSCLC. Patient data are summarized in Table 2. Measurements for WT and I21R *HLTF* were considered reliable based on ICC values (0.984 and 0.846, respectively). As in NSCLC cell lines, the level of WT *HLTF* expression was significantly higher than the level of I21R *HLTF* expression in tumours of patients with NSCLC (Fig. 3) when considering all patients (median 20.6 vs. 2.2 respectively, Wilcoxon signed-rank test, $p = 2.2 \times 10^{-16}$).

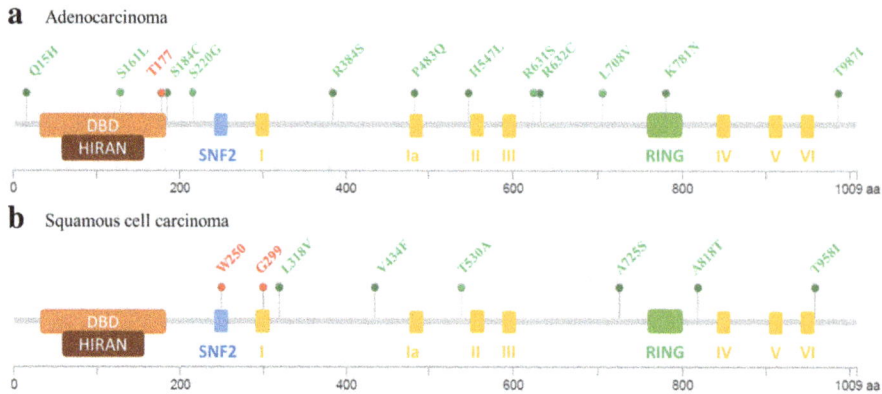

Fig. 2 HLTF mutations in NSCLC. **a**. Lung adenocarcinoma. **b**. Lung squamous cell carcinoma. Mutation data were retrieved from TCGA and COSMIC databases. HLTF protein is depicted as a grey line with its functional domains: DNA binding domain (DBD, orange box), HIRAN (brown box), SNF2 (blue box), Helicase/ATPase I–III (yellow boxes), zinc finger RING (green box). Under the protein is a scale showing the amino-acid size. Mutation are depicted by colored dots (missense: green; spliced or stop mutation: red) with their position and the residue change

There was no difference between SCC and ADC for WT and I21R *HLTF* expressions ($p = 0.09$ and 0.17, respectively). Overall, the level of *HLTF* expression was lower in tumours from patients than in cell lines (WT *HLTF*: 20.6 vs. 71.5, $p = 9.3 \times 10^{-11}$ and I21R *HLTF*: 2.2 vs. 18.3, $p = 2.8 \times 10^{-12}$, Wilcoxon rank-sum test; Fig. 3).

HLTF and clinical characteristics
WT and I21R *HLTF* expressions were first tested for their association with patient clinical characteristics (age, sex, histology, and stage). There was no association with these characteristics and *HLTF* expression (Table 2).

Second, we considered a composite covariate combining WT and I21R *HLTF* expressions dichotomized at their median levels. Four groups were built accordingly. There was no association with patient clinical characteristics (Table 3).

HLTF expression and outcome
A univariate analysis (Cox proportional hazard regression model and log-rank test) was first performed to assess the association between WT and I21R *HLTF* expression levels, and OS and DFS. The mRNA expression measures were sequentially considered as continuous and as dichotomous variables. There was no

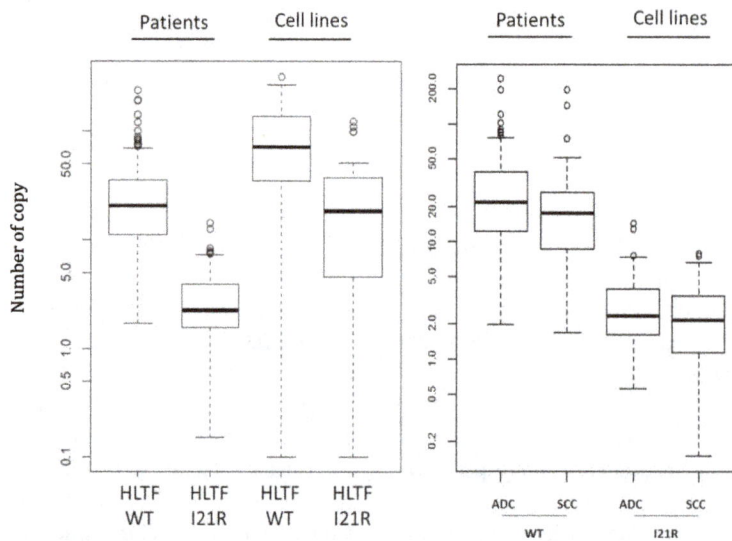

Fig. 3 Distribution of WT and I21R HLTF expressions (number of copy) in lung adenocarcinoma (ADC) (left panel) and squamous cell carcinoma (SCC) (right panel) patients and cell lines. RNA from cell lines and tumors was extracted and reverse transcribed. A ddPCR was performed to detect WT and I21R HLTF expression by using specific primer sets. The high sensitivity of ddPCR provides an absolute count of RNA copies for each sample, displayed in Y-axis

Table 2 Association of WT HLTF and I21R HLTF expressions with patient clinical characteristics

Clinical factor	Categories	n	Summary WT HLTF Median (range)	p-value	Summary I21R HLTF Median (range)	p-value
Age	Age < 65	57	20.7 (2–193)	0.63	2.1 (0.7–12.7)	0.54
	Age > =65	114	20.5 (1.7–240)		2.3 (0.2–14.3)	
Sex	F	78	20.4 (2–121)	0.84	2.4 (0.2–8.4)	0.71
	M	93	20.6 (1.7–240)		2.2 (0.6–14.3)	
Stage	I	121	19.6 (1.7–240)	0.46	2.1 (0.2–14.3)	0.91
	II	50	23.8 (3.5–195)		2.3 (0.6–7.6)	
Histology	ADC	122	21.5 (2–240)	0.061	2.3 (0.6–14.3)	0.19
	OTH	49	17.5 (1.7–195)		2.1 (0.2–8.4)	
	ADC	122	21.5 (2–240)	0.09	2.3 (0.6–14.3)	0.17
	SCC	42	17.5 (1.7–195)		2.1 (0.2–7.9)	

ADC Adenocarcinoma, OTH Other histology types, SCC Squamous cell carcinoma. The Mann-Whitney test was used. A cut-off of $p \leq 0.05$ was used for statistical significance

significant association of each variable with OS and DFS (Table 4).

The association of the combined covariates of WT and I21R *HLTF* expression with OS and DFS were analyzed by the log-rank test. When considering the four groups, the « Low WT *HLTF*-High I21R *HLTF* » group showed a trend for a poorer DFS, but did not reach statistical significance (DFS at 5 years = 25%, log-rank $p = 0.067$), compared with the three other groups. We thus compared this group (Low WT *HLTF*-High I21R *HLTF*) to the three other groups combined. There was no statistical difference in OS (HR 1.26, CI 0.67–2.34; $p = 0.48$), but the DFS was significantly worse in this group (HR 1.96, CI 1.17–3.30; $p = 0.011$) (Table 4 and Fig. 4d).

A multivariate analysis (Cox proportional hazard regression model) was performed to include age, sex, stage, histology, and *HLTF* expression; WT alone (model 1), I21R alone (model 2) and the 2 composite groups (model 3) were considered (Table 5). *HLTF* expression (for each model) was not associated with OS. The

expressions of WT (model 1) and I21R *HLTF* (model 2) were not associated with DFS. However, the shorter DFS of the group « Low WT *HLTF*-High I21R *HLTF* » (model 3) as compared with the other groups remained significant (HR 1.98, CI 1.15–3.4, $p = 0.014$; Table 5).

Discussion

The purpose of this study was to assess the expression of WT and variant forms of *HLTF* mRNAs in NSCLC and evaluate their clinical relevance. Our hypothesis was that the expression of *HLTF* mRNA variant I21R has a poor prognosis on patients with NSCLC. In head and neck, cervix and thyroid cancers, the expression of HLTF truncated protein has been associated with poor outcome [16–20]. The present study showed that in a cohort of 171 patients, the combination of low expression of WT *HLTF* transcript and high expression of I21R *HLTF* transcript was associated with poor prognosis in early stage NSCLC.

Table 3 Association of the composite covariate combining WT HLTF and I21R HLTF expression levels (n, %) with patient clinical characteristics

Clinical factor	Categories	n	WT < =20.6 Mut < =2.23	WT < =20.6 Mut > 2.23	WT > 20.6 Mut < =2.23	WT > 20.6 Mut > 2.23	p-value
Age	Age < 65	57	20 (32.8%)	8 (32%)	10 (45.5%)	19 (30.2%)	0.62
	Age > =65	114	41 (67.2%)	17 (68%)	12 (54.5%)	44 (69.8%)	
Sex	F	78	26 (42.6%)	13 (52%)	11 (50%)	28 (44.4%)	0.85
	M	93	35 (57.4%)	12 (48%)	11 (50%)	35 (55.6%)	
Stage	I	121	46 (75.4%)	17 (68%)	15 (68.2%)	43 (68.3%)	0.81
	II	50	15 (24.6%)	8 (32%)	7 (31.8%)	20 (31.7%)	
Histology	ADC	122	40 (65.6%)	16 (64%)	17 (77.3%)	49 (77.8%)	0.78
	OTH	49	21 (34.4%)	9 (36%)	5 (22.7%)	14 (22.2%)	
	ADC	122	20 (32.8%)	8 (32%)	10 (45.5%)	19 (30.2%)	0.35
	SCC	42	41 (67.2%)	17 (68%)	12 (54.5%)	44 (69.8%)	

ADC Adenocarcinoma, OTH Other histology types, SCC Squamous cell carcinoma. The Mann-Whitney test was used. A cut-off of $p \leq 0.05$ was used for statistical significance

Table 4 Univariate analyses of the association of HLTF expression with overall survival and disease-free survival

Outcome			Overall survival (OS)				Disease-free survival (DFS)			
Category		n	Estimate at 5 years	Logrank p-value	HR (95% CI)[a]	Wald p-value	Estimate at 5 years	Logrank p-value	HR (95% CI)[a]	Wald p-value
WT	<=20.6	86	61%	0.63	1.03 (0.97–1.1)	0.34	48%	0.14	1.01 (0.95–1.08)	0.72
	> 20.6	85	64%				61%			
I21R	<=2.23	83	63%	0.65	1.03 (0.92–1.15)	0.61	58%	0.73	1.02 (0.93–1.13)	0.64
	> 2.23	88	61%				49%			
Composite covariable	Wt > 20.6 or Mut < =2.23	146	65%	0.47	1.26 (0.67–2.34)	0.48	59%	0.0096	1.96 (1.17–3.3)	0.011
	Wt < =20.6 and Mut > 2.23	25	50%				25%			

Cox proportional hazard regression model and log-rank test were used. A cut-off of $p \leq 0.05$ was used for statistical significance
[a]Note: HRs for WT HLTF represent the increase of the hazard for 10 units increase in the WT HLTF

Overall, in silico analysis showed that *HLTF* alterations, including gene amplifications, high expression, and methylation occurred more frequently in SCC than in ADC. Mutations in *HLTF* were rare in both ADC and SCC; however, the mutations observed in ADC were different from those found in SCC. In ADC, mutations occur in DNA binding domain and DNA repair domains (Fig. 2), which might alter HLTF transcriptional and

DNA repair abilities. Conversely, in SCC, mutations did not occur in functional domains but there are 2 nonsense mutations leading to the expression of a shorter protein containing only the DBD. This suggests that these shorter proteins would only have transcriptional activity. Further investigations are required to assess the functional consequence and potential clinical impact of these mutations in cancer. Copy number alterations

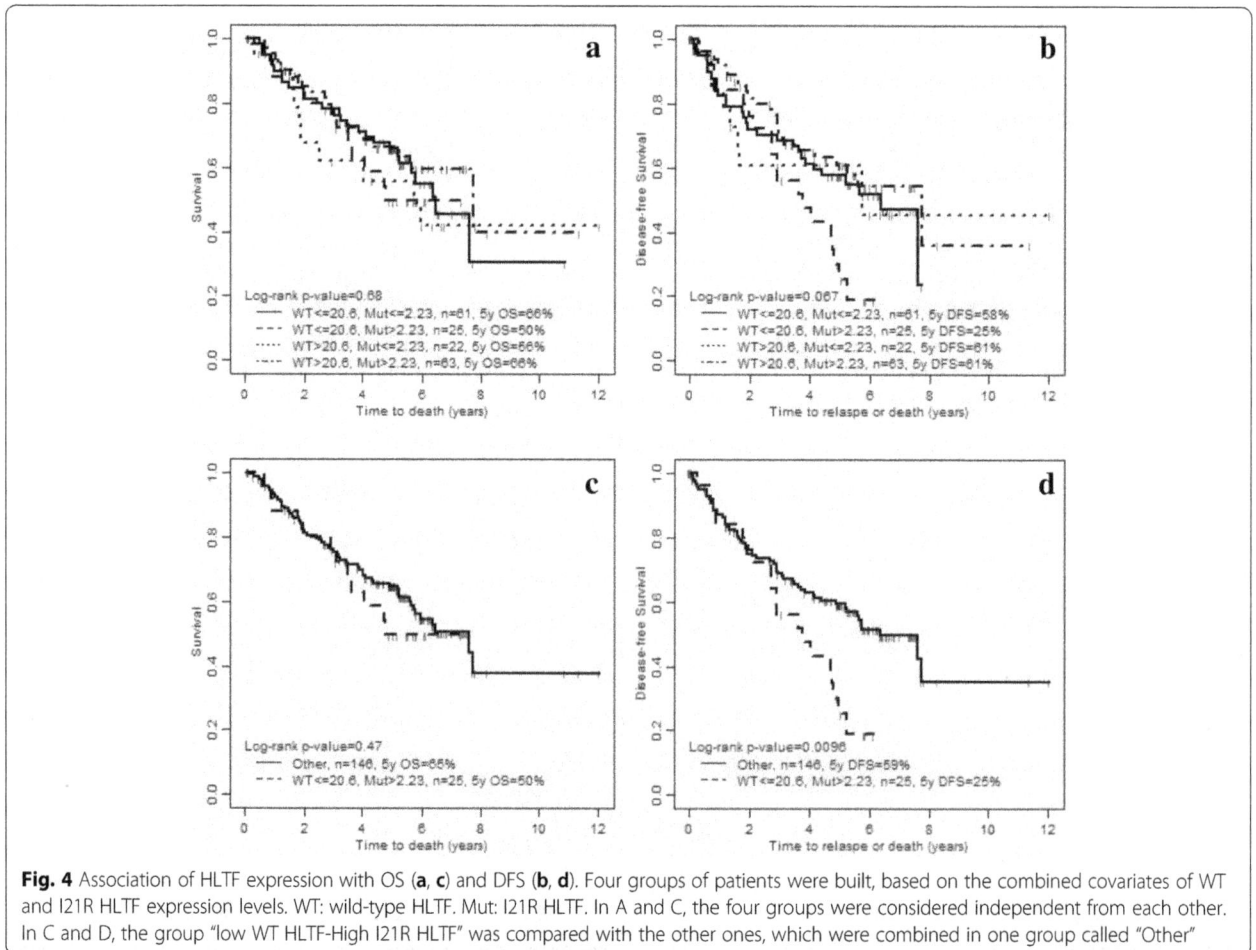

Fig. 4 Association of HLTF expression with OS (**a**, **c**) and DFS (**b**, **d**). Four groups of patients were built, based on the combined covariates of WT and I21R HLTF expression levels. WT: wild-type HLTF. Mut: I21R HLTF. In A and C, the four groups were considered independent from each other. In C and D, the group "low WT HLTF-High I21R HLTF" was compared with the other ones, which were combined in one group called "Other"

Table 5 Multivariate analyses of the association of HLTF expression with survival and disease-free survival

Models[a]	Overall survival (OS)			Disease-free survival (DFS)		
	HR	95% CI	p-value	HR	95% CI	p-value
Model 1: adjusted effect of WT HLTF (for 10 units)	1.02	0.96–1.08	0.58	1	0.94–1.06	0.94
Model 2: adjusted effect of I21R HLTF	1.01	0.9–1.13	0.84	1	0.9–1.11	0.97
Model 3: adjusted effect of HLTF WT < =20.6 & I21R > 2.23 vs. the rest	1.21	0.64–2.28	0.56	1.98	1.15–3.4	0.014

Cox proportional hazard regression model was used. A cut-off of $p \leq 0.05$ was used for statistical significance
[a]All models are adjusted for age, sex, stage and histology

were also found to be different between ADC and SCC; high amplifications were rare in ADC, but 83% of SCC have either a gain (57%) or an amplification (26%) of *HLTF*. These observations are consistent with the fact that *HLTF* is located on chromosome 3q, which is frequently amplified in SCC. We also analyzed the association of *HLTF* expression with its methylation status in both NSCLC types. In both ADC and SCC, there was a negative correlation between methylation and *HLTF* expression, but a high expression was more frequently seen in SCC, which might be related to the higher frequency of gene copy number. Intriguingly, we did not notice any difference in *HLTF* expression levels (WT and I21R) between ADC and SCC by RT-ddPCR. This discrepancy may be possibly explained by the fact that we assessed *HLTF* mRNA variants separately, while data reported in cBioportal considered only WT *HLTF* expression without distinguishing the variants.

In the available online data, only WT *HLTF* expression was assessed. To our knowledge, to date the expression of the *HLTF* spliced variants with intron 21 retention (I21R) has not been assessed. Using the RT-ddPCR with specific primers that we constructed, we were able to evaluate the expression of WT *HLTF* mRNA and its spliced variants I21R. Spliced variants I21R lead to the expression of shorter protein forms, which are thought to disturb WT HLTF function and act as oncogene proteins [16]. Studies in head and neck, cervix and thyroid cancers showed that the expression of such shorter proteins was associated with poor prognosis [17–20]. They replace WT HLTF progressively and accumulate along the carcinogenic process, most likely due to their higher stability compared with WT HLTF. It was reported that the I21R transcripts have a lower abundance than the WT *HLTF* transcript in mouse heart and brain transcriptomes [7, 24]. We analyzed RNA-seq data from TCGA for the presence of the intron 21 sequence and found that its expression was a rare event in NSCLC. In both the NSCLC cell lines and the 171 resected NSCLC from patients, WT *HLTF* levels were significantly higher than I21R *HLTF*.

Castro et al. studied the methylation for several genes including *HLTF* in NSCLC and reported that patients

with *HLTF* methylation have shorter survival [21]; this study represents the only study of *HLTF* in lung cancer. They reported *HLTF* methylation frequency for NSCLC and did not observe any significant difference for *HLTF* methylation between ADC and SCC (12/33 vs. 9/20, respectively; $p = 0.57$, Fisher exact test). cBioportal does not provide gene methylation frequency but only correlations with the expression of a given gene. In both ADC and SCC, we observed a negative correlation between *HLTF* expression and methylation. Interestingly, *HLTF* expression was affected more by the variation in *HLTF* copy number than its promoter methylation status.

Conclusion

So far to our knowledge, our study is the first to assess the clinical impact of WT and variant forms of *HLTF* expression in patients with NSCLC. TCGA in silico analysis of *HLTF* alterations including mutations, amplification, and mRNA expression modifications were more frequent in SCC than in ADC. In NSCLC cell lines and patient samples, both the expressions of WT and spliced I21R *HLTF* mRNAs were detected, but with the latter at lower levels. In a cohort of 171 patients with resected stage I-II NSCLC, the combination of a low WT *HLTF* expression with a high I21R *HLTF* expression was associated with shorter DFS both in univariate and multivariate analyses. Surgically resected early stage NSCLC are very heterogeneous and no prognostic factor has been clinically validated for the risk of relapse. Very likely, a panel of several biomarkers will be necessary to predict tumour with poor prognostic; that would therefore require more intensive follow-up and treatment. If validated in independant cohorts, the combination of low WT and high I21R *HLTF* might belong to this biomarker panel for the prognostic of surgically resected NSCLC. As detailed in a review article we published recently [16], the *HLTF* gene could be involved in various ways during the stages of tumour initiation and progression, by its ability to alternatively express proteins of different sizes with distinct functions ranging from tumour suppressor to oncoprotein. The involvement of alternative RNA splicing in producing tumour promoting proteins is a process that does not require inactivating mutation of a tumour suppressor gene and might be an underestimated carcinogenic mechanism. Further studies should precisely investigate the functions of these HLTF protein forms and their role in cancer development.

Abbreviations
ADC: Adenocarcinoma; CNA: Copy number alteration; DFS: Disease-free survival; HLTF: Helicase-like transcription factor; HR: Hazard ratio; ICC: Intraclass coefficient; NSCLC: Non-small cell lung cancer; OS: Overall survival; RT-ddPCR: Reverse transcription-droplet digital PCR; SCC: Squamous cell carcinoma; WT: Wild-type

Acknowledgements
We acknowledge Dr. Claude Lachance for his help in ddPCR design.

Funding
This work was supported by funds from F. R. S.-FNRS (doctoral research fellowship) (L.D.), Télévie (AI.B., C.M.), FRMH (Fonds pour la Recherche Médicale dans le Hainaut, Belgium) (L.D.) and research grant from Canadian Cancer Society (grant #701595, MS.T.). C.M. was supported by research funds from Boehringer-Ingelheim Canada. The funding bodies had no role in the design of the study and collection, analysis and interpretation of the data.

Authors' contributions
LD and CM designed the study and wrote the manuscript. LD performed RNA extractions with RN and ST, ddPCR, and in silico analyses with EK. MP performed statistical analyses. ArB, FS, AIB, and MST supervised the study and drafted the manuscript. All authors read and approved the final manuscript.

Competing interests
The authors declare that they have no competing interests.

Author details
[1]Laboratory of Molecular Biology, Research Institute for Health Sciences and Technology, Université de Mons, Mons, Belgium. [2]Princess Margaret Research Institute, Princess Margaret Cancer Centre, University Health Network, Toronto, Canada. [3]Cellular and Molecular Epigenetics, Université de Liège-GIGA, Liège, Belgium. [4]Biostatistics Department, University of Toronto, Toronto, Canada. [5]Université Libre de Bruxelles (ULB), Bruxelles, Belgium. [6]Division of Medical Oncology and Hematology, Princess Margaret Cancer Centre, University Health Network, Toronto, Canada. [7]Laboratory of Medicine and Pathobiology, University of Toronto, Toronto, Canada. [8]Department of Muldisciplinary Oncology and Therapeutic Innovations, Assistance Publique des Hôpitaux de Marseille (AP-HM), Aix-Marseille University, Chemin des Bourrely, 13195 Marseille, Cedex 20, France. [9]Centre de Recherche en Cancérologie de Marseille (CRCM, Cancer Research Center of Marseille), Inserm UMR1068, CNRS UMR7258 and Aix-Marseille University UM105, Marseille, France.

References
1. Siegel R, Ma J, Zou Z, Jemal A. Cancer statistics, 2014. CA Cancer J Clin. 2014;64:9–29.
2. Goldstraw P, Crowley J, Chansky K, Giroux DJ, Groome PA, Rami-Porta R, Postmus PE, Rusch V, Sobin L, International Association for the Study of Lung Cancer International Staging Committee, et al. The IASLC lung Cancer staging project: proposals for the revision of the TNM stage groupings in the forthcoming (seventh) edition of the TNM classification of malignant tumours. J Thorac Oncol. 2007;2:706–14.
3. Pujol JL, Breton JL, Gervais R, Tanguy M-L, Quoix E, David P, Janicot H, Westeel V, Gameroff S, Genève J, et al. Phase III double-blind, placebo-controlled study of thalidomide in extensive-disease small-cell lung cancer after response to chemotherapy: an intergroup study FNCLCC cleo04 IFCT 00-01. J Clin Oncol. 2007;25:3945–51.
4. Tanaka F, Yoneda K. Adjuvant therapy following surgery in non-small cell lung cancer (NSCLC). Surg Today. 2016;46(1):25–37.
5. Mascaux C, Feser WJ, Lewis MT, Barón AE, Coldren CD, Merrick DT, Kennedy TC, Eckelberger JI, Rozeboom LM, Franklin WA, et al. Endobronchial miRNAs as biomarkers in lung cancer chemoprevention. Cancer Prev Res Phila. 2013;6:100–8.
6. Ding H, Benotmane AM, Suske G, Collen D, Belayew A. Functional interactions between Sp1 or Sp3 and the helicase-like transcription factor mediate basal expression from the human plasminogen activator inhibitor-1 gene. J Biol Chem. 1999;274:19573–80.
7. Helmer RA, Martínez-Zaguilán R, Dertien JS, Fulford C, Foreman O, Peiris V, Chilton BS. Helicase-like transcription factor (hltf) regulates g2/m transition, wt1/gata4/hif-1a cardiac transcription networks, and collagen biogenesis. PLoS One. 2013;8:e80461.
8. Blastyák A, Hajdú I, Unk I, Haracska L. Role of double-stranded DNA translocase activity of human HLTF in replication of damaged DNA. Mol Cell Biol. 2010;30:684–93.
9. Motegi A, Liaw H-J, Lee K-Y, Roest HP, Maas A, Wu X, Moinova H, Markowitz SD, Ding H, Hoeijmakers JHJ, et al. Polyubiquitination of proliferating cell nuclear antigen by HLTF and SHPRH prevents genomic instability from stalled replication forks. Proc Natl Acad Sci U S A. 2008;105:12411–6.
10. Sandhu S, Wu X, Nabi Z, Rastegar M, Kung S, Mai S, Ding H. Loss of HLTF function promotes intestinal carcinogenesis. Mol Cancer. 2012;11:18.
11. Moinova HR, Chen W-D, Shen L, Smiraglia D, Olechnowicz J, Ravi L, Kasturi L, Myeroff L, Plass C, Parsons R, et al. HLTF gene silencing in human colon cancer. Proc Natl Acad Sci U S A. 2002;99:4562–7.
12. Bai AHC, Tong JHM, To K-F, Chan MWY, Man EPS, Lo K-W, Lee JFY, Sung JJY, Leung WK. Promoter hypermethylation of tumor-related genes in the progression of colorectal neoplasia. Int J Cancer. 2004;112:846–53.
13. Hibi K, Nakao A. Highly-methylated colorectal cancers show poorly-differentiated phenotype. Anticancer Res. 2006;26:4263–6.
14. Hibi K, Nakayama H, Kanyama Y, Kodera Y, Ito K, Akiyama S, Nakao A. Methylation pattern of HLTF gene in digestive tract cancers. Int J Cancer. 2003;104:433–6.
15. Philipp AB, Stieber P, Nagel D, Neumann J, Spelsberg F, Jung A, Lamerz R, Herbst A, Kolligs FT. Prognostic role of methylated free circulating DNA in colorectal cancer. Int J Cancer. 2012;131:2308–19.
16. Dhont L, Mascaux C, Belayew A. The helicase-like transcription factor (HLTF) in cancer: loss of function or oncomorphic conversion of a tumor suppressor? Cell Mol Life Sci. 2015;73:129–45.
17. Capouillez A, Decaestecker C, Filleul O, Chevalier D, Coppée F, Leroy X, Belayew A, Saussez S. Helicase-like transcription factor exhibits increased expression and altered intracellular distribution during tumor progression in hypopharyngeal and laryngeal squamous cell carcinomas. Virchows Arch. 2008;453:491–9.
18. Capouillez A, Debauve G, Decaestecker C, Filleul O, Chevalier D, Mortuaire G, Coppée F, Leroy X, Belayew A, Saussez S. The helicase-like transcription factor is a strong predictor of recurrence in hypopharyngeal but not in laryngeal squamous cell carcinomas. Histopathology. 2009;55:77–90.
19. Capouillez A, Noël J-C, Arafa M, Arcolia V, Mouallif M, Guenin S, Delvenne P, Belayew A, Saussez S. Expression of the helicase-like transcription factor and its variants during carcinogenesis of the uterine cervix: implications for tumour progression. Histopathology. 2011;58:984–8.
20. Arcolia V, Paci P, Dhont L, Chantrain G, Sirtaine N, Decaestecker C, Remmelink M, Belayew A, Saussez S. Helicase-like transcription factor: a new

marker of well-differentiated thyroid cancers. BMC Cancer. 2014;14:492.

21. Castro M, Grau L, Puerta P, Gimenez L, Venditti J, Quadrelli S, Sánchez-Carbayo M. Multiplexed methylation profiles of tumor suppressor genes and clinical outcome in lung cancer. J Transl Med. 2010;8:86.

22. Forbes SA, Beare D, Gunasekaran P, Leung K, Bindal N, Boutselakis H, Ding M, Bamford S, Cole C, Ward S, et al. COSMIC: exploring the world's knowledge of somatic mutations in human cancer. Nucleic Acids Res. 2015;43:D805–11.

23. Liu C, Tsao MS. In vitro and in vivo expressions of transforming growth factor-alpha and tyrosine kinase receptors in human non-small-cell lung carcinomas. Am J Pathol. 1993;142:1155–62.

24. Helmer RA, Foreman O, Dertien JS, Panchoo M, Bhakta SM, Chilton BS. Role of helicase-like transcription factor (hltf) in the G2/m transition and apoptosis in brain. PLoS One. 2013;8:e66799.

17

An inflammation-related nomogram for predicting the survival of patients with non-small cell lung cancer after pulmonary lobectomy

Ying Wang[1,4†], Xiao Qu[1†], Ngar-Woon Kam[4], Kai Wang[1], Hongchang Shen[3], Qi Liu[1*] and Jiajun Du[1,2*]

Abstract

Background: Emerging inflammatory response biomarkers are developed to predict the survival of patients with cancer, the aim of our study is to establish an inflammation-related nomogram based on the classical predictive biomarkers to predict the survivals of patients with non-small cell lung cancer (NSCLC).

Methods: Nine hundred and fifty-two NSCLC patients with lung cancer surgery performed were enrolled into this study. The cutoffs of inflammatory response biomarkers were determined by Receiver operating curve (ROC). Univariate and multivariate analysis were conducted to select independent prognostic factors to develop the nomogram.

Results: The median follow-up time was 40.0 months (range, 1 to 92 months). The neutrophil to lymphocyte ratio (cut-off: 3.10, HR:1.648, $P = 0.045$) was selected to establish the nomogram which could predict the 5-year OS probability. The C-index of nomogram was 0.72 and the 5-year OS calibration curve displayed an optimal agreement between the actual observed outcomes and the predictive results.

Conclusions: Neutrophil to lymphocyte ratio was shown to be a valuable biomarker for predicting survival of patients with NSCLC. The addition of neutrophil to lymphocyte ratio could improve the accuracy and predictability of the nomogram in order to provide reference for clinicians to assess patient outcomes.

Keywords: Non-small cell lung cancer, Inflammatory response biomarker, Nomogram

Background

Lung cancer remains the leading cause of cancer-related death worldwide and 85% of lung cancers diagnosis are non-small cell lung cancer (NSCLC). Numerous studies investigated the prognostic factors in the early stage patients in order to establish a more efficient model to assess patient prognosis. In the seventh edition of the American Joint Committee on Cancer TNM classification, tumor extent, lymph node involvement and distant metastasis contributed significantly to individualized survival predictions [1]. In recent years, more studies reported that tumor characteristics were not the only determinants to predict the outcomes of patients with cancer. As inflammation emerged as a hallmark of cancer, inflammatory response biomarkers have shown to be promising prognostic factors for improving the predictive accuracy in cancer research. In 1986, Shoenfeld et al. demonstrated that high level of white blood cells in peripheral blood was associated with poor outcomes in patients who suffered from non-hematological malignancies [2]. Neutrophil to lymphocyte ratio [3–9], calculated by the ratio of absolute neutrophil counts to absolute lymphocyte counts in whole blood, was established by Walsh et al. who reported its potential prognostic value in colorectal cancer [10]. Additionally, derived neutrophil to lymphocyte ratio [5, 11, 12], lymphocyte to monocyte ratio [13, 14], platelet to lymphocyte ratio [3, 7] and systematic immune-inflammation index [15] were considered as potential systematic inflammatory response biomarkers for survival prediction.

* Correspondence: liuqi66@sdu.edu.cn; dujiajun@sdu.edu.cn
†Ying Wang and Xiao Qu contributed equally to this work.
[1]Institute of Oncology, Shandong Provincial Hospital Affiliated to Shandong University, 324 Jingwu Road, Jinan 250021, People's Republic of China
Full list of author information is available at the end of the article

Although some articles have studied the prognostic or predictive value of these inflammatory response biomarkers, inflammation-related nomogram on NSCLC remains undefined.

Nomogram is a relative novel and convenient model to predict survivals of patients with cancer. It could generate an intuitive graph by integrating diverse determinant variables and reflect an individual probability of a clinical event. Postoperative nomograms can assist patients and physicians to get more information about the prognosis.

In this study, we have evaluated the prognostic values of various inflammatory response biomarkers and selected the most significant factors to establish our nomogram model. The established nomogram was compared with traditional TMN staging system to validate its effectiveness.

Methods

From January 2006 to December 2011, 1454 patients with lung cancer (including adenocarcinoma or squamous cell carcinoma) who underwent surgery in Shandong Provincial Hospital Affiliated to Shandong University were retrospectively reviewed and consecutively selected. The clinical stages of all patients were identified according to the seventh edition TNM classification. The exclusion criteria included: Patients with incomplete clinical and pathological data; patients with distant metastasis or stage IV; Patients whose primary cancers were not lung cancer; Patients who received radiotherapy or chemotherapy before surgery. We reviewed the hospital records of 952 patients who met the criteria. All patients underwent lung resection and systematic lymph node sampling. Demographic data (age, gender), clinical characteristics (biochemical index, smoking history), histopathological results (pathological type, differentiation, pathological stage of tumor and involved lymph nodes according to TNM system staging), postoperative outcomes and survival data were collected and recorded. Tumor size was assessed using the longest diameter of the tumor. The information of tumor size, nodal metastases and distant metastasis were collected from the pathological and medical image reports.

Ethics statement

All patients provided written informed consent for their information to be stored in the hospital database and used for research. Ethical approval was obtained from Provincial Hospital Affiliated to Shandong University ethics committee, and the study was carried out in accordance with the approved guidelines.

Postoperative Treatment and Follow-up

All patients involved in our study were followed up from surgery to July 2014. The minimal follow-up period was 36.0 months (range, 1 to 92 months) and median follow-up time was 40.0 months. Routine examinations such as CT scan postoperatively were performed every 3 months for the first year, every 6 months for the second year and then once a year thereafter.

Candidate biomarkers

The hematological variables were obtained from blood tests routinely performed 1–3 days before surgery. Inflammatory response biomarkers included: neutrophil to lymphocyte ratio, absolute neutrophil counts to absolute lymphocyte counts, lymphocyte to monocyte ratio, platelet to lymphocyte ratio and systematic immune-inflammation index, which were calculated in the analysis. Neutrophil to lymphocyte ratio is defined as the ratio of absolute neutrophil count to absolute lymphocyte count in whole blood. Absolute neutrophil counts to absolute lymphocyte counts is defined as the ratio of absolute neutrophil count to the absolute white cell count minus the absolute count of neutrophils in whole blood. Platelet to lymphocyte ratio is defined as the ratio of absolute platelet count to absolute lymphocyte count in whole blood. Lymphocyte to monocyte ratio is defined as the ratio of absolute lymphocyte count to the absolute monocyte count in whole blood. Systematic immune-inflammation index is defined as the results of the peripheral platelet count multiplied by neutrophil count and divided by lymphocyte counts in whole blood.

Statistical analysis

Demographic characteristics were showed through descriptive statistics. Normally distributed continuous data was presented as mean ± standard deviation, while discrete data was presented as count and proportion. Overall survival (OS) was defined as the period from surgery to death or the last date of follow-up for patients alive. The optimal cut-off levels of neutrophil to lymphocyte ratio, absolute neutrophil counts to absolute lymphocyte counts, lymphocyte to monocyte ratio and platelet to lymphocyte ratio were obtained by ROC analysis based on OS. Survival curves were derived by the Kaplan-Meier method and were assessed by log-rank test univariately. A Cox proportional hazards model was used to conduct multivariate analysis, with a significance level set at two-sided 0.05. Multivariable stepwise Cox models were performed to select final variables for prognostic factors. Above steps were performed with the statistical software SPSS version 20.0.

Based on the results of the multivariable analysis, a nomogram was established by R 3.2.0 software (Institute for Statistics and Mathematics, Vienna, Austria) with the rms and survival package. Internal validation of the nomogram was conducted and it was subjected to 1000 bootstrap resamples. Then we compared this nomogram with traditional TNM system staging by Harrell's concordance index (c-index) to validate the accuracy of the nomogram. After bias correction, calibration curves on 5-year OS were generated by comparison between the predicted survival and observed survival [16].

Results
Clinicopathological features
Totally 952 eligible NSCLC patients, 674 men and 278 women, were enrolled into this study, with a mean age of 59 years (range, 20 to 79 years old). The primary tumor size ranged from 3 to 130.0 mm with a mean size of 38.6 mm, while the pathologic T stage showed 300 patients were in pathologic T1, 515 in pathologic T2,79 in pathologic T3 and 58 in pathologic T4. According to TNM system staging, pathological N stages were divided into three levels, and among them there were 530 pathologic N0 patients, 204 pathologic N1 patients, 213 pathologic N2 patients and 5 pathologic N3 patients. There were 416 patients with squamous cell carcinoma and 536 patients with adenocarcinoma respectively. Regarding degree of tumor differentiation, 131 patients were identified as well differentiated, 676 patients were identified as moderately differentiated and 145 patients were identified as poorly differentiated. Among the enrolled patients, 772 patients had the smoking experience and 180 patients did not have the experience. There were 483 patients received adjuvant chemotherapy after surgery and 483 patients did not receive chemotherapy. The characteristic information based on neutrophil to lymphocyte ratio was shown in Table 1. The optimal cut-offs obtained from ROC curves of neutrophil to lymphocyte ratio, absolute neutrophil counts to absolute lymphocyte counts, lymphocyte to monocyte ratio and platelet to lymphocyte ratio and systematic immune-inflammation index were shown in Table 2. Patients were divided into groups on the basis of optimal cut-offs.

Independent prognostic factors screened for nomogram
Kaplan-Meier survival analysis was conducted to evaluate the relationship between inflammatory response biomarkers and survival outcomes. Patients were divided into two groups based on the optimal cutoffs of inflammatory response biomarkers (in Table 3),and all groups

Table 1 The clinicopathological characteristics based on neutrophil to lymphocyte ratio

	Total (n = 952)	NLR <3.1(n = 732)	>3.1(n = 220)
Gender			
Male	674	486	188
Female	278	246	32
Age	59(20–79)	59(20–79)	60(27–78)
Smoking history			
N	180	126	54
Y	772	606	166
pT category			
pT1	300	233	67
pT2	515	391	124
pT3	79	61	18
pT4	58	47	11
pN category			
pN0	530	416	114
pN1	204	150	54
pN2	213	163	50
pN3	5	3	2
Histology			
ADC	536	453	83
SCC	416	279	137
PGTD			
I	131	111	20
II	676	508	168
III	145	113	32
Chemotherapy			
N	469	371	98
Y	483	361	122

pT category pathologcial T category
pN category pathological N category
ADC adenocarcinoma
SCC squamous cell carcinoma
PGTD pathological grading of tumor differentiation
NLR neutrophil to lymphocyte ratio

Table 2 The optimal cut-off point based on OS

	Median values	Range	AUC	Cut-off
NLR	2.49	0.33–12.40	0.584	3.1
dNLR	0.68	0.21–9.79	0.423	0.499
PLR	140.43	31.22–450.00	0.553	170.58
LMR	4.72	0.66–195.00	0.428	3.53
SII	614.99	76.26–3954.03	0.582	781.82

NLR neutrophil to lymphocyte ratio
dNLR derived neutrophil to lymphocyte ratio
PLR platelet to lymphocyte ratio
LMR lymphocyte to monocyte ratio
SII systematic immune-inflammation index

Table 3 Univariable analysis and cox proportional hazards regression analysis

Variable	Univariable analysis			Multivariable analysis		
	Hazard ratio	95% CI	P	Hazard ratio	95% CI	P
Age	1.388	1.112–1.733	0.004	1.649	1.306–2.081	<0.001
Gender						
Female	R					
Male	1.243	0.965–1.601	0.092			
Smoking history						
N	R					
Y	1.426	1.120–1.815	0.004	1.157	0.878–1.524	0.300
pT category						
T1–2	R			R		0.007
T3–4	2.030	1.558–2.645	<0.001	1.455	1.097–1.930	0.009
pN category						
N0	R		<0.001	R		<0.001
N1	2.414	1.808–3.22	<0.001	2.277	1.690–3.067	<0.001
N2	4.097	3.153–5.323	<0.001	4.233	3.216–5.570	<0.001
N3	6.170	1.953–19.493	0.002	5.121	1.530–17.144	0.008
Histology						
Histology ADC	R			R		
Histology CC	1.311	1.050–1.636	0.017	0.965	0.744–1.252	0.789
PGTD						
PGTD I	R		<0.001	R		0.008
PGTD II	0.174	0.091–0.332	<0.001	2.671	1.433–4.979	0.002
PGTD III	0.789	0.594–1.049	0.103	2.563	1.315–4.999	0.006
Chemotherapy						
N	R					
Y	1.166	0.934–1.457	0.175			
NLR						
<3.1	R					
>3.1	1.845	1.457–2.337	<0.001	1.648	1.010–2.687	0.045
dNLR						
<0.499	R					
>0.499	0.627	0.497–0.790	<0.001	1.470	0.936–2.309	0.095
PLR						
<170.58	R					
>170.58	1.636	1.284–2.085	<0.001	1.201	0.895–1.621	0.221
LMR						
<3.53	R					
>3.53	0.619	0.496–0.772	<0.001	1.020	0.770–1.351	0.890
SII						
<781.82	R					
>781.82	1.852	1.463–2.344	<0.001	1.412	0.955–2.090	0.084

pT category pathologcial T category
pN category pathologcial N category
R reference
ADC adenocarcinoma
SCC squamous cell carcinoma
PGTD pathological grading of tumor differentiation
NLR neutrophil to lymphocyte ratio
dNLR derived neutrophil to lymphocyte ratio
PLR platelet to lymphocyte ratio
LMR lymphocyte to monocyte ratio
SII systematic immune-inflammation index

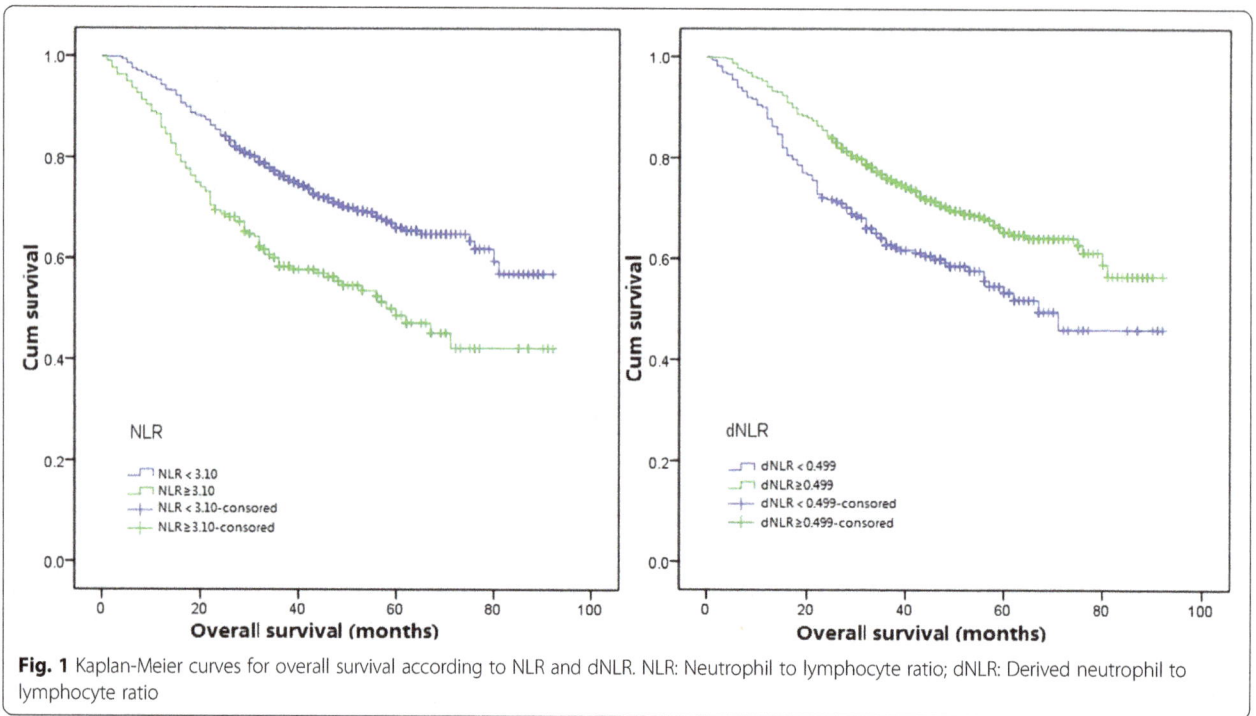

Fig. 1 Kaplan-Meier curves for overall survival according to NLR and dNLR. NLR: Neutrophil to lymphocyte ratio; dNLR: Derived neutrophil to lymphocyte ratio

had significantly different survival ends(in Figs. 1 and 2). The univariate analysis indicated that age, neutrophil to lymphocyte ratio, absolute neutrophil counts to absolute lymphocyte counts, lymphocyte to monocyte ratio and platelet to lymphocyte ratio and systematic immune-inflammation index, pathologic T staging, pathologic N staging, tumor differentiation and smoking history were associated with OS (in Table 4). Multivariate analysis suggested that age, pathologic T and N staging, tumor differentiation, neutrophil to lymphocyte ratio were significantly associated with patients with reduced OS.

Prognostic nomogram on OS

A nomogram was established which embraced the significant prognostic factors, age, pathologic T and N staging, tumor differentiation, and neutrophil to lymphocyte ratio and had the ability to reflect the 5-year OS (in Fig. 3). The nomogram evinced that neutrophil to lymphocyte ratio made a significant contribution to survival outcomes.

Internal validation and calibration plot

The C-index was 0.72 in the nomogram, higher than that of TNM system staging (0.69). Afterwards, the 5-year OS calibration curves of our nomogram displayed an optimal agreement between the actual observed outcomes and the predictions (in Fig. 4), compared with

TNM system staging. The nomogram of our model was validated by the sample size of 100, while TNM system staging was validated by the sample size of 300 for its fewer variates. In the same time, The ROC of the nomogram was performed and the AUC of our nomogram was 0.767 (Fig. 5).

Discussion

Although there have been several nomograms used to select individual therapy for patients with lung cancer [16, 17], a nomogram incorporated with inflammatory response biomarkers has not been put forward. The aim of our study is to investigate the impact of inflammatory response biomarkers on survival outcomes and to establish an inflammation-related nomogram in patients with NSCLC who underwent surgery.

In our study, both classical and novel inflammatory response biomarkers are the candidates for nomogram including: neutrophil to lymphocyte ratio, absolute neutrophil counts to absolute lymphocyte counts, lymphocyte to monocyte ratio and platelet to lymphocyte ratio and systematic immune-inflammation index. All the biomarkers show their predictive ability on survival outcomes and among them, only the neutrophil to lymphocyte ratio has been selected to be included in the nomogram after survival analysis through Kaplan-Meier curves, univariate and multivariate method. For

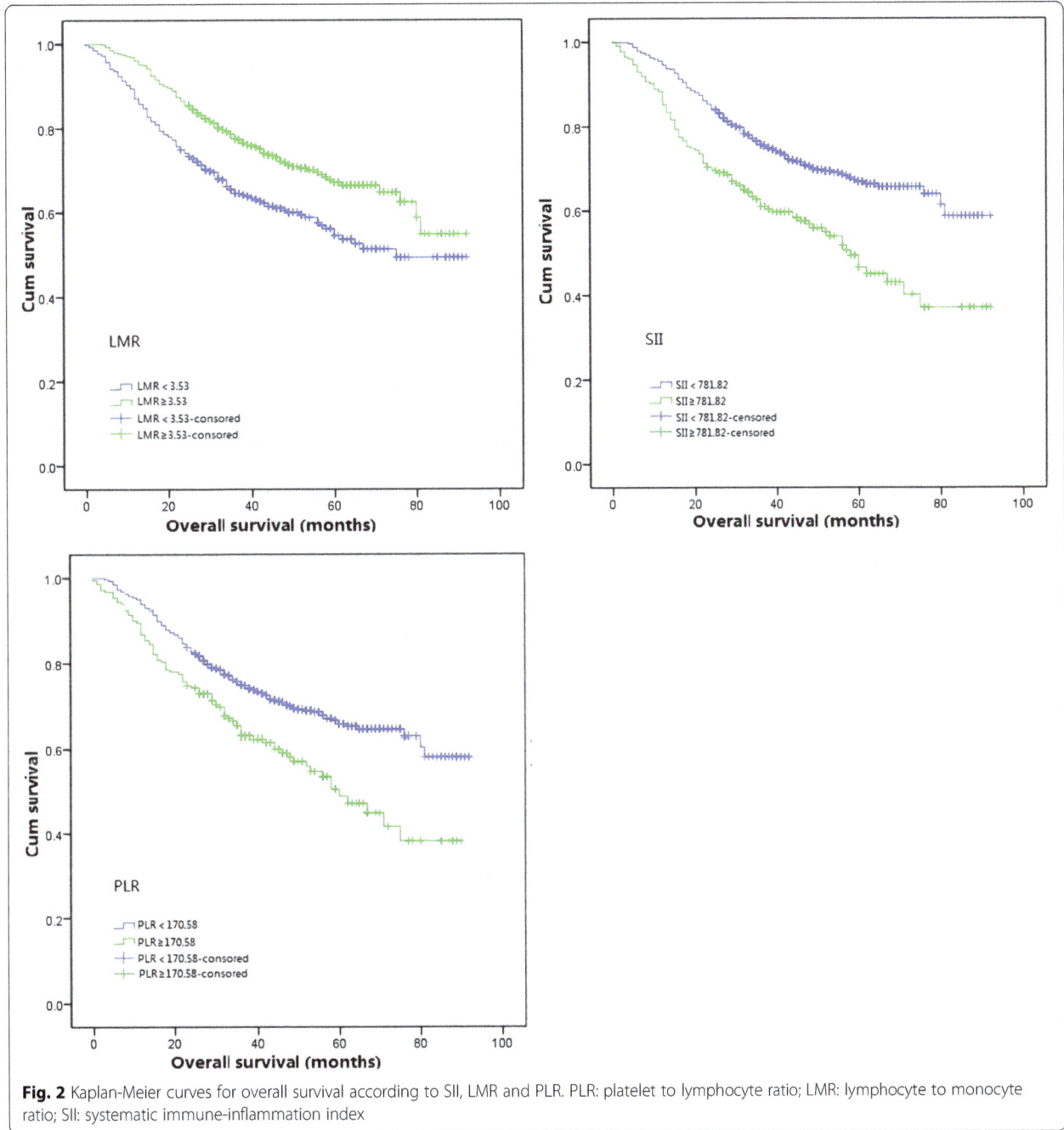

Fig. 2 Kaplan-Meier curves for overall survival according to SII, LMR and PLR. PLR: platelet to lymphocyte ratio; LMR: lymphocyte to monocyte ratio; SII: systematic immune-inflammation index

non-inflammatory biomarkers, pathologic T and N staging, age and tumor differentiation are also considered as independent prognostic factors which could be incorporated into the nomogram. In the nomogram, neutrophil to lymphocyte ratio is the third most important prognostic factors following pathologic N staging and age to predict the survival. Internal validation and calibration curve are performed to test the repeatability and reliability of the nomogram. Compared with TNM traditional system staging, the nomogram has a higher C-index (0.72) through internal validation, indicating

that the nomogram has a better ability to discriminate survival outcomes. Calibration curves for the nomogram of 5-year OS disclose an excellent agreement between prediction and actual observation and is superior to those of TNM system staging. Based on the above results, we believe that inflammatory response biomarkers should be incorporated into the predictive models as independent prognostic factors of patients with lung cancer, and the inflammation-related nomogram have been shown to provide more precise prediction compared with traditional TNM classification.

Table 4 The survival data of subgroups according to inflammation response biomarkers

Groups	Cutoff	Patients	3-year OS	5-year OS	P
NLR					<0.001
	<3.10	732	76.50%	66.10%	
	>3.10	220	58.40%	48.80%	
dNLR					<0.001
	<0.499	262	79.50%	62.80%	
	>0.499	690	65.30%	53.40%	
PLR					<0.001
	<170.58	738	75.00%	63.00%	
	>170.58	214	65.70%	48.80%	
LMR					<0.001
	<3.53	388	64.60%	77.60%	
	>3.53	564	54.60%	57.20%	
SII					<0.001
	<781.82	729	75.70%	61.00%	
	>781.82	233	66.90%	46.70%	

NLR neutrophil to lymphocyte ratio
dNLR derived neutrophil to lymphocyte ratio
PLR platelet to lymphocyte ratio
LMR lymphocyte to monocyte ratio
SII systematic immune-inflammation index

Cancer-related inflammation has been referred as local inflammation and systemic inflammation which could promote tumorigenesis and metastasis [18] in a broad range of cancers [19]. Increasing novel inflammatory response biomarkers are therefore developed to better refine the stratification of patients. Recently, increasing attention is being paid to the biomarkers derived from innate immune cells in peripheral blood. Neutrophil to lymphocyte ratio is a simple index of the systemic inflammatory response, and the increased level of neutrophil to lymphocyte ratio has been shown to predict worse overall survival in patients with NSCLC [3, 4, 6–8]. Additionally, it has been reported that the perioperative use of nonsteroidal anti-inflammatory drugs (NSAIDs), such as celecoxib and ketorolac, could change the tumor microenvironment and reduce migration and invasion of circulating malignant cells [4, 20–22]. Taken together, these findings demonstrate the importance of perioperative inflammation and immune suppression on oncological outcomes.

Neutrophils could be stimulated to proliferate by cancer-related inflammatory factors, such as Tumor necrosis factor-alpha and Interleukin-6, which subsequently secrete reactive oxygen species and pro-angiogenic factors, and therefore favors tumorigenesis and tumor microenvironment [23, 24]. Also, bone marrow could lead to an abnormal release of neutrophils precursors upon inflammation. Regarding lymphocytes, they have shown to exert a vital role in cell-mediated immunity against host cancer cells, and the decreases in lymphocytes count have worse survival outcomes Nomograms possess their own merits of predicting oncologic prognosis, such as intuitive graphs and numerical probability of clinical events, so they are identified as reliable tools to quantify risks. Given the importance of neutrophils and lymphocytes in tumor development, we therefore seek to integrate the neutrophil to lymphocyte ratio into the nomogram for improving the accuracy of the predictive model. Our results indicate that the contribution of neutrophil to lymphocyte ratio

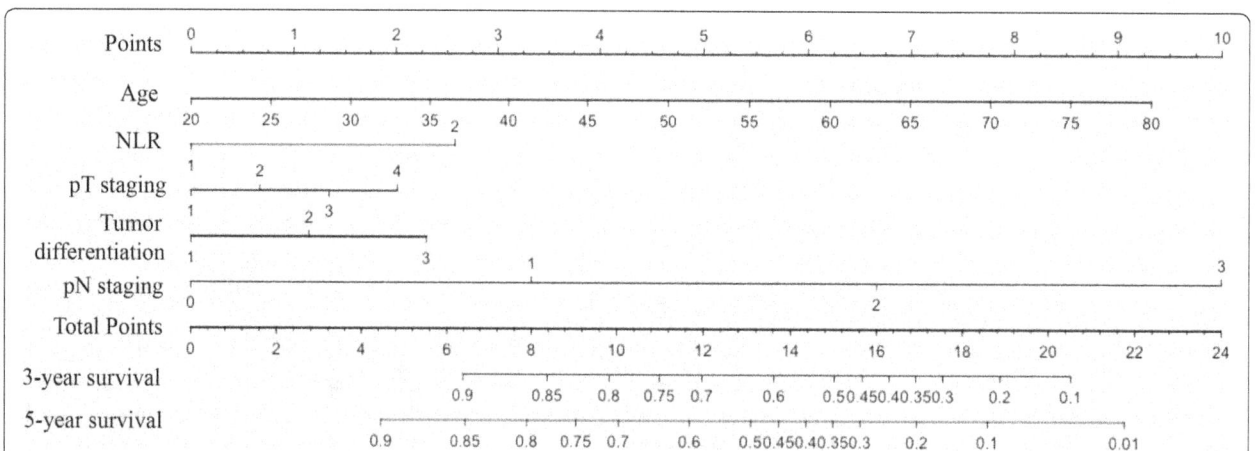

Fig. 3 Postoperative prognostic nomogram predicted the probability of patients with resected NSCLC for 3- and 5-year overall survival. To use the nomogram, each patient was assigned a score on each variable axis, and the sum of these numbers could determine the location on total points axis. A line is drawn downward to the survival axes to determine the 3- or 5-year overall survival

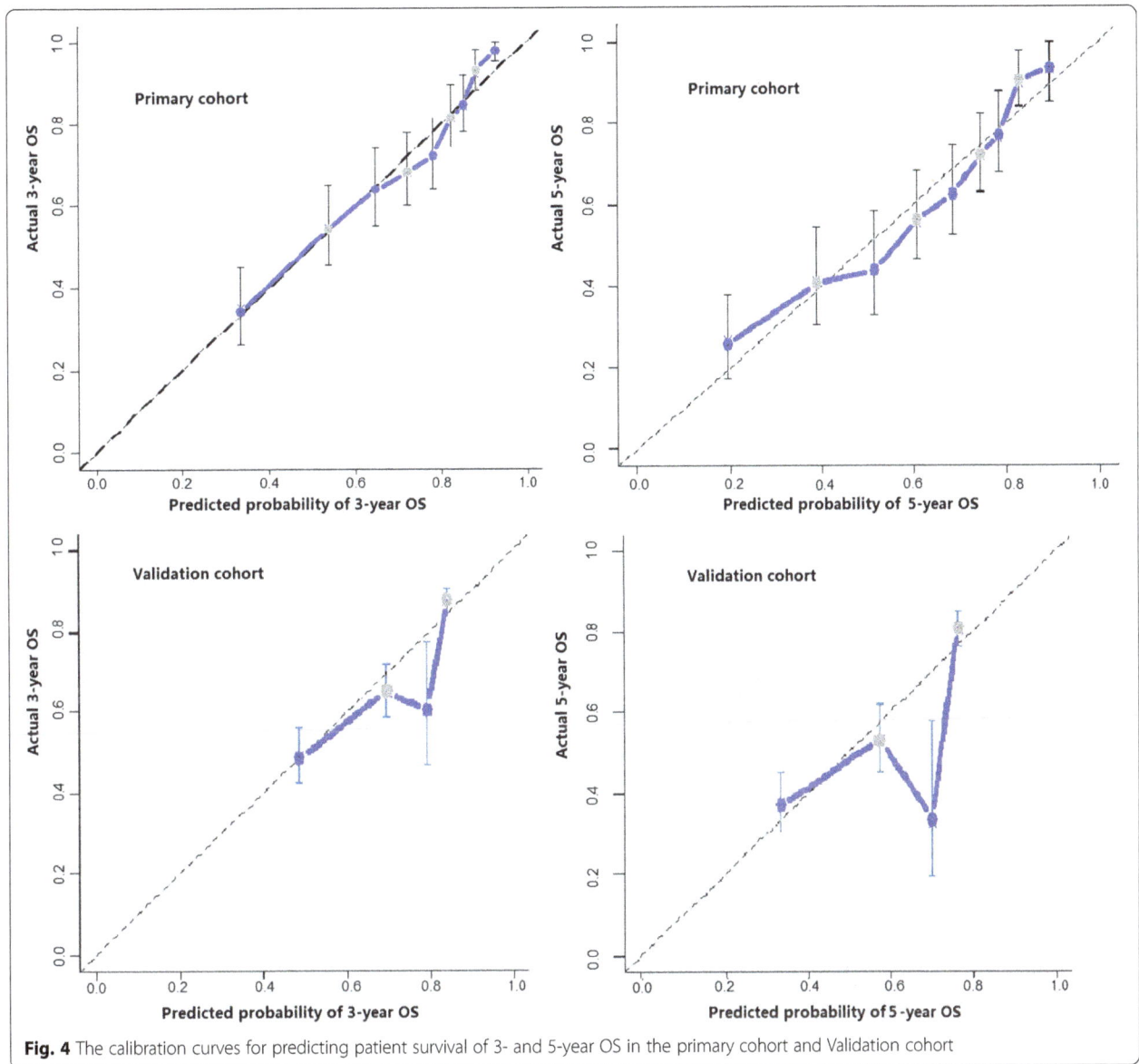

Fig. 4 The calibration curves for predicting patient survival of 3- and 5-year OS in the primary cohort and Validation cohort

is at the third place as a predictor, following pathologic N staging and age. Our proposed nomogram highlights the significant predictive role of neutrophil to lymphocyte ratio in prognosis.

Apart from inflammatory response biomarkers, age, tumor differentiation, pathologic T stage and pathologic N stage are the other independent prognostic factors which reveal a significant influence on survival. The nomogram incorporated with neutrophil to lymphocyte ratio might have the ability to predict the prognosis of patients undergoing surgery according to their inflammatory status, pathologic T and pathologic N stages and other tumor characteristics. Moreover, our nomogram could also assist clinicians in developing tailored treatment for

individual patients based on their inflammatory status.

Our nomogram has some limitations. First, the analysis is conducted retrospectively which creates intrinsic drawbacks. Second, some prognostic parameters (such as carcinoembryonic levels) and other important molecular factors (such as Epithelial growth factor receptor mutation) are not included in our analysis due to lack of data.

Conclusions

In conclusion, we have established an inflammation-related prognostic nomogram predicting individual survival in patients with NSCLC after surgery. Additionally, neutrophil to lymphocyte ratio can be considered as an

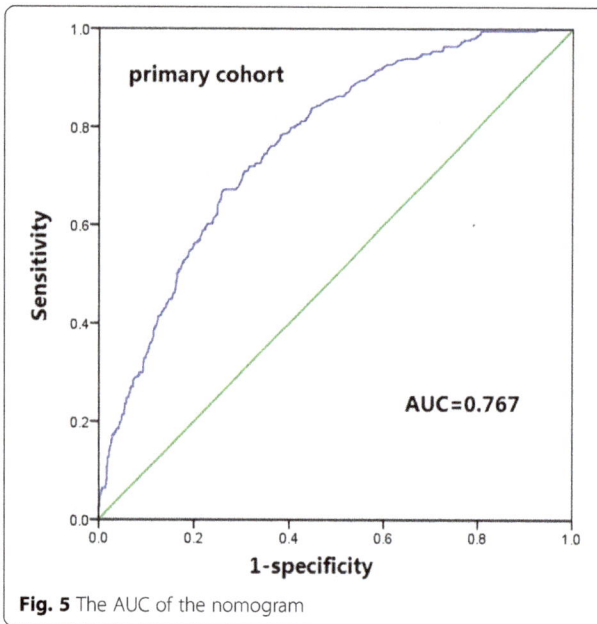

Fig. 5 The AUC of the nomogram

independent prognostic factor. The proposed nomogram in this study provides better predictive accuracy and confirms the predictive value of inflammation response biomarkers. It offers a useful tool for providing reference for clinicians to assess the survival of individual patients after surgery.

Abbreviations
ADC: Adenocarcinoma; dNLR: Derived neutrophil to lymphocyte ratio; LMR: Lymphocyte to monocyte ratio; NLR: Neutrophil to lymphocyte ratio; NSAID: Nonsteroidal anti-inflammatory drug; NSCLC: Non-small cell lung cancer; OS: Overall survival; PGTD: Pathological grading of tumor differentiation; PLR: Platelet to lymphocyte ratio; pN category: pathologcial N category; pT category: pathologcial T category; R: Reference; ROC: Receiver operating curve; SCC: Squamous cell carcinoma; SII: Systematic immune-inflammation index

Funding
The work was supported by National Natural Science Foundation of China (81301728) and Provincial Natural Science Foundation of Shandong (ZR2013HZ001) and (ZR2014HM100). The funding body had no role in the design of the study and collection, analysis, and interpretation of data and in writing the manuscript.

Authors' contributions
JJD and QL have full access to all of the data in the study and take responsibility for the integrity of the data and the accuracy of the data analysis. YW and XQ: contributed to the study design, definition of the inclusion and exclusion criteria, data analysis and interpretation, and drafting and revision the manuscript. NWK, HCS, KW: contributed to the study design and revision the manuscript. All the authors read and approved the final manuscript.

Competing interests
The authors declare that they have no competing interests.

Author details
Institute of Oncology, Shandong Provincial Hospital Affiliated to Shandong University, 324 Jingwu Road, Jinan 250021, People's Republic of China. [2]Department of Thoracic Surgery, Shandong Provincial Hospital Affiliated to Shandong University, 324 Jingwu Road, Jinan 250021, People's Republic of China. [3]Department of Oncology, Shandong Provincial Hospital Affiliated to Shandong University, 324 Jingwu Road, Jinan 250021, People's Republic of China. [4]Department of Clinical Oncology, The University of Hong Kong, Laboratory block, 21 Sassoon, Pokfulam, Hong Kong, People's Republic of China.

References
1. Groome PA, Bolejack V, Crowley JJ, Kennedy C, Krasnik M, Sobin LH, Goldstraw P. The IASLC lung Cancer staging project: validation of the proposals for revision of the T, N, and M descriptors and consequent stage groupings in the forthcoming (seventh) edition of the TNM classification of malignant tumours. J Thorac Oncol. 2007;2(8):694–705.
2. Shoenfeld Y, Tal A, Berliner S, Pinkhas J. Leukocytosis in non hematological malignancies–a possible tumor-associated marker. J Cancer Res Clin Oncol. 1986;111(1):54–8.
3. Cannon NA, Meyer J, Iyengar P, Ahn C, Westover KD, Choy H, Timmerman R. Neutrophil-lymphocyte and platelet-lymphocyte ratios as prognostic factors after stereotactic radiation therapy for early-stage non-small-cell lung cancer. J Thorac Oncol. 2015;10(2):280–5.
4. Choi JE, Villarreal J, Lasala J, Gottumukkala V, Mehran RJ, Rice D, Yu J, Feng L, Cata JP. Perioperative neutrophil:lymphocyte ratio and postoperative NSAID use as predictors of survival after lung cancer surgery: a retrospective study. Cancer Med. 2015;4(6):825–33.
5. Dirican A, Kucukzeybek BB, Alacacioglu A, Kucukzeybek Y, Erten C, Varol U, Somali I, Demir L, Bayoglu IV, Yildiz Y, et al. Do the derived neutrophil to lymphocyte ratio and the neutrophil to lymphocyte ratio predict prognosis in breast cancer? Int J Clin Oncol. 2015;20(1):70–81.
6. Huang C, Yue J, Li Z, Li N, Zhao J, Qi D. Usefulness of the neutrophil-to-lymphocyte ratio in predicting lymph node metastasis in patients with non-small cell lung cancer. Tumour Biol. 2015;36(10):7581–9.
7. Kemal Y, Yucel I, Ekiz K, Demirag G, Yilmaz B, Teker F, Ozdemir M. Elevated serum neutrophil to lymphocyte and platelet to lymphocyte ratios could be useful in lung cancer diagnosis. Asian Pac J Cancer Prev. 2014;15(6):2651–4.
8. Lin GN, Peng JW, Liu PP, Liu DY, Xiao JJ, Chen XQ. Elevated neutrophil-to-lymphocyte ratio predicts poor outcome in patients with advanced non-small-cell lung cancer receiving first-line gefitinib or erlotinib treatment. Asia-Pacific journal of clinical oncology 2017;13(5):e189–e194.
9. Sarraf KM, Belcher E, Raevsky E, Nicholson AG, Goldstraw P, Lim E. Neutrophil/lymphocyte ratio and its association with survival after complete resection in non-small cell lung cancer. J Thorac Cardiovasc Surg. 2009; 137(2):425–8.
10. Walsh SR, Cook EJ, Goulder F, Justin TA, Keeling NJ. Neutrophil-lymphocyte ratio as a prognostic factor in colorectal cancer. J Surg Oncol. 2005;91(3):181–4.
11. Absenger G, Szkandera J, Pichler M, Stotz M, Arminger F, Weissmueller M, Schaberl-Moser R, Samonigg H, Stojakovic T, Gerger A. A derived neutrophil to lymphocyte ratio predicts clinical outcome in stage II and III colon cancer patients. Br J Cancer. 2013;109(2):395_400.
12. Szkandera J, Gerger A, Liegl-Atzwanger B, Stotz M, Samonigg H, Friesenbichler J, Stojakovic T, Leithner A, Pichler M. The derived neutrophil/lymphocyte ratio predicts poor clinical outcome in soft tissue sarcoma patients. Am J Surg. 2014;210(1):111_6.
13. Huang Y, Feng JF. Low preoperative lymphocyte to monocyte ratio predicts poor cancer-specific survival in patients with esophageal squamous cell carcinoma. OncoTargets Ther. 2015;8:137_45.
14. Lin GN, Peng JW, Xiao JJ, Liu DY, Xia ZJ. Prognostic impact of circulating monocytes and lymphocyte-to-monocyte ratio on previously untreated metastatic non-small cell lung cancer patients receiving platinum-based doublet. Med Oncol. 2014;31(7):70.
15. Hu B, Yang XR, Xu Y, Sun YF, Sun C, Guo W, Zhang X, Wang WM, Qiu SJ, Zhou J, et al. Systemic immune-inflammation index predicts prognosis of patients after curative resection for hepatocellular carcinoma. Clin Cancer Res. 2014;20(23):6212–22.

16. Liang W, Zhang L, Jiang G, Wang Q, Liu L, Liu D, Wang Z, Zhu Z, Deng Q, Xiong X, et al. Development and validation of a nomogram for predicting survival in patients with resected non-small-cell lung cancer. J Clin Oncol. 2015;33(8):861–9.

17. Keam B, Kim DW, Park JH, Lee JO, Kim TM, Lee SH, Chung DH, Heo DS. Nomogram predicting clinical outcomes in non-small cell lung Cancer patients treated with epidermal growth factor receptor tyrosine kinase inhibitors. Cancer Res Treat. 2014;46(4):323–30.

18. Hu P, Shen H, Wang G, Zhang P, Liu Q, Du J. Prognostic significance of systemic inflammation-based lymphocyte- monocyte ratio in patients with lung cancer: based on a large cohort study. PLoS One. 2014;9(9):e108062.

19. Qu X, Pang Z, Yi W, Wang Y, Wang K, Liu Q, Du J. High percentage of alpha1-globulin in serum protein is associated with unfavorable prognosis in non-small cell lung cancer. Med Oncol. 2014;31(10):238.

20. Yuan D, Zhu K, Li K, Yan R, Jia Y, Dang C. The preoperative neutrophil-lymphocyte ratio predicts recurrence and survival among patients undergoing R0 resections of adenocarcinomas of the esophagogastric junction. J Surg Oncol. 2014;110(3):333–40.

21. Forget P, Machiels JP, Coulie PG, Berliere M, Poncelet AJ, Tombal B, Stainier A, Legrand C, Canon JL, Kremer Y, et al. Neutrophil:lymphocyte ratio and intraoperative use of ketorolac or diclofenac are prognostic factors in different cohorts of patients undergoing breast, lung, and kidney cancer surgery. Ann Surg Oncol. 2013;20(Suppl 3):S650–60.

22. Zhang S, Da L, Yang X, Feng D, Yin R, Li M, Zhang Z, Jiang F, Xu L. Celecoxib potentially inhibits metastasis of lung cancer promoted by surgery in mice, via suppression of the PGE2-modulated beta-catenin pathway. Toxicol Lett. 2014;225(2):201–7.

23. Kusumanto YH, Dam WA, Hospers GA, Meijer C, Mulder NH. Platelets and granulocytes, in particular the neutrophils, form important compartments for circulating vascular endothelial growth factor. Angiogenesis. 2003;6(4):283–7.

24. McGuire L, Kiecolt-Glaser JK, Glaser R. Depressive symptoms and lymphocyte proliferation in older adults. J Abnorm Psychol. 2002;111(1):192–7.

18

Gefitinib provides similar effectiveness and improved safety than erlotinib for east Asian populations with advanced non–small cell lung cancer

Wenxiong Zhang, Yiping Wei* (iD), Dongliang Yu, Jianjun Xu and Jinhua Peng

Abstract

Background: The first-generation epidermal growth factor receptor tyrosine kinase inhibitors gefitinib and erlotinib have both been proven effective for treating advanced non–small cell lung cancer (NSCLC), especially in East Asian patients. We conducted this meta-analysis to compare their efficacy and safety in treating advanced NSCLC in this population.

Methods: We systematically searched PubMed, ScienceDirect, The Cochrane Library, Scopus, Ovid MEDLINE, Embase, Web of Science, and Google Scholar for the relevant studies. Overall survival (OS), progression-free survival (PFS), objective response rate (ORR), disease control rate (DCR), and adverse effects (AEs) were analyzed as primary endpoints.

Results: We identified 5829 articles, among which 31 were included in the final analysis. Both gefitinib and erlotinib were effective for treating advanced NSCLC, with comparable PFS (95% confidence interval [CI]: 0.97–1.10, $p = 0.26$), OS (95% CI: 0.89–1.21, $p = 0.61$), ORR (95% CI: 1.00–1.18, $p = 0.06$), and DCR (95% CI: 0.93–1.05, $p = 0.68$). Erlotinib induced a significantly higher rate of dose reduction (95% CI: 0.13–0.65, $p = 0.002$) and grade 3–5 AEs (95% CI: 0.27–0.71, $p = 0.0008$). In subgroup analysis of AEs, the erlotinib group had a significantly higher rate and severity of skin rash, nausea/vomiting, diarrhea, fatigue and stomatitis.

Conclusions: With equal anti-tumor efficacy and fewer AEs compared with erlotinib, gefitinib is more suitable for treating advanced NSCLC in East Asian patients. Further large-scale, well-designed randomized controlled trials are warranted to confirm our findings.

Keywords: Gefitinib, Erlotinib, Non-small cell lung cancer, East Asian populations, Targeted therapy, Meta-analysis

Background

In Asia, lung cancer is the most common cancer in men (age-standardized rate [ASR; per 100,000] = 35.2) and the third most common cancer in women (ASR = 12.7). The number of patients with lung cancer has increased rapidly by the year [1, 2]. The discovery and development of therapeutics targeting epidermal growth factor receptor (EGFR), namely tyrosine kinase inhibitors (TKIs), in the past decade was an important clinical advance in non–small cell lung cancer (NSCLC) treatment

* Correspondence: weiyiping2015@163.com
Department of thoracic surgery, The second affiliated hospital of Nanchang University, 1 Min De Road, Nanchang 330006, China

[3, 4]. Recommended by clinical guidelines, both gefitinib (Iressa) and erlotinib (Tarceva) are now widely accepted as standard-of-care therapy for patients with NSCLC whose tumors harbor activating *EGFR* mutations, especially patients with certain clinical characteristics (Asian descent, female gender, never-smoker, adenocarcinoma) [5–8]. The EGFR TKIs gefitinib and erlotinib both achieve a higher response rate for treating NSCLC in East Asian countries than in the Western countries [9]. However, which EGFR TKI can achieve better efficacy is controversial. In a phase III randomized controlled trial (RCT), Urata reported a higher incidence of grade 3–4 skin rash but less alanine aminotransferase/aspartate

aminotransferase elevation in the erlotinib arm. Progression-free survival (PFS), overall survival (OS), and objective response rate (ORR) were similar between the two groups [10]. In another phase III RCT, Yang reported that gefitinib and erlotinib had similar efficacy (PFS, OS, ORR) in NSCLC, with similar toxicities [11]. Some studies have shown that gefitinib has better anti-tumor efficacy or less toxicity for NSCLC [12, 13]. However, other studies have reported opposite results and have suggested that erlotinib is more effective [14, 15].

To resolve this controversy, we conducted a meta-analysis of related studies to compare the anti-tumor efficacy and adverse effects (AEs) of gefitinib and erlotinib for treating East Asian populations with NSCLC.

Methods
We conducted this meta-analysis according to PRISMA (Preferred Reporting Items for Systematic Review and Meta-Analysis) guidelines.

Search strategy
The relevant literature was retrieved using the following electronic databases: (1) PubMed; (2) ScienceDirect; (3) The Cochrane Library; (4) Scopus; (5) Web of Science; (6) Embase; (7) Ovid MEDLINE; and (8) Google Scholar. The last search was on February 14, 2018. The following terms were used: "gefitinib", "erlotinib", and "Lung cancer". The complete search we used for PubMed was: (gefitinib [MeSH Terms] OR gefitinib [Text Word] OR IRESSA [Text Word] OR ZD1839 [Text Word]) AND (erlotinib [MeSH Terms] OR erlotinib [Text Word] OR Tarceva [Text Word] OR OSI-774 [Text Word]) AND (lung cancer [MeSH Terms] OR lung cancer [Text Word] OR lung carcinoma [Text Word] OR lung neoplasm [Text Word] OR NSCLC [Text Word]). The references of retrieved articles were also searched for further eligible articles. No language restriction was imposed.

Selection criteria
Articles that met the following criteria were included: (1) East Asian population with histologically or cyto-logically confirmed NSCLC based on the Eastern Cooperative Oncology Group; (2) compared gefitinib versus erlotinib; (3) outcomes were PFS, OS, ORR, disease control rate (DCR), and AEs. We excluded reviews without original data, meta-analyses, animal experiments, abstracts only, and studies with duplicated data.

Data extraction
Two investigators extracted the following data independently: first author, publication year, country, number of participants, participant characteristics (age, sex, stage of cancer, pathological type, line of treatment), anti-tumor efficacy indices (PFS, OS, ORR, DCR), and number of AEs (total AEs, grade 3–5 AEs). A third investigator resolved disagreements on all terms.

Quality assessment
The quality of RCTs was assessed using the 5-point Jadad scale, which contains questions on three main items: randomization, masking, and accountability of all patients. High-quality studies score ≥ 3 points [16].

The quality of cohort studies was assessed using the Newcastle-Ottawa Scale (NOS, 9 points), which also contains questions on three main items: selection, comparability, and exposure. High-quality studies score 8–9 points; medium-quality studies score 6–7 points [17].

Statistical analysis
The meta-analysis was conducted using Review Manager (version 5.3, The Nordic Cochrane Centre) and STATA (version 12.0, Stata Corp). Hazard ratios (HR) with 95% confidence intervals (CI) were used to analyze the PFS and OS (HR > 1 favors the erlotinib group; HR < 1 favors the gefitinib group). The HR data were extracted directly from some studies or from Kaplan–Meier curves according to Tierney et al. [18] from other studies. Pooled risk ratios (RR) with 95% CIs were used to analyze the ORR, DCR, and AEs (RR > 1 favors the gefitinib group; RR < 1 favors the erlotinib group). Subgroup analysis of PFS, OS, and ORR was conducted to determine whether the results would change according to *EGFR* mutation status, ethnicity, line of treatment, histology, tumor stage, and study design. Heterogeneity was evaluated using the χ^2 test and I^2 statistic. If $I^2 > 50\%$ or $p < 0.1$ for the χ^2 test, reflecting significant heterogeneity, the random-effects model was used; otherwise, the fixed-effects model was used. Publication bias was explored using Begg's rank correlation and Egger's linear regression tests. $P < 0.05$ indicated statistical significance.

Results
Search results and study quality assessment
We initially identified 5829 potentially eligible studies. After screening, 31 studies involving 8054 patients (gefitinib group, 4907 patients; erlotinib group, 3147 patients) were included for the final analysis (Fig. 1) [10–15, 19–43]. Of the 31 studies, three were RCTs and 28 were retrospective studies. Twenty-two studies were of high quality (three RCTs scored 4–5 points, five retrospective studies scored 9 points, 14 retrospective studies scored 8 points) and nine studies were of medium quality (seven retrospective studies scored 7 points, two retrospective studies scored 6 points) (Table 1). Table 2 summarizes the baseline characteristics and main evaluation indices of the included studies.

```
┌──────────────────────────────────────────────────────────────────────────────────────┐
│  ┌─────────────────────────────────────┐      ┌─────────────────────────────┐          │
│  │ Records were identified though      │      │ Additional records were     │          │
│  │ database searching from PubMed,     │      │ identified through Google   │          │
│  │ Ovid Medline, Embase, Web of        │      │ Scholar.                    │          │
│  │ Science, ScienceDirect, the         │      │ n = 46                      │          │
│  │ Cochrane Library, Scopus.           │      └─────────────────────────────┘          │
│  │ n = 5783 (Duplicates removed)       │                                                │
│  └─────────────────────────────────────┘                                               │
│                                                                                        │
│              ┌─────────────────────────────────────┐                                   │
│              │ Title and abstracts screened for     │                                   │
│              │ eligibility. n = 5829                │                                   │
│              └─────────────────────────────────────┘                                   │
│                              │           ┌──────────────────────────────┐              │
│                              │───────────│ 5615 articles were excluded. │              │
│              ┌───────────────▼──────────┐└──────────────────────────────┘              │
│              │ Full retrieved for        │   ┌──────────────────────────────────┐       │
│              │ detailed assessment.      │   │ 183 articles were excluded.      │       │
│              │ n = 214                   │───│ Reasons for exclusion:           │       │
│              └───────────────┬──────────┘   │ 63 non-comparative studies       │       │
│                              │              │ 43 not compare gefitinib and     │       │
│                              │              │ erlotinib                        │       │
│                              │              │ 42 not published in English      │       │
│              ┌───────────────▼──────────┐   │ 21 only abstract                 │       │
│              │ 31 articles included in   │   │ 9 not only East Asian patients   │       │
│              │ meta-analysis.            │   │ 5 duplicate centres              │       │
│              │ For PFS: n = 24           │   └──────────────────────────────────┘       │
│              │ For OS: n = 21            │                                              │
│              │ For ORR: n = 13           │                                              │
│              │ For DCR: n = 11           │                                              │
│              │ For AEs: n=14             │                                              │
│              └───────────────────────────┘                                             │
└──────────────────────────────────────────────────────────────────────────────────────┘
```

Fig. 1 Flow chart of study selection

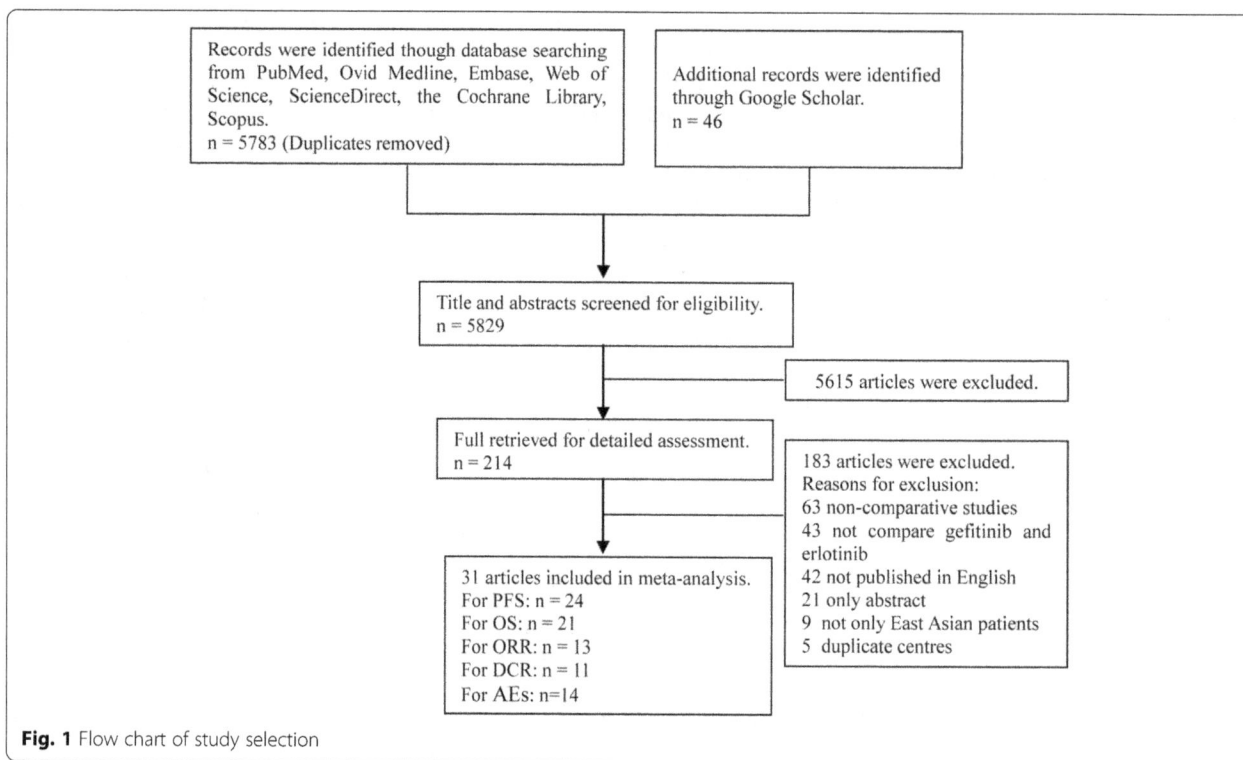

Anti-tumor efficacy

We assessed anti-tumor efficacy between the gefitinib and erlotinib groups based on PFS, OS, ORR, and DCR.

Twenty-four studies compared PFS (heterogeneity: $p = 0.03$, $I^2 = 38\%$). No significant difference was found between the two groups (95% CI: 0.97–1.10, $p = 0.26$; Fig. 2).

Twenty-one studies compared OS (heterogeneity: $p = 0.0004$, $I^2 = 58\%$). No significant difference was found between the two groups (95% CI: 0.89–1.21, $p = 0.61$; Fig. 3).

Thirteen studies compared ORR (heterogeneity: $p = 0.24$, $I^2 = 20\%$). No significant difference was found between the two groups (95% CI: 1.00–1.18, $p = 0.06$; Fig. 4a).

Eleven studies compared DCR (heterogeneity: $p = 0.17$, $I^2 = 29\%$). No significant difference was found between the two groups (95% CI: 0.93–1.05, $p = 0.68$; Fig. 4b).

Toxicity

We compared toxicity between the gefitinib and erlotinib groups based on total AEs, grade 3–5 AEs, and subgroup analysis of the 10 most reported AEs.

Five studies compared total AEs (heterogeneity: $p = 0.0007$, $I^2 = 79\%$). No significant difference was found between the two groups (95% CI: 0.87–1.13, $p = 0.94$; Fig. 5a).

Seven studies compared grade 3–5 AEs (heterogeneity: $p = 0.001$, $I^2 = 73\%$). The gefitinib group had a significantly lower incidence rate of grade 3–5 AEs than the erlotinib group (95% CI: 0.27–0.71, $p = 0.0008$; Fig. 5b). Some patients had drug discontinuations/reductions due to the occurrence of serious AEs. Two studies compared drug discontinuations; there was no significant difference between the two groups (95% CI: 0.40–1.80, $p = 0.68$; Fig. 6a). Four studies compared drug reductions; the erlotinib group had more drug reductions (95% CI: 0.13–0.65, $p = 0.002$; Fig. 6b).

In subgroup analysis of the 10 most reported AEs (skin rash, diarrhea, nausea/vomiting, fatigue, anorexia, interstitial lung disease, stomatitis, elevated liver enzymes, infection, neutropenia), the results for all-grade AEs showed no significant differences in anorexia, interstitial lung disease, elevated liver enzymes, infection, neutropenia and nausea/vomiting between the two groups. For all-grade AEs, erlotinib induced significantly higher rates of skin rash (95% CI: 0.74–0.94, $p = 0.003$), diarrhea (95% CI: 0.73–0.95, $p = 0.005$), fatigue (95% CI: 0.23–0.95, $p = 0.04$), and stomatitis (95% CI: 0.15–0.54, $p = 0.0001$) (Table 3). The results for grade 3–5 AEs showed no significant differences in anorexia, interstitial lung disease, elevated liver enzymes, infection, and neutropenia between the two groups. For grade 3–5 AEs, erlotinib induced significantly higher rates of skin rash (95% CI: 0.12–0.41, $p < 0.00001$), diarrhea (95% CI: 0.29–0.74, $p = 0.001$), nausea/vomiting (95% CI: 0.11–0.49, $p = 0.0001$), fatigue (95% CI: 0.09–0.87, $p = 0.03$), and stomatitis (95% CI: 0.08–0.99, $p = 0.05$) (Table 4).

Table 1 Quality assessment of all included studies

Study		Selection	Comparability	Exposure	Randomization	Masking	Accountability of all patients	Quality (score)
Randomized controlled trial								
2012	Kim [26]				★★	★	★	4
2016	Urata [10]				★★	★★	★	5
2017	Yang [11]				★★	★★	★	5
Retrospective study								
2010	Kim [19]	★★★	★★	★★				7
2010	Hotta [20]	★★★★	★★	★★★				9
2010	Hong [21]	★★★	★★	★★				7
2011	Wu [22]	★★★★	★★	★★★				9
2011	Shin [12]	★★★	★★	★★				7
2011	Togashi [23]	★★★★	★★	★★				8
2011	Fan [14]	★★★★	★★	★★				8
2011	Jung [24]	★★★	★★	★				6
2012	Wu [25]	★★★★	★★	★★				8
2012	Suzumura [27]	★★★	★★	★★★				8
2013	Yoshida [28]	★★★★	★★	★★				8
2013	Shao [29]	★★★★	★★	★★★				9
2013	Lee [30]	★★★★	★★	★★				8
2013	Yu [31]	★★★★	★★	★★				8
2014	Lim [32]	★★★★	★★	★★★				9
2014	Sato [13]	★★★★	★★	★★				8
2014	Lin [33]	★★★	★★	★★				7
2014	Ren [34]	★★★★	★★	★★				8
2014	Li [35]	★★★	★★	★★★				8
2014	Takeda [36]	★★★	★★	★				6
2015	Otsuka [37]	★★★★	★★	★★★				9
2015	Song [38]	★★★	★★	★★				7
2015	Koo [39]	★★★★	★★	★				7
2016	Ruan [40]	★★★	★★	★★★				8
2016	Hirano [41]	★★★	★★	★★★				8
2016	Suh [42]	★★★	★★	★★				7
2016	Kashima [43]	★★★	★★	★★★				8
2017	Kuan [15]	★★★★	★★	★★				8

Subgroup analysis

To determine whether the anti-tumor efficacy of gefitinib versus erlotinib was consistent across subgroups, the pooled efficacy for PFS, OS, and ORR was estimated within each category of the following classification variables: country, tumor stage, histology, line of treatment, *EGFR* mutation status, and study design. All subgroup differences were not statistically significant in terms of PFS, OS, and ORR between the gefitinib and erlotinib groups (Table 5).

Sensitivity analysis

Significant heterogeneity was found in the analysis of OS, total AEs and grade 3–5 AEs. The influence of each study on the pooled results was evaluated to evaluate stability and sensitivity. The results suggested that the outcomes of OS, total AEs and grade 3–5 AEs were reliable and stable (Fig. 7).

Cumulative meta-analysis

Analyses of PFS (Additional file 1: Figure S1), OS (Additional file 2: Figure S2), ORR (Additional file 3:

Table 2 Characteristics of included studies

Study	Country	Groups	Patients (n)	Median age (year)	Stage	Treatment line	EGFR mutations	Adenocarcinoma (%)	Design	Quality (score)
2010 Kim [19]	Korea	G vs. E	171/171	58/59	IIIb, IV	2, 3	–	86	RS	7
2010 Hotta [20]	Japan	G vs. E	330/209	68/68	II–IV or recurrent	2, 3	–	76	RS	9
2010 Hong [21]	Keroa	G vs. E	20/17	61/67	IIIb, IV	2, 3	–	75	RS	7
2011 Wu [22]	Taiwan	G vs. E	440/276	67/67	IIIb, IV	1 or later	Partial	85	RS	9
2011 Shin [12]	Keroa	G vs. E	100/82	65/65	III, IV	2	Partial	0	RS	7
2011 Togashi [23]	Japan	G vs. E	85/69	65/68	IIIb, IV	1 or later	Partial	82	RS	8
2011 Fan [14]	Taiwan	G vs. E	715/407	–	IIIb, IV	1 or later	Partial	77	RS	8
2011 Jung [24]	Korea	G vs. E	72/51	55/55	IIIb, IV	1 or later	Partial	59	RS	6
2012 Wu [25]	Taiwan	G vs. E	124/100	–	IIIb, IV	1 or later	Partial	100	RS	8
2012 Kim [26]	Keroa	G vs. E	48/48	59/60	IIIb, IV	2	Partial	91	RCT	4
2012 Suzumura [27]	Japan	G vs. E	232/86	67/66	IIIb, IV	–	Partial	95	RS	8
2013 Yoshida [28]	Japan	G vs. E	107/35	64/67	III, IV or recurrent	1 or later	Partial	84	RS	8
2013 Shao [29]	Taiwan	G vs. E	655/329	61/63	IIIb, IV or recurrent	3	–	80	RS	9
2013 Lee [30]	Korea	G vs. E	11/14	49/58	IV	1 or later	Partial	92	RS	8
2013 Yu [31]	China	G vs. E	16/22	54/52	–	3	Partial	100	RS	8
2014 Lim [32]	Korea	G vs. E	121/121	58/58	IIIb, IV	1 or later	All	98	RS	9
2014 Sato [13]	Japan	G vs. E	213/69	66/66	IIIb, IV or recurrent	–	Partial	86	RS	8
2014 Lin [33]	China	G vs. E	57/24	–	IIIb, IV	1	All	59	RS	7
2014 Ren [34]	China	G vs. E	60/142	59/59	IV	1 or later	Partial	66	RS	8
2014 Li [35]	China	G vs. E	53/97	59/59	IIIb, IV	2	Partial	67	RS	8
2014 Takeda [36]	Japan	G vs. E	57/11	69/69	III, IV or recurrent	1 or later	All	99	RS	6
2015 Otsuka [37]	Japan	G vs. E	35/9	70/62	IIIb, IV	1 or later	All	91	RS	9
2015 Song [38]	China	G vs. E	37/65	75/75	IIIb, IV	2 or later	Partial	83	RS	7
2015 Koo [39]	Korea	G vs. E	166/56	–	IV	1, 2, 3	All	87	RS	7
2016 Ruan [40]	China	G vs. E	63/134	59/60	III, IV	–	All	–	RS	8
2016 Hirano [41]	Japan	G vs. E	10/16	71/71	IB–IV or recurrent	–	All	81	RS	8
2016 Urata [10]	Japan	G vs. E	279/280	68/67	IIIb, IV or recurrent	2, 3	Partial	100	RCT	5
2016 Suh [42]	Korea	G vs. E	146/5	65/65	IIIb, IV	1	All	97	RS	7
2016 Kashima [43]	Japan	G vs. E	52/11	68/68	IV	–	All	–	RS	8
2017 Yang [11]	China	G vs. E	128/128	–	IIIb, IV	1, 2	All	96	RCT	5
2017 Kuan [15]	Taiwan	G vs. E	304/63	65/67	IIIb, IV	1	All	–	RS	8

Abbreviations: G gefitinib, E erlotinib, EGFR epidermal growth factor receptor, RS retrospective study, RCT randomized controlled trial, –: not available

Figure S3), DCR (Additional file 4: Figure S4) and total AEs (Additional file 5: Figure S5) demonstrated that the RRs of the final results became robust within a narrow range and remained not significant as publication years increased and as recent high-quality studies were included. After inclusion of Shin et al.'s study [12], the RR and 95% CI for grade 3–5 AEs decreased to < 1 and became stable (Additional file 6: Figure S6). Although there was no significantly reduced risk in ORR, clear evidence showed that the confidence interval was becoming narrow, and trended toward significance (favors gefitinib).

Publication bias

There was no evidence of publication bias for PFS (Begg's test $p = 0.585$; Egger's test $p = 0.477$, Fig. 8a) and OS (Begg's test $p = 0.880$; Egger's test $p = 0.798$, Fig. 8b).

				Hazard Ratio		Hazard Ratio
Study or Subgroup	log[Hazard Ratio]	SE	Weight	IV, Fixed, 95% CI	Year	IV, Fixed, 95% CI
Kim 2010	-0.2157	0.1152	7.2%	0.81 [0.64, 1.01]	2010	
Hong 2010	0.0392	0.0514	36.2%	1.04 [0.94, 1.15]	2010	
Wu 2011	-0.5447	0.3338	0.9%	0.58 [0.30, 1.12]	2011	
Jung 2011	-0.3567	0.865	0.1%	0.70 [0.13, 3.81]	2011	
Shin 2011	0.088	0.153	4.1%	1.09 [0.81, 1.47]	2011	
Fan 2011	0.2351	0.0976	10.0%	1.27 [1.04, 1.53]	2011	
Kim 2012	-0.1863	0.192	2.6%	0.83 [0.57, 1.21]	2012	
Wu 2012	-0.1165	0.1546	4.0%	0.89 [0.66, 1.21]	2012	
Yu 2013	-0.12783	0.3612	0.7%	0.88 [0.43, 1.79]	2013	
Yoshida 2013	-0.1098	0.3458	0.8%	0.90 [0.45, 1.76]	2013	
Li 2014	-0.2219	0.207	2.2%	0.80 [0.53, 1.20]	2014	
Takeda 2014	0.0392	0.4741	0.4%	1.04 [0.41, 2.63]	2014	
Lin 2014	-1.4271	1.0675	0.1%	0.24 [0.03, 1.94]	2014	
Ren 2014	0.088	0.1788	3.0%	1.09 [0.77, 1.55]	2014	
Lim 2014	-0.1278	0.1461	4.5%	0.88 [0.66, 1.17]	2014	
Koo 2015	-0.1508	0.1831	2.9%	0.86 [0.60, 1.23]	2015	
Song 2015	-0.4463	0.5243	0.3%	0.64 [0.23, 1.79]	2015	
Otsuka 2015	1.1086	0.5274	0.3%	3.03 [1.08, 8.52]	2015	
Urata 2016	0.1178	0.0918	11.3%	1.13 [0.94, 1.35]	2016	
Hirano 2016	0.0583	0.4502	0.5%	1.06 [0.44, 2.56]	2016	
Suh 2016	-0.4385	0.5243	0.3%	0.65 [0.23, 1.80]	2016	
Kashima 2016	1.1151	0.6585	0.2%	3.05 [0.84, 11.09]	2016	
Kuan 2017	0.5621	0.2239	1.9%	1.75 [1.13, 2.72]	2017	
Yang 2017	0.2107	0.1344	5.3%	1.23 [0.95, 1.61]	2017	
Total (95% CI)			100.0%	1.04 [0.97, 1.10]		

Heterogeneity: Chi² = 37.29, df = 23 (P = 0.03); I² = 38%
Test for overall effect: Z = 1.12 (P = 0.26)

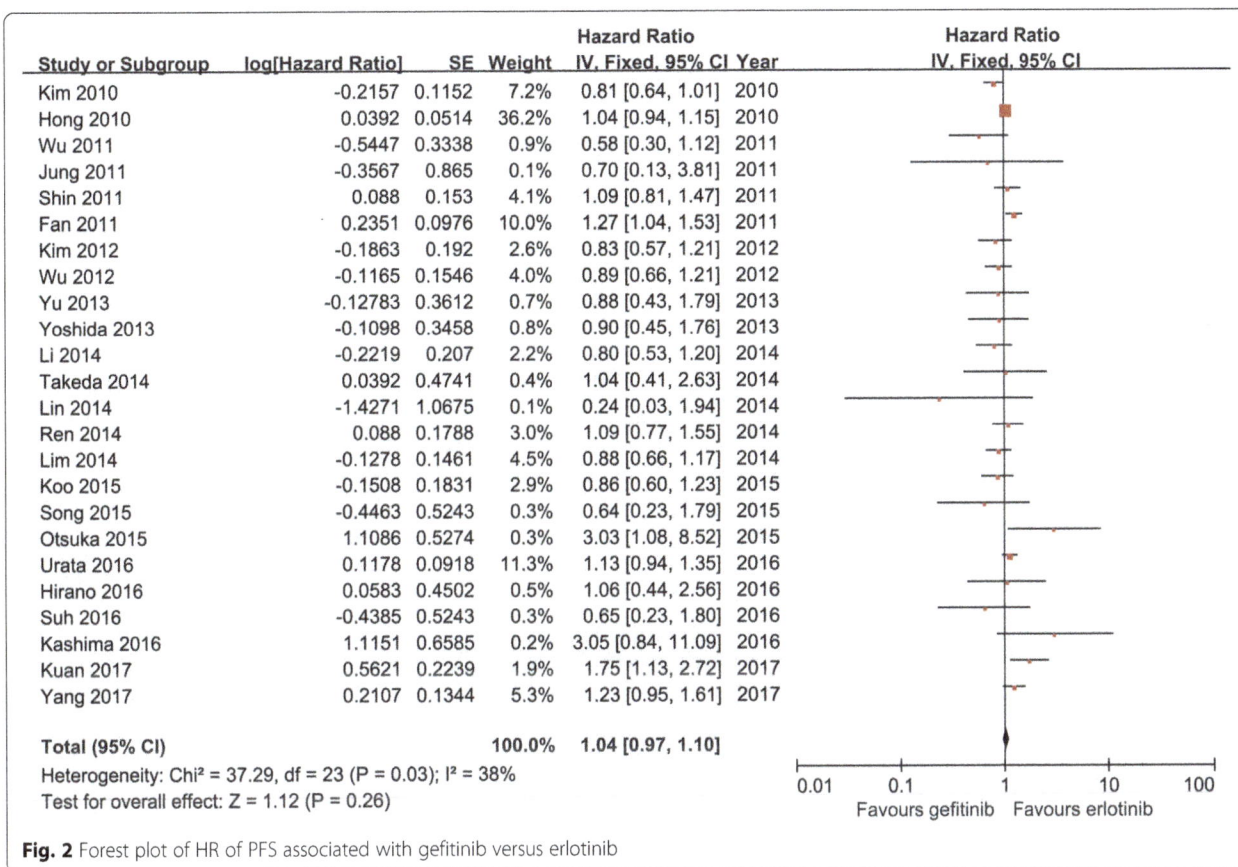

Fig. 2 Forest plot of HR of PFS associated with gefitinib versus erlotinib

				Hazard Ratio	Hazard Ratio
Study or Subgroup	log[Hazard Ratio]	SE	Weight	IV, Random, 95% CI	IV, Random, 95% CI
Fan 2011	0.39	0.1183	8.9%	1.48 [1.17, 1.86]	
Hirano 2016	0.1222	0.4617	2.3%	1.13 [0.46, 2.79]	
Hong 2010	-0.3425	0.7357	1.0%	0.71 [0.17, 3.00]	
Jung 2011	0.4055	0.6019	1.5%	1.50 [0.46, 4.88]	
Kashima 2016	0.2927	0.5137	1.9%	1.34 [0.49, 3.67]	
Kim 2010	-0.004	0.13	8.6%	1.00 [0.77, 1.29]	
Kim 2012	0.793	0.6096	1.4%	2.21 [0.67, 7.30]	
Koo 2015	-0.0943	0.2027	6.4%	0.91 [0.61, 1.35]	
Lee 2013	0.108	0.4181	2.7%	1.11 [0.49, 2.53]	
Li 2014	0.0733	0.2252	5.8%	1.08 [0.69, 1.67]	
Lin 2014	-2.4079	0.7394	1.0%	0.09 [0.02, 0.38]	
Ren 2014	-0.0263	0.1727	7.2%	0.97 [0.69, 1.37]	
Shao 2013	-0.0392	0.0875	9.8%	0.96 [0.81, 1.14]	
Shin 2011	0.3192	0.2702	4.8%	1.38 [0.81, 2.34]	
Suh 2016	-0.587	0.5164	1.9%	0.56 [0.20, 1.53]	
Takeda 2014	-0.462	0.5619	1.6%	0.63 [0.21, 1.90]	
Urata 2016	0.0373	0.1124	9.1%	1.04 [0.83, 1.29]	
Wu 2011	-0.4463	0.1323	8.5%	0.64 [0.49, 0.83]	
Wu 2012	0.6387	0.2324	5.6%	1.89 [1.20, 2.99]	
Yang 2017	0.1744	0.149	8.0%	1.19 [0.89, 1.59]	
Yu 2013	-0.0124	0.5098	1.9%	0.99 [0.36, 2.68]	
Total (95% CI)			100.0%	1.04 [0.89, 1.21]	

Heterogeneity: Tau² = 0.05; Chi² = 48.00, df = 20 (P = 0.0004); I² = 58%
Test for overall effect: Z = 0.50 (P = 0.61)

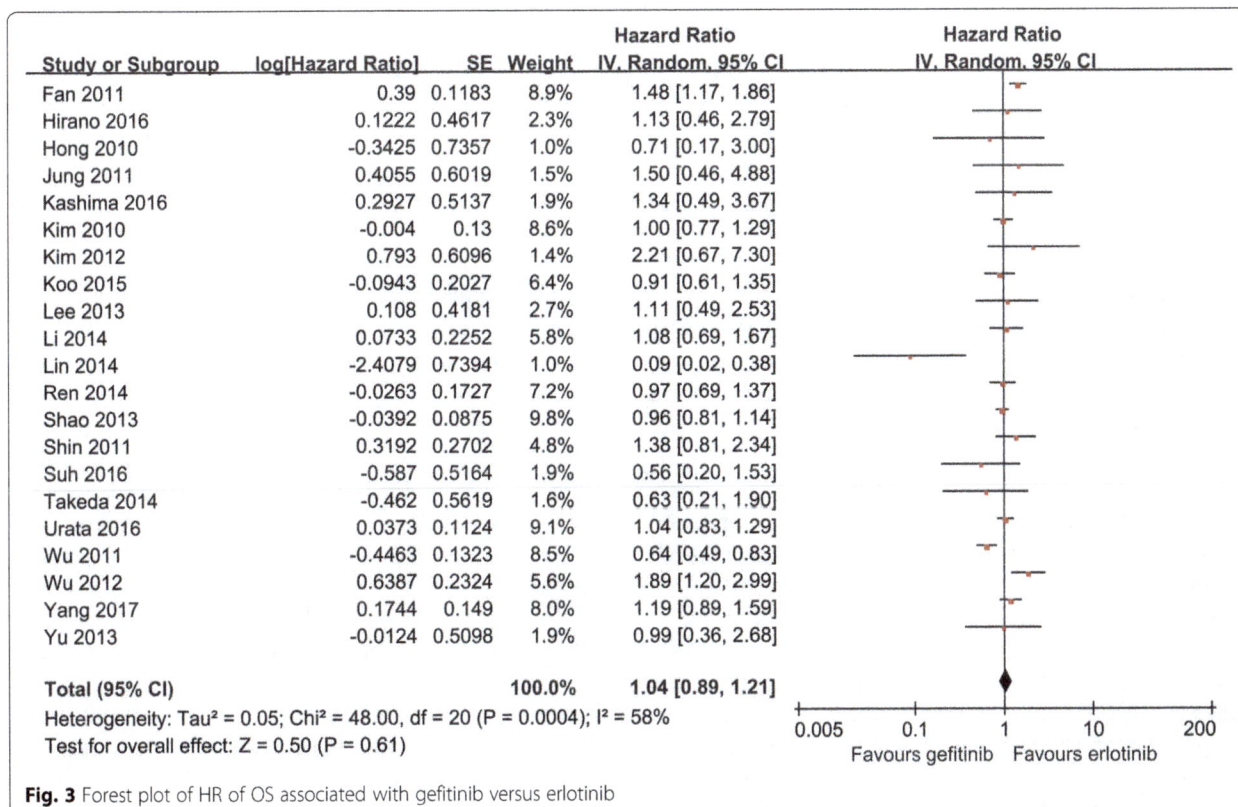

Fig. 3 Forest plot of HR of OS associated with gefitinib versus erlotinib

A

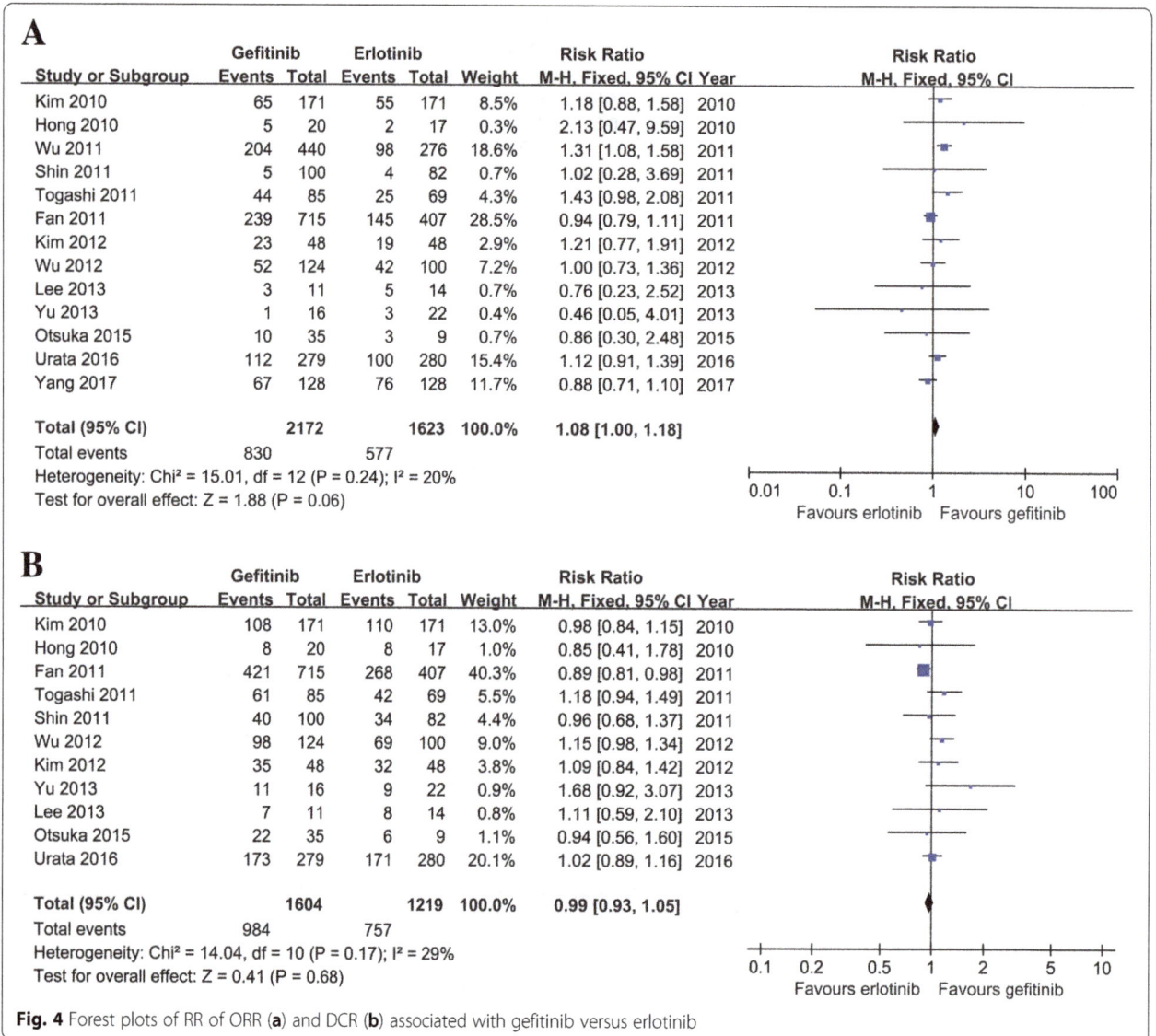

Study or Subgroup	Gefitinib Events	Total	Erlotinib Events	Total	Weight	Risk Ratio M-H, Fixed, 95% CI	Year
Kim 2010	65	171	55	171	8.5%	1.18 [0.88, 1.58]	2010
Hong 2010	5	20	2	17	0.3%	2.13 [0.47, 9.59]	2010
Wu 2011	204	440	98	276	18.6%	1.31 [1.08, 1.58]	2011
Shin 2011	5	100	4	82	0.7%	1.02 [0.28, 3.69]	2011
Togashi 2011	44	85	25	69	4.3%	1.43 [0.98, 2.08]	2011
Fan 2011	239	715	145	407	28.5%	0.94 [0.79, 1.11]	2011
Kim 2012	23	48	19	48	2.9%	1.21 [0.77, 1.91]	2012
Wu 2012	52	124	42	100	7.2%	1.00 [0.73, 1.36]	2012
Lee 2013	3	11	5	14	0.7%	0.76 [0.23, 2.52]	2013
Yu 2013	1	16	3	22	0.4%	0.46 [0.05, 4.01]	2013
Otsuka 2015	10	35	3	9	0.7%	0.86 [0.30, 2.48]	2015
Urata 2016	112	279	100	280	15.4%	1.12 [0.91, 1.39]	2016
Yang 2017	67	128	76	128	11.7%	0.88 [0.71, 1.10]	2017
Total (95% CI)		2172		1623	100.0%	1.08 [1.00, 1.18]	
Total events	830		577				

Heterogeneity: Chi² = 15.01, df = 12 (P = 0.24); I² = 20%
Test for overall effect: Z = 1.88 (P = 0.06)

B

Study or Subgroup	Gefitinib Events	Total	Erlotinib Events	Total	Weight	Risk Ratio M-H, Fixed, 95% CI	Year
Kim 2010	108	171	110	171	13.0%	0.98 [0.84, 1.15]	2010
Hong 2010	8	20	8	17	1.0%	0.85 [0.41, 1.78]	2010
Fan 2011	421	715	268	407	40.3%	0.89 [0.81, 0.98]	2011
Togashi 2011	61	85	42	69	5.5%	1.18 [0.94, 1.49]	2011
Shin 2011	40	100	34	82	4.4%	0.96 [0.68, 1.37]	2011
Wu 2012	98	124	69	100	9.0%	1.15 [0.98, 1.34]	2012
Kim 2012	35	48	32	48	3.8%	1.09 [0.84, 1.42]	2012
Yu 2013	11	16	9	22	0.9%	1.68 [0.92, 3.07]	2013
Lee 2013	7	11	8	14	0.8%	1.11 [0.59, 2.10]	2013
Otsuka 2015	22	35	6	9	1.1%	0.94 [0.56, 1.60]	2015
Urata 2016	173	279	171	280	20.1%	1.02 [0.89, 1.16]	2016
Total (95% CI)		1604		1219	100.0%	0.99 [0.93, 1.05]	
Total events	984		757				

Heterogeneity: Chi² = 14.04, df = 10 (P = 0.17); I² = 29%
Test for overall effect: Z = 0.41 (P = 0.68)

Fig. 4 Forest plots of RR of ORR (**a**) and DCR (**b**) associated with gefitinib versus erlotinib

Discussion

Gefitinib and erlotinib are two similar small molecules with different binding capabilities and pharmacokinetic and pharmacodynamic properties related to their differing molecular structures [44–46]. Whether the differences between these first-generation EGFR TKIs can cause different anti-tumor efficacy is controversial [10, 11, 47]. By analyzing 31 high-quality studies, we directly compared the anti-tumor efficacy and safety of gefitinib and erlotinib for treating NSCLC [10–15, 19–43]. Our meta-analysis provides the most current medical evidence and shows that anti-tumor efficacy (PFS, OS, ORR, DCR) is comparable between gefitinib and erlotinib for treating East Asian patients with NSCLC. Subgroup analysis according to country, tumor stage, histology, line of treatment, EGFR mutation, and study design did not change the results. However, erlotinib toxicity was significantly greater than

that of gefitinib, especially in all-grade/grade 3–4 skin rash, nausea/vomiting, fatigue, and stomatitis.

The greater drug toxicity is an critical problem regarding erlotinib. In our analysis, we found high incidences of drug reduction, skin rash, diarrhea, nausea/vomiting, fatigue, and stomatitis in the erlotinib arm. Although it might not decrease survival time, it greatly reduces patients' quality of life [48, 49]. We believe there are two reasons for these results: (1) the oral dose of erlotinib (150 mg/day) was closer to the maximum tolerated dose (150 mg/day) as compared with gefitinib (oral dose, 250 mg/day; maximum tolerated dose, 600 mg/day) [50, 51]; (2) The two EGFR TKIs have different pharmacokinetics. After absorption, more gefitinib accumulates in tumor tissue than in plasma; the opposite is true for erlotinib [52]. In the published literature, more severe AEs have been reported in East Asian patients as

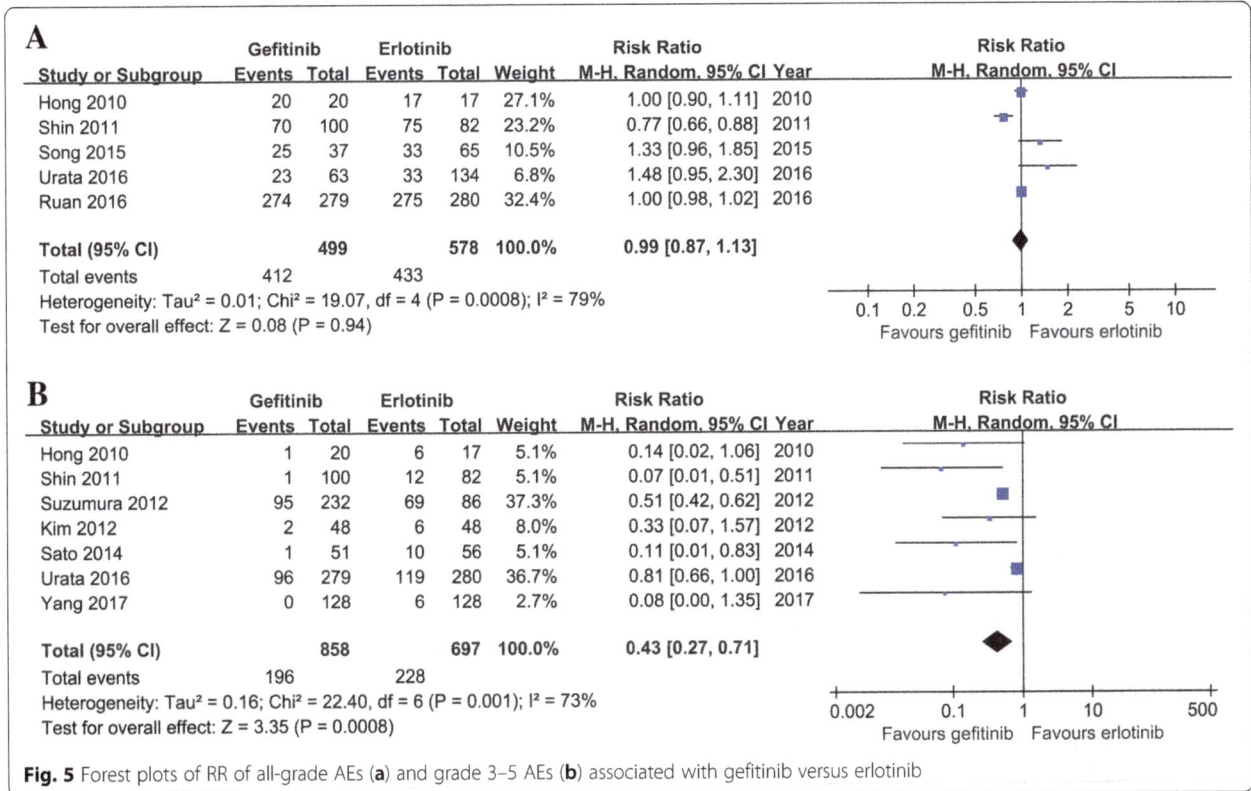

Fig. 5 Forest plots of RR of all-grade AEs (**a**) and grade 3–5 AEs (**b**) associated with gefitinib versus erlotinib

compared with patients from Europe and America [9, 53]. Interstitial lung disease is one of the most important AEs, and can cause worse prognosis and increased risk of death [54]. However, our analysis and other published studies show that most cases of interstitial lung disease are reported in East Asian populations and that it is rare in Western populations. This might be attributed to the smaller physiques of Asians in general. In a retrospective study, Yeo reduced the erlotinib dose to 25 mg/day and achieved similar or even better prognosis as compared with the standard dose [55]. Other retrospective studies have reported similar results [13, 56–58]. Accordingly, we

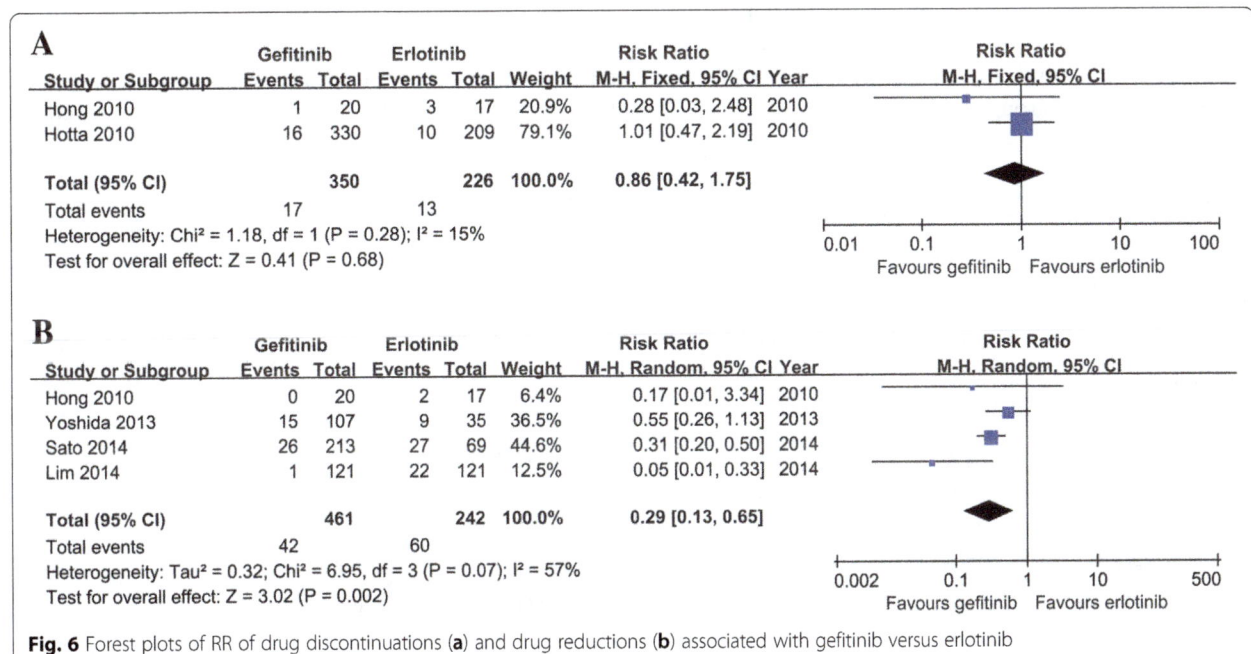

Fig. 6 Forest plots of RR of drug discontinuations (**a**) and drug reductions (**b**) associated with gefitinib versus erlotinib

Table 3 Top 10 adverse effects (all grade) associated with gefitinib versus erlotinib

Adverse effects	Gefitinib group (event/total)	Erlotinib group (event/total)	RR (95% CI)	P value	Heterogeneity I^2 (%)	P value
Skin rash	673/1099	650/944	0.83 (0.74–0.94)	0.003	68	0.0009
Diarrhea	298/999	273/745	0.83 (0.73–0.95)	0.005	47	0.06
Nausea/Vomiting	107/639	139/531	0.71 (0.32–1.57)	0.4	74	0.002
Fatigue	124/639	149/531	0.47 (0.23–0.95)	0.04	81	< 0.0001
Anorexia	53/403	40/310	0.98 (0.40–2.42)	0.97	78	0.001
Interstitial lung disease	35/949	19/723	1.38 (0.78–2.44)	0.26	0	0.65
Stomatitis	12/260	29/169	0.29 (0.15–0.54)	0.0001	24	0.27
Elevated liver enzymes	366/931	264/680	1.16 (0.85–0.1.56)	0.35	61	0.04
Infection	45/686	23/466	1.53 (0.93–2.51)	0.1	23	0.27
Neutropenia	61/399	51/379	1.19 (0.85–1.66)	0.32	0	0.55

suggest that individualized drug dose based on weight or body surface area might be more appropriate than a fixed oral dose for treating advanced NSCLC. More large-sample, well-designed RCTs are needed to confirm the best dose of gefitinib and erlotinib for East Asian patients with advanced NSCLC.

Almost all of the included studies did not show any differences in all anti-tumor efficacy indices, which formed the basis of our results. Only one study reported an unfavorable result for erlotinib, with both lower PFS and OS, which might relate to the erlotinib group having more patients with non-adenocarcinoma NSCLC as based on government regulations [14]. Our results also showed a trend for prolonged median PFS (gefitinib group, 7.1 months vs. 4.9 months; erlotinib group, 7.7 months vs. 3.4 months) and OS (gefitinib group, 19.1 months vs. 14.0 months; erlotinib group, 15.5 months vs. 12.7 months) in patients with adenocarcinoma as compared with squamous-included NSCLC. However, no difference was found between gefitinib and erlotinib in this subgroup.

In the *EGFR* mutation status subgroup, we also found no difference between the anti-tumor efficacy of gefitinib and erlotinib. However, our results indirectly prove that both gefitinib and erlotinib are more suitable for treating *EGFR* mutation–positive NSCLC. Both median PFS (gefitinib group, 11.4 months vs. 4.9 months; erlotinib group, 9.6 months vs. 3.1 months) and OS (gefitinib group, 22.6 months vs. 16.0 months; erlotinib group, 20.9 months vs. 12.0 months) were longer in the *EGFR* mutation–positive subgroup than in the partial *EGFR* mutation–positive subgroup. Accordingly, we observed that the proportion of *EGFR* mutations increased by the year in EGFR TKI treatment (Table 1). Multiple *EGFR* mutation isoforms (exon 19, exon 21, others) were found, although the isoform most susceptible to gefitinib or erlotinib remains unclear. A phase III RCT compared gefitinib and erlotinib treatment in *EGFR* mutation–positive NSCLC and found significantly higher RR and longer median OS for patients with *EGFR* exon 19 mutations than for patients with *EGFR* exon 21 mutations following erlotinib or gefitinib treatment. However, no

Table 4 Top 10 adverse effects (grade 3–5) associated with gefitinib versus erlotinib

Grade 3–5 Adverse effects	Gefitinib group (event/total)	Erlotinib group (event/total)	RR (95% CI)	P value	Heterogeneity I^2 (%)	P value
Skin rash	72/999	163/745	0.22 (0.12–0.41)	< 0.00001	73	0.0006
Diarrhea	31/892	38/710	0.46 (0.29–0.74)	0.001	0	0.46
Nausea/Vomiting	8/639	27/531	0.23 (0.11–0.49)	0.0001	20	0.29
Fatigue	18/639	40/531	0.28 (0.09–0.87)	0.03	74	0.02
Anorexia	3/403	4/310	0.25 (0.06–1.04)	0.06	NA	NA
Interstitial lung disease	7/619	3/514	1.05 (0.27–4.06)	0.95	17	0.3
Stomatitis	3/260	8/169	0.28 (0.08–0.99)	0.05	24	0.27
Elevated liver enzymes	80/652	23/400	1.50 (0.97–2.31)	0.07	0	0.64
Infection	9/454	7/380	1.12 (0.46–2.69)	0.8	20	0.28
Neutropenia	2/399	3/379	0.67 (0.11–3.97)	0.66	NA	NA

Table 5 Subgroup analysis for progression-free survival, overall survival and objective response rate

Group	PFS				OS				ORR			
	No.of studies	HR (95% CI)	P	I² (%)	No.of studies	RR (95% CI)	P	I² (%)	No.of studies	RR (95% CI)	P	I² (%)
Total	24	1.04 (0.97–1.10)	0.26	38	21	1.04 (0.89–1.21)	0.61	58	13	1.08 (1.00–1.18)	0.06	20
Nation												
Korea	8	0.89 (0.78–1.02)	0.09	18	8	1.03 (0.85–1.23)	0.79	0	5	1.18 (0.94–1.49)	0.16	0
China	6	1.05 (0.88–1.25)	0.63	20	5	0.92 (0.62–1.36)	0.67	67	2	0.87 (0.70–1.08)	0.21	0
Japan	6	1.15 (0.98–1.36)	0.09	20	4	1.04 (0.84–1.27)	0.74	0	3	1.18 (0.98–1.41)	0.08	0
Taiwan	4	1.09 (0.77–1.54)	0.62	74	4	1.12 (0.75–1.67)	0.59	90	3	1.07 (0.86–1.35)	0.54	71
Tumor stage												
IIIb-IV	22	1.04 (0.98–1.10)	0.23	40	18	1.08 (0.92–1.26)	0.34	53	12	1.09 (1.00–1.18)	0.05	24
I-IV	2	0.77 (0.39–1.51)	0.45	25	3	0.54 (0.18–1.63)	0.27	80	1	0.46 (0.05–4.01)	0.48	NA
History												
Non-squamous	13	1.04 (0.96–1.14)	0.88	51	11	1.06 (0.86–1.31)	0.58	68	9	1.08 (0.99–1.17)	0.09	42
Squamous included	10	1.02 (0.94–1.12)	0.6	11	9	0.98 (0.86–1.13)	0.81	48	4	1.19 (0.81–1.77)	0.38	0
Unclear	1	3.05 (0.84–11.09)	0.09	NA	1	1.34 (0.49–3.67)	0.57	NA				
Treatment line												
First line included	14	1.09 (0.98–1.20)	0.11	46	11	0.97 (0.72–1.30)	0.82	77	7	1.06 (0.90–1.25)	0.52	52
Second line or later	8	1.01 (0.93–1.08)	0.89	22	8	1.02 (0.91–1.14)	0.78	0	6	1.15 (0.98–1.35)	0.08	0
First line only	3	0.89 (0.32–2.49)	0.82	66	2	0.24 (0.04–1.43)	0.12	75				
Second line only	3	0.93 (0.76–1.14)	0.5	0	2	1.25 (0.90–1.73)	0.19	0	2	1.18 (0.76–1.82)	0.47	0
Third line only	1	0.88 (0.43–1.79)	0.72	NA	2	0.96 (0.81–1.14)	0.47	0	1	0.46 (0.05–4.01)	0.48	NA
Unclear	2	1.48 (0.72–3.08)	0.29	43	2	1.22 (0.62–2.39)	0.56	0				
EGFR mutation												
Partial mutation	11	1.02 (0.91–1.15)	0.68	21	11	1.15 (0.91–1.45)	0.24	68	9	1.10 (1.00–1.21)	0.05	21
All mutation	9	1.11 (0.90–1.36)	0.33	50	7	0.82 (0.54–1.25)	0.36	59	2	0.88 (0.71–1.09)	0.24	0
Unclear	4	0.98 (0.76–1.26)	0.88	57	3	0.97 (0.84–1.13)	0.67	0	2	1.22 (0.92–1.62)	0.18	2
Study design												
Retrospective study	21	1.02 (0.95–1.09)	0.37	40	18	1.01 (0.84–1.21)	0.92	63	10	1.10 (1.00–1.22)	0.06	19
RCT	3	1.11 (0.96–1.27)	0.15	32	3	1.11 (0.93–1.32)	0.25	0	3	1.04 (0.90–1.20)	0.62	36

Abbreviations: PFS progression-free survival, OS overall survival, ORR objective response rate, HR hazard ratio, RR relative risk, RCT randomized controlled trial, NA not available

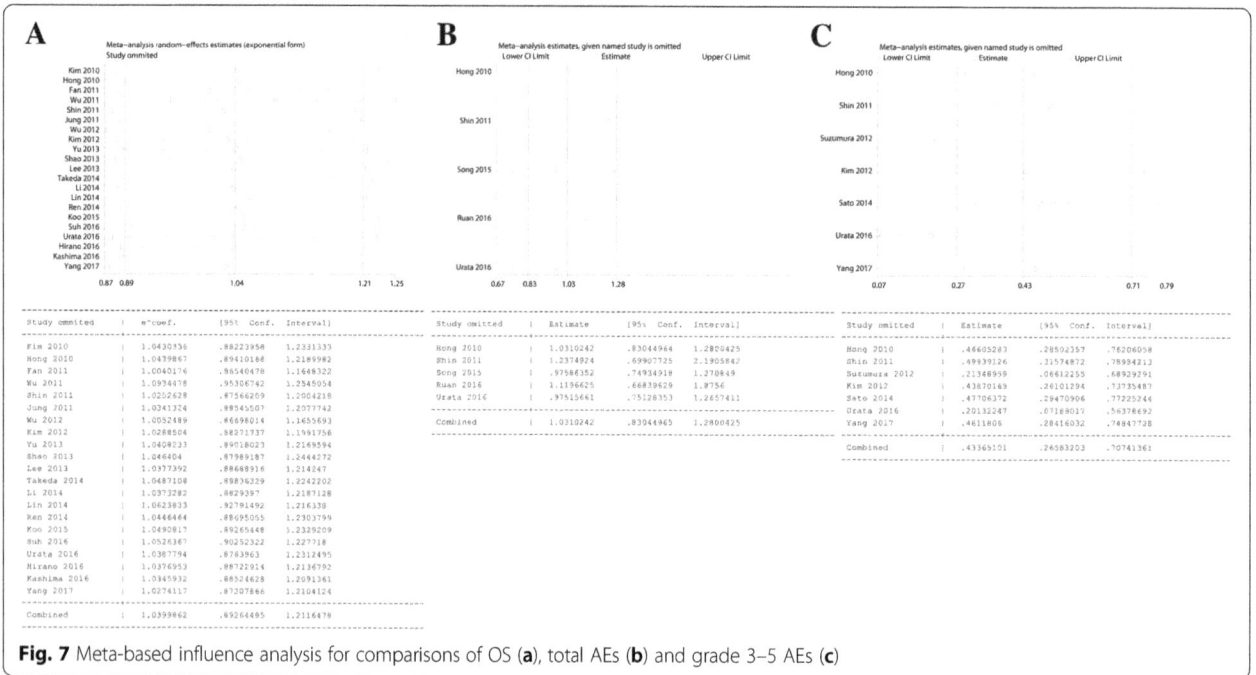

Fig. 7 Meta-based influence analysis for comparisons of OS (**a**), total AEs (**b**) and grade 3–5 AEs (**c**)

difference was found between gefitinib and erlotinib for both mutations [11]. Another RCT involving more *EGFR* mutation isoforms (exon 19, exon 21, T790 M) reported similar results [10]. However, Kuan suggested that erlotinib is associated with significantly longer PFS and lower risk of progression than gefitinib in patients with *EGFR* exon 19 deletions [15]. Limited by the quantity of published studies and included patients, further large-sample, well-designed RCTs focusing on single *EGFR* mutations are warranted to identify the best EGFR TKIs.

The line of treatment in which EGFR TKIs should be used in NSCLC remains controversial. Mainstream thinking considers EGFR TKIs second-line or later treatment after chemotherapy failure or first-line treatment for patients unable to tolerate chemotherapy. However, Table 1 shows that an increasing number of studies have used gefitinib and erlotinib as first-line treatment for advanced NSCLC [15, 33, 42]. However, no differences were found for PFS, OS, and ORR between gefitinib and erlotinib in each line of treatment subgroup. Wu et al. conducted a phase III RCT and suggested that first-line

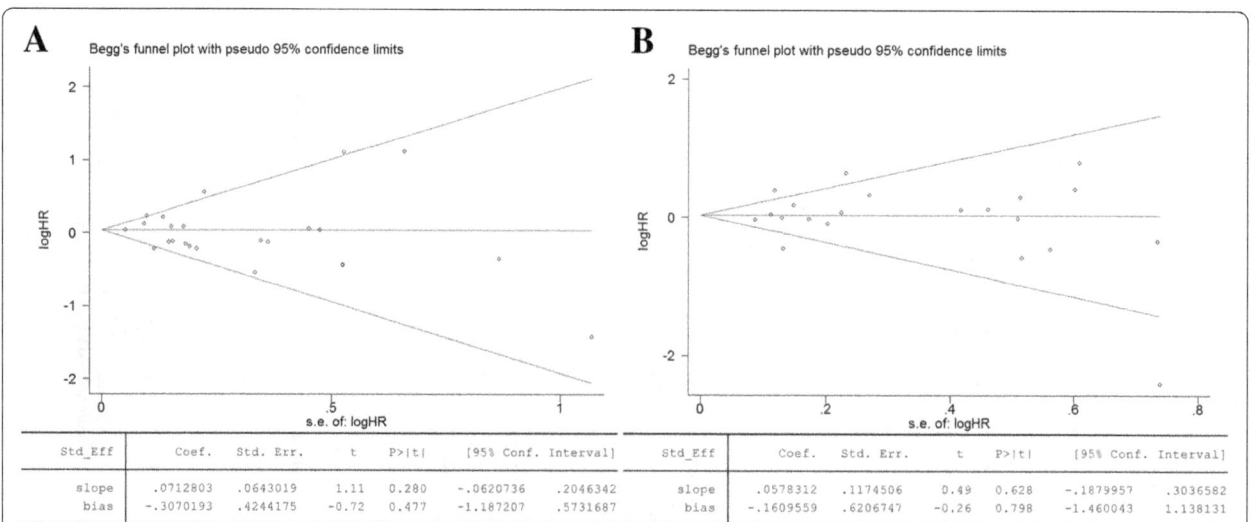

Fig. 8 Begg's and Egger's tests for comparisons of PFS (**a**) and OS (**b**)

erlotinib can significantly improve PFS as compared to gemcitabine+cisplatin in patients with *EGFR* mutation–positive NSCLC [59]. Another phase III RCT suggested that PFS is significantly longer with gefitinib treatment in patients with mutation-positive NSCLC as compared with carboplatin+paclitaxel [60]. Several other high-quality RCTs have reported similar results [61–63]. Based on these positive results, the US Food and Drug Administration approved gefitinib as first-line treatment for *EGFR* mutation–positive NSCLC [64]. In the 2017 National Comprehensive Cancer Network (NCCN) guideline on NSCLC, both gefitinib and erlotinib are suggested as first-line treatment for *EGFR* mutation–positive NSCLC [65].

Several limitations should considered when interpreting our results. First, only high-quality studies published in English were included, which might result in language bias. Second, only three RCTs were included, which would weaken the quality of the results. Third, there was significant heterogeneity for some comparisons (OS and total/grade 3–5 AEs), which would weaken the reliability of these results. Fourth, the type and rate of *EGFR* mutations differed between the included studies, which might increase heterogeneity and weaken the quality of the results. Fifth, we obtained data from only three East Asian countries (China [Mainland and Taiwan], Japan, Korea), which might reduce the representativeness of the study. Sixth, quality of life and survival time are two equally important evaluating indicators for a treatment. Quality of life cannot simply be replaced by the number of AEs. However, the included studies did not compare quality of life between treatment with the two EGFR TKIs. Accordingly, we suggest that quality of life be considered an essential indicator in future drug evaluation studies.

Conclusion

Our results show that both gefitinib and erlotinib are effective for treating advanced NSCLC in East Asian patients, with comparable PFS, OS, ORR, and DCR. Erlotinib induces a significantly higher rate and severity of skin rash, nausea/vomiting, fatigue, and stomatitis, which might cause a higher rate of dose reduction. Therefore, we suggest that individualized drug dose based on weight or body surface area might be more appropriate than a fixed oral dose for both agents in treating East Asian patients with advanced NSCLC. However, due to the inherent limitations of our meta-analysis, more large-scale, high-quality RCTs are warranted to confirm this conclusion.

Additional files

Additional file 1: Figure S1. Cumulative meta-analysis related to PFS associated with gefitinib versus erlotinib. (TIFF 1895 kb)

Additional file 2: Figure S2. Cumulative meta-analysis related to OS associated with gefitinib versus erlotinib. (TIFF 1885 kb)

Additional file 3: Figure S3. Cumulative meta-analysis related to ORR associated with gefitinib versus erlotinib. (TIFF 1498 kb)

Additional file 4: Figure S4. Cumulative meta-analysis related to DCR associated with gefitinib versus erlotinib. (TIF 1379 kb)

Additional file 5 Figure S5. Cumulative meta-analysis related to total AEs associated with gefitinib versus erlotinib. (TIFF 999 kb)

Additional file 6: Figure S6. Cumulative meta-analysis related to grade 3–5 AEs associated with gefitinib versus erlotinib. (TIFF 1104 kb)

Abbreviations
AEs: Adverse effects; ASR: Age-standardized rate; CI: Confidence interval; DCR: Disease control rate; EGFR TKIs: Epidermal growth factor receptor tyrosine kinase inhibitors; HR: Hazard ratios; NOS: Newcastle-Ottawa Scale; NSCLC: Non-small cell lung cancer; ORR: Objective response rate; OS: Overall survival; PFS: Progression-free survival; PRISMA: Preferred Reporting Items for Systematic Review and Meta-Analysis; RR: Risk ratios

Acknowledgements
The authors would like to thank Dr. Han Jiang for the data collection, Professor Yanhua Tang for her advice and assistance in language improvement, and all the patients who participated in this study.

Funding
This study was supported by National Natural Science Foundation of China (NSFC), with no commercial entity involved, number of grants (81560345). Role of the Funding: The NSFC had no role in the design and conduct of the study; collection, management, analysis, and interpretation of the data; preparation, review, or approval of the manuscript; and decision to submit the manuscript for publication.

Authors' contributions
WXZ conceived of the idea, designed the study, searched the relevant database and wrote the manuscript. DLY interpreted the data and performed the study through STATA. JHP interpreted the data and other relevant information. JJX analyzed quality of each study and confirmed statistical analyses. YW provided the examination for the methodology, reviewed and revised our manuscript. All authors read and approved the final manuscript.

Competing interests
The authors declare that they have no competing interests.

References
1. Siegel RL, Miller KD, Jemal A. Cancer statistics, 2018. CA Cancer J Clin. 2018; 68(1):7–30.
2. Chen W, Zheng R, Baade PD, Zhang S, Zeng H, Bray F, et al. Cancer statistics in China, 2015. CA Cancer J Clin. 2016;66(2):115–32.
3. Liu TC, Jin X, Wang Y, Wang K. Role of epidermal growth factor receptor in lung cancer and targeted therapies. Am J Cancer Res. 2017;7(2):187–202.
4. Malik PS, Jain D, Kumar L. Epidermal growth factor receptor tyrosine inhibitors in advanced non-small cell lung cancer. Oncology. 2016;91(1):26–34.
5. NICE, EGFR-TK mutation testing in adults with locally advanced or metastatic non-small-cell lung cancer. http://www.nice.org.uk/guidance/dg9, (Accessed 2 Aug 2016).
6. National Comprehensive Cancer Network Practice guidelines in oncology-version V.4.2016 (non-small-cell lung cancer). https://www.nccn.org/professionals/physician_gls/pdf/nscl.pdf. Accessed 2 Aug 2016.

7. Dearden S, Stevens J, Wu YL, Blowers D. Mutation incidence and coincidence in non small-cell lung cancer: meta-analyses by ethnicity and histology (mutMap). Ann Oncol. 2013;24(9):2371–6.

8. Wu YL, Saijo N, Thongprasert S, Yang JC, Han B, Margono B, et al. Efficacy according to blind independent central review: post-hoc analyses from the phase III, randomized, multicenter, IPASS study of first-line gefitinib versus carboplatin/paclitaxel in Asian patients with EGFR mutation-positive advanced NSCLC. Lung Cancer. 2017;104:119–25.

9. Chang GC, Tsai CM, Chen KC, Yu CJ, Shih JY, Yang TY, et al. Predictive factors of gefitinib antitumor activity in east Asian advanced non-small cell lung cancer patients. J Thorac Oncol. 2006;1(6):520–5.

10. Urata Y, Katakami N, Morita S, Kaji R, Yoshioka H, Seto T, et al. Randomized phase III study comparing gefitinib with erlotinib in patients with previously treated advanced lung adenocarcinoma: WJOG 5108L. J Clin Oncol. 2016;34(27):3248–57.

11. Yang JJ, Zhou Q, Yan HH, Zhang XC, Chen HJ, Tu HY, et al. A phase III randomised controlled trial of erlotinib vs gefitinib in advanced non-small cell lung cancer with EGFR mutations. Br J Cancer. 2017;116(5):568–74.

12. Shin HJ, Kim TO, Kang HW, Chi SY, Ban HJ, Kim SO, et al. Comparison of therapeutic efficacy of gefitinib and erlotinib in patients with squamous cell lung cancer. Tuberculosis & Respiratory Diseases. 2011;71(1):15–23.

13. Sato S, Kurishima K, Miyazaki K, Kodama T, Ishikawa H, Kagohashi K, et al. Efficacy of tyrosine kinase inhibitors in non-small-cell lung cancer patients undergoing dose reduction and those with a low body surface area. Mol Clin Oncol. 2014;2(4):604–8.

14. Fan WC, Yu CJ, Tsai CM, Huang MS, Lai CL, Hsia TC, et al. Different efficacies of erlotinib and gefitinib in taiwanese patients with advanced non-small cell lung cancer: a retrospective multicenter study. J Thorac Oncol. 2011;6(1):148–55.

15. Kuan FC, Li SH, Wang CL, Lin MH, Tsai YH, Yang CT. Analysis of progression-free survival of first-line tyrosine kinase inhibitors in patients with non-small cell lung cancer harboring leu858Arg or exon 19 deletions. Oncotarget. 2017;8(1):1343–53.

16. Jadad AR, Moore RA, Carroll D, Jenkinson C, Reynolds DJ, Gavaghan DJ, et al. Assessing the quality of reports of randomized clinical trials: is blinding necessary? Control Clin Trials. 1996;17(1):1–12.

17. Wells GA, Shea BJ, O'Connell D, Peterson J, Welch V, Losos M, et al. The Newcastle–Ottawa scale (nos) for assessing the quality of non-randomized studies in meta-analysis. Appl Eng Agric. 2014;18(6):727–34.

18. Tierney JF, Stewart LA, Ghersi D, Burdett S, Sydes MR. Practical methods for incorporating summary time-to-event data into meta-analysis. Trials. 2007;8:16.

19. Kim ST, Lee J, Kim JH, Won YW, Sun JM, Yun J, et al. Comparison of gefitinib versus erlotinib in patients with non-small cell lung cancer who failed previous chemotherapy. Cancer. 2010;116(12):3025–33.

20. Hotta K, Kiura K, Takigawa N, Yoshioka H, Harita S, Kuyama S, et al. Comparison of the incidence and pattern of interstitial lung disease during erlotinib and gefitinib treatment in Japanese patients with non-small cell lung cancer: the Okayama lung Cancer study group experience. J Thorac Oncol. 2010;5(2):179–84.

21. Hong J, Kyung SY, Lee SP, Park JW, Jung SH, Lee JI, et al. Pemetrexed versus gefitinib versus erlotinib in previously treated patients with non-small cell lung cancer. Korean J Intern Med. 2010;25(3):294–300.

22. Wu JY, Wu SG, Yang CH, Chang YL, Chang YC, Hsu YC, et al. Comparison of gefitinib and erlotinib in advanced NSCLC and the effect of EGFR mutations. Lung Cancer. 2011;72(2):205–12.

23. Togashi Y, Masago K, Fujita S, Hatachi Y, Fukuhara A, Nagai H, et al. Differences in adverse events between 250 mg daily gefitinib and 150 mg daily erlotinib in Japanese patients with non-small cell lung cancer. Lung Cancer. 2011;74(1):98–102.

24. Jung M, Kim SH, Lee YJ, Hong S, Kang YA, Kim SK, et al. Prognostic and predictive value of CEA and CYFRA 21-1 levels in advanced non-small cell lung cancer patients treated with gefitinib or erlotinib. Exp Ther Med. 2011;2(4):685.

25. Wu WS, Chen YM, Tsai CM, Shih JF, Chiu CH, Chou KT, et al. Erlotinib has better efficacy than gefitinib in adenocarcinoma patients without EGFR-activating mutations, but similar efficacy in patients with EGFR-activating mutations. Exp Ther Med. 2012;3(2):207–13.

26. Kim ST, Uhm JE, Lee J, Sun JM, Sohn I, Kim SW, et al. Randomized phase II study of gefitinib versus erlotinib in patients with advanced non-small cell lung cancer who failed previous chemotherapy. Lung Cancer. 2012;75(1):82–8.

27. Suzumura T, Kimura T, Kudoh S, Umekawa K, Nagata M, Matsuura K, et al. Reduced CYP2D6 function is associated with gefitinib-induced rash in patients with non-small cell lung cancer. BMC Cancer. 2012;12:568.

28. Yoshida T, Yamada K, Azuma K, Kawahara A, Abe H, Hattori S, et al. Comparison of adverse events and efficacy between gefitinib and erlotinib in patients with non-small-cell lung cancer: a retrospective analysis. Med Oncol. 2013;30(1):349.

29. Shao YY, Shau WY, Lin ZZ, Chen HM, Kuo R, Yang JC, et al. Comparison of gefitinib and erlotinib efficacies as third-line therapy for advanced non-small-cell lung cancer. Eur J Cancer. 2013;49(1):106–14.

30. Lee E, Keam B, Kim DW, Kim TM, Lee SH, Chung DH, et al. Erlotinib versus gefitinib for control of leptomeningeal carcinomatosis in non-small-cell lung cancer. J Thorac Oncol. 2013;8(8):1069–74.

31. Yu S, Wang Y, Li J, Hao X, Wang B, Wang Z, et al. Gefitinib versus erlotinib as salvage treatment for lung adenocarcinoma patients who benefited from the initial gefitinib: a retrospective study. Thoracic Cancer. 2013;4(2):109–16.

32. Lim SH, Lee JY, Sun JM, Ahn JS, Park K, Ahn MJ. Comparison of clinical outcomes following gefitinib and erlotinib treatment in non-small-cell lung cancer patients harboring an epidermal growth factor receptor mutation in either exon 19 or 21. J Thorac Oncol. 2014;9(4):506–11.

33. Lin GN, Peng JW, Liu PP, Liu DY, Xiao JJ, Chen XQ. Elevated neutrophil-to-lymphocyte ratio predicts poor outcome in patients with advanced non-small-cell lung cancer receiving first-line gefitinib or erlotinib treatment. Asia Pac J Clin Oncol. 2014;110(7):2696–703.

34. Ren S, Su C, Wang Z, Li J, Fan L, Li B, et al. Epithelial phenotype as a predictive marker for response to EGFR-TKIs in non-small cell lung cancer patients with wild-type EGFR. Int J Cancer. 2014;135(12):2962–71.

35. Li J, Li X, Ren S, Chen X, Zhang Y, Zhou F, et al. miR-200c overexpression is associated with better efficacy of EGFR-TKIs in non-small cell lung cancer patients with EGFR wild-type. Oncotarget. 2014;5(17):7902–16.

36. Takeda M, Okamoto I, Nakagawa K. Survival outcome assessed according to tumor response and shrinkage pattern in patients with EGFR mutation–positive non–small cell lung cancer treated with gefitinib or erlotinib. J Thorac Oncol. 2014;9(2):200–4.

37. Otsuka T, Mori M, Yano Y, Uchida J, Nishino K, Kaji R, et al. Effectiveness of tyrosine kinase inhibitors in Japanese patients with non-small cell lung cancer harboring minor epidermal growth factor receptor mutations: results from a multicenter retrospective study (HANSHIN oncology group 0212). Anticancer Res. 2015;35(7):3885–91.

38. Song Z, Zhang Y. Efficacy of gefitinib or erlotinib in patients with squamous cell lung cancer. Arch Med Sci. 2015;11(1):164–8.

39. Koo DH, Kim KP, Choi CM, Lee DH, Lee JC, Lee JS, et al. EGFR-TKI is effective regardless of treatment timing in pulmonary adenocarcinoma with EGFR mutation. Cancer Chemother Pharmacol. 2015;75(1):197–206.

40. Ruan Y, Jiang J, Guo L, Li Y, Huang H, Shen L, et al. Genetic association of curative and adverse reactions to tyrosine kinase inhibitors in Chinese advanced non-small sell lung cancer patients. Sci Rep. 2016;6:23368.

41. Hirano R, Uchino J, Ueno M, Fujita M, Watanabe K. Low-dose epidermal growth factor receptor (EGFR)-tyrosine kinase inhibition of EGFR mutation-positive lung cancer: therapeutic benefits and associations between dosage, efficacy and body surface area. Asian Pac J Cancer Prev. 2016;17(2):785−9.

42. Suh KJ, Keam B, Kim M, Park YS, Kim TM, Jeon YK, et al. Serum neuron-specific enolase levels predict the efficacy of first-line epidermal growth factor receptor (EGFR) tyrosine kinase inhibitors in patients with non-small cell lung cancer harboring EGFR mutations. Clin Lung Cancer. 2016;17(4):245–52.

43. Kashima J, Okuma Y, Miwa M, Hosomi Y. Survival of patients with brain metastases from non-small-cell lung cancer harboring EGFR mutations treated with epidermal growth factor receptor tyrosine kinase inhibitors. Med Oncol. 2016;33(11):129.

44. Yun CH, Boggon TJ, Li Y, Woo MS, Greulich H, Meyerson M, et al. Structures of lung cancer-derived EGFR mutants and inhibitor complexes: mechanism of activation and insights into differential inhibitor sensitivity. Cancer Cell. 2007;11(3):217–27.

45. Ling J, Fettner S, Lum BL, Riek M, Rakhit A. Effect of food on the pharmacokinetics of erlotinib, an orally active epidermal growth factor receptor tyrosine-kinase inhibitor, in healthy individuals. Anti-Cancer Drugs. 2008;19(2):209–16.

46. Cantarini MV, McFarquhar T, Smith RP, Bailey C, Marshall AL. Relative bioavailability and safety profile of gefitinib administered as a tablet or as a dispersion preparation via drink or nasogastric tube: results of a

randomized, open-label, three-period crossover study in healthy volunteers. Clin Ther. 2004;26(10):1630–6.

47. Russo A, Franchina T, Ricciardi GR, Picone A, Ferraro G, Zanghì M, et al. A decade of EGFR inhibition in EGFR-mutated non small cell lung cancer (NSCLC): old successes and future perspectives. Oncotarget. 2015;6(29): 26814–25.

48. Yang SC, Lai WW, Hsiue TR, Su WC, Lin CK, Hwang JS, et al. Health-related quality of life after first-line anti-cancer treatments for advanced non-small cell lung cancer in clinical practice. Qual Life Res. 2016;25(6):1441–9.

49. Wu YL, Fukuoka M, Mok TS, Saijo N, Thongprasert S, Yang JC, et al. Tumor response and health-related quality of life in clinically selected patients from Asia with advanced non-small-cell lung cancer treated with first-line gefitinib: post hoc analyses from the IPASS study. Lung Cancer. 2013;81(2):280–7.

50. Baselga J, Rischin D, Ranson M, Calvert H, Raymond E, Kieback DG, et al. Phase I safety, pharmacokinetic, and pharmacodynamic trial of ZD1839, a selective oral epidermal growth factor receptor tyrosine kinase inhibitor, in patients with five selected solid tumor types. J Clin Oncol. 2002;20(21): 4292–302.

51. Hidalgo M, Siu LL, Nemunaitis J, Rizzo J, Hammond LA, Takimoto C, et al. Phase I and pharmacologic study of OSI-774, an epidermal growth factor receptor tyrosine kinase inhibitor, in patients with advanced solid malignancies. J Clin Oncol. 2001;19(13):3267–79.

52. Rukazenkov Y, Speake G, Marshall G, Anderton J, Davies BR, Wilkinson RW, et al. Epidermal growth factor receptor tyrosine kinase inhibitors: similar but different? Anti-Cancer Drugs. 2009;20(10):856–66.

53. Mok T, Wu YL, Au JS, Zhou C, Zhang L, Perng RP, Park K. Efficacy and safety of erlotinib in 1242 east/south-east Asian patients with advanced non-small cell lung cancer. J Thorac Oncol. 2010;5(10):1609–15.

54. Ando M, Okamoto I, Yamamoto N, Takeda K, Tamura K, Seto T, et al. Predictive factors for interstitial lung disease, antitumor response, and survival in non-small-cell lung cancer patients treated with gefitinib. J Clin Oncol. 2006;24(16):2549–56.

55. Yeo WL, Riely GJ, Yeap BY, Lau MW, Warner JL, Bodio K, et al. Erlotinib at a dose of 25 mg daily for non-small cell lung cancers with EGFR mutations. J Thorac Oncol. 2010;5(7):1048–53.

56. Takashima N, Kimura T, Watanabe N, Umemura T, Katsuno S, Arakawa K, et al. Prognosis in patients with non-small cell lung cancer who received erlotinib treatment and subsequent dose reduction due to skin rash. Onkologie. 2012;35(12):747–52.

57. Satoh H, Inoue A, Kobayashi K, Maemondo M, Oizumi S, Isobe H, et al. Low-dose gefitinib treatment for patients with advanced non-small cell lung cancer harboring sensitive epidermal growth factor receptor mutations. J Thorac Oncol. 2011;6(8):1413–7.

58. Sim SH, Keam B, Kim DW, Kim TM, Lee SH, Chung DH, et al. The gefitinib dose reduction on survival outcomes in epidermal growth factor receptor mutant non-small cell lung cancer. J Cancer Res Clin Oncol. 2014;140(12): 2135–42.

59. Wu YL, Zhou C, Liam CK, Wu G, Liu X, Zhong Z, et al. First-line erlotinib versus gemcitabine/cisplatin in patients with advanced EGFR mutation-positive non-small-cell lung cancer: analyses from the phase III, randomized, open-label. ENSURE study Ann Oncol. 2015;26(9):1883–9.

60. Fukuoka M, Wu YL, Thongprasert S, Sunpaweravong P, Leong SS, Sriuranpong V, et al. Biomarker analyses and final overall survival results from a phase III, randomized, open-label, first-line study of gefitinib versus carboplatin/paclitaxel in clinically selected patients with advanced non-small-cell lung cancer in Asia (IPASS). J Clin Oncol. 2011;29(21):2866–74.

61. Fiala O, Pesek M, Finek J, Benesova L, Bortlicek Z, Minarik M. Comparison of EGFR-TKI and chemotherapy in the first-line treatment of advanced EGFR mutation-positive NSCLC. Neoplasma. 2013;60(4):425–31.

62. Zhou C, Wu YL, Chen G, Feng J, Liu XQ, Wang C, et al. Erlotinib versus chemotherapy as first-line treatment for patients with advanced EGFR mutation-positive non-small-cell lung cancer (OPTIMAL, CTONG-0802): a multicentre, open-label, randomised, phase 3 study. Lancet Oncol. 2011;12(8):735–42.

63. Rosell R, Carcereny E, Gervais R, Vergnenegre A, Massuti B, Felip E, et al. Erlotinib versus standard chemotherapy as first-line treatment for European patients with advanced EGFR mutation-positive non-small-cell lung cancer

(EURTAC): a multicentre, open-label, randomised phase 3 trial. Lancet Oncol. 2012;13(3):239–46.

64. Kazandjian D, Blumenthal GM, Yuan W, He K, Keegan P, Pazdur R. FDA approval of gefitinib for the treatment of patients with metastatic EGFR mutation-positive non-small-cell lung cancer. Clin Cancer Res. 2016;22(6):1307–12.

65. National Comprehensive Cancer Network. (NCCN) Clinical Practice Guidelines in Oncology. Small Cell Lung Cancer (Version 5. 2017). Available at https://www.nccn.org/professionals/physician_gls/pdf/sclc.pdf. Accessed 16 Mar 2017.

19

Body mass index and lung cancer risk in never smokers

Hongjun Zhu[1] and Shuanglin Zhang[2*]

Abstract

Background: Obesity is found to increase the risk of most cancer types, but reduce lung cancer risk in many studies. However, the association between obesity and lung cancer is still controversial, mainly owing to the confounding effect of smoking.

Methods: Eligible studies were identified from electric databases to July 1, 2017. Relevant data were extracted and pooled using random-effects models; dose-response and subgroup analyses were also performed.

Results: Twenty-nine studies with more than 10,000 lung cancer cases in15 million never smokers were included. Compared with normal weight, the summary relative risk (RR) was 0.77(95% confidence interval [CI]: 0.68–0.88, $P < 0.01$) for excess body weight (body mass index [BMI] $\geq$ 25 kg/m^2). An inverse linear dose-response relationship was observed between BMI and lung cancer risk in never smokers, with an RR of 0.89(95% CI: 0.84–0.95, $P < 0.01$) per 5 kg/m^2 increment in BMI. The results remained stable in most subgroup analyses. However, when stratified by sex, a significant inverse association existed in women but not in men. Similar results were found in analyses for other categories of BMI.

Conclusion: Our results indicate that higher BMI is associated with lower lung cancer risk in never smokers.

Keywords: Lung cancer, Obesity, Risk factor, Smoking, Meta-analysis

Background

Obesity is one of the most important risk factors for several major non-communicable diseases, including cardiovascular diseases, diabetes, and cancer, and the widespread prevalence of obesity is becoming a major threat to global public health [1]. Accumulating evidence suggest that excess body weight not only increases the overall cancer incidence but is also associated with worse outcomes in certain types of cancer [2–4].

As one of the most common cancers in both men and women, lung cancer causes more deaths than any other cancer [5]. Curiously, the association between obesity and lung cancer seems to be different from other cancer types, which has been disputed for years [6–9]. Many previous epidemiological studies found that higher body mass index (BMI) was associated with lower overall lung cancer risk, which was further confirmed in several

meta-analyses [10–12] However, the results were always explained by the confounding effect of smoking, which was also associated with lower BMI [7]. Preclinical weight loss and socioeconomic status were also considered to be involved in the association [3, 13]. Hence, the true relationship between obesity and lung cancer risk remains to be clarified, and interpretation of data in only never smokers might be the best approach to reveal the real picture. Interestingly, several recent studies also reported that higher BMI was associated with better survival in patients with non-small cell lung cancer [14–16].

Lung cancer in never-smokers accounts for approximately 10–15% of all lung cancer patients and causes more than 15,000 deaths annually [17]. Concerning the association between obesity and lung cancer risk in never smokers, inconsistent results were also reported. In fact, subgroup analyses in previous meta-analyses have reported pooled results for the association. In the first meta-analysis performed by Yang Y, et al., found an significant inverse association between excess weight and lung cancer incidence in non-smokers based on 11

* Correspondence: zhangshuanglinhn@163.com
[2]Department of Thoracic and Cardiovascular Surgery, the First Affiliated Hospital of Henan University, No. 357 Ximen Street, Kaifeng City 475000, Henan Province, China
Full list of author information is available at the end of the article

studies, while the association become insignificant for obesity and overweight categories [11]. Then Duan, et, al. also reported an attenuated linear dose-response association between BMI and lung cancer risk (including both incidence and mortality) in non-smokers, without statistical significance [12]. In the meta-analysis for lung cancer mortality by Shen N, et, al. in 2017, only 2 studies was included in subgroup analysis for never smokers, and the result was 0.95 (95%CI: 0.88–1.02) [10]. However, the results from the above three meta-analyses were sub-group analyses and based on only a small number of original studies included. To clarify the intrinsic association between obesity and the risk of lung cancer, and avoid the influence of confounding factors, we carried out an updated meta-analysis between body mass index and lung cancer risk in only never smokers, with a more complete literature search, which included both incidence and mortality to increase the sample size and statistical power.

Methods
Study selection
We searched the PubMed database to find relevant studies from January 1, 1966, to July 1, 2017.The following key words were used: *obesity, overweight, body mass index, body size, leanness,* or *anthropometric* in combination with *lung cancer, lung carcinoma,* or *lung neoplasm*. Our literature search was restricted to the full-text publications, and no language restriction was applied. The reference lists of identified articles and other similar meta-analyses were also checked to find additional studies.

Eligibility criteria
Two independent investigators reviewed all the records and included studies that met the following criteria: 1) study population was never (or non-) smokers, current and former (past or ex-) smokers were not considered in this study, never smokers are defined as those who have not smoked greater than 100 cigarettes in their lifetimes and do not currently smoke; 2) the exposure of interest was BMI (kg/m^2), including the categories of obesity, overweight, underweight or excess weight; 3) relative risk (RR) estimates (or hazard ratios or odds ratios) and 95% confidence intervals (CIs) for never smokers were reported or could be calculated from the data. 4) the outcome was the incidence or mortality of lung cancer; 5) observational studies with a cohort or case-control design. When duplicated studies were reported from the same population, the ones with the longest follow-up were included.

Data extraction and quality assessment
For each study, the following data were extracted: the first author's name, publication date, country, design,

study population, BMI measurement, cancer ascertainment, sex, BMI categories with estimated midpoints, cases and participants per category, RRs with 95%CIs, and adjusted variables. RRs adjusted for the largest number of confounding variables were adopted. Quality of original studies was assessed by the Newcastle-Ottawa scale [18], which was widely used in observational studies, with a final score ≥ 7 considered as high quality.

Statistical methods
Obesity and overweight were defined as BMI ≥30 and 25–29.99 kg/m^2, in accordance with the definitions by of the World Health Organization, whereas excess weight combines the two categories. Normal weight was defined as 18.5–24.99 kg/m^2, which was considered as the reference level. When the RRs with 95%Cis were reported by different BMI categories, the estimates for alternative comparisons were converted using the methods by Hamling et al. [19]. A fixed-effects model was employed to pool the results separated by sex. For some studies, we extracted the RR estimates from the figures presented in the manuscripts, using the software Engauge Digitizer version 2.11 (free software downloaded from http://sourceforge.net). A random-effects model was used to pool the individual RRs, considering the heterogeneity among studies, which was evaluated by the Q and I^2 statistics [20].

Only studies that reported RRs with 95% CIs for at least 3categories were included into the dose-response analysis using the method proposed by Greenland [21] and Orsiniet al. [22]. For each BMI category, the average between the lower and upper boundary was assigned to the corresponding RR. When the extreme category was open-ended, the boundary was assumed to be the same amplitude as adjacent categories. RR trend estimates with 95%CIs in each study were calculated per 5 kg/m^2increment in BMI and pooled together using a random-effects model. To compute the study-specific slope from the correlated log RR estimates across BMI levels, a two-stage generalized least-squares method with fractional-polynomial regression models was employed [22]. To test for nonlinearity, a likelihood ratio test was used to investigate the difference between nonlinear and linear models.

We also carried out subgroup analyses stratified by potential confounding factors, including study design, outcome, sex, diagnosis method, ethnicity, and quality. Meta-regression analyses were performed to explore the sources of heterogeneity. To evaluate the stability of the results, sensitivity analysis was employed to examine the change of pooled results after removing one study each time. Publication bias was assessed by funnel plot and Egger's test, $p < 0.10$ was regarded as statistically significant, and the trim-and-fill method was used to adjust for potential bias. All statistical analyses were done with the STATA version 12.0 software (Stata Corporation, College Station, TX).

Results

Literature search and study characteristics

In total, 3937 articles were identified from the databases, and after removing the ineligible studies, 29 studies were included in the meta-analysis, including 21 cohort studies and 8 case-control studies (Fig. 1). Among these studies, 24 reported the RRs for lung cancer incidence and 5 provided mortality data. Twelve were from America, 7 from Europe, 10 from Asia. Two studies in Chinese were included in our study [23, 24]. 2studies were excluded because of multiple reports of the same population [7, 25].

In general, the quality scores ranged from 4 to 9 with an average of 7 points (7.3 for cohort studies and 6.2 for case-control studies). Among all studies, 21 were considered as high quality (≥7 points). The most common confounders adjusted in original studies included age, sex, alcohol consumption, vegetable/fruit intake, and physical activity; however, few studies were controlled for total calorie intake, other chronic diseases, concomitant medication, or environmental status. The baseline characteristics of all studies are shown in Additional file 1: Table S1 and the quality scores are listed in Additional file 2: Table S2 and Additional file 3: Table S3.

Overall analyses

Overall analyses showed that there was an inverse association between BMI and lung cancer risk in never

smokers. Eighteen and 15 studies reported the data for obesity and overweight categories, respectively. After pooling all results, RRs were 0.78(95% CI: 0.65–0.94, $P = 0.01$) and 0.76(95% CI: 0.65–0.87, $P < 0.01$) compared with the normal category. Combined analysis of 23 studies showed that the RR was 0.77(95% CI: 0.68–0.88, $P < 0.01$) for the excess weight category (Fig. 2). Substantial heterogeneity was observed among the included studies, I^2 was 54.30, 50.60, and 62.40% for obesity, overweight, and excess weight categories, respectively.

Subgroup analyses suggested that RRs did not differ significantly by design, outcome, cancer ascertainment, BMI assessment, quality, or whether important confounders were adjusted for in original studies, although some results were statistically negative, mainly owing to the small number of studies included. When stratified by sex, some differences were observed; the results for women were consistently significant for all categories, whereas no positive associations were found for men (Table 1). To avoid the disturbance by preclinical weight loss caused by early lung cancer itself, studies were ruled out in which BMI was measured < 5 years before the diagnosis of lung cancer [12, 23, 25–28], and the pooled analysis of remaining studies gave an RR of 0.79 (95% CI: 0.70–0.91, $P < 0.01$) for the excess weight category.

Dose-response analyses

Finally, 28 studies were included in the dose-response analysis; the summary RR was 0.89(95% CI: 0.84–0.95, $P < 0.01$) per 5 kg/m^2 increase in BMI, with a high

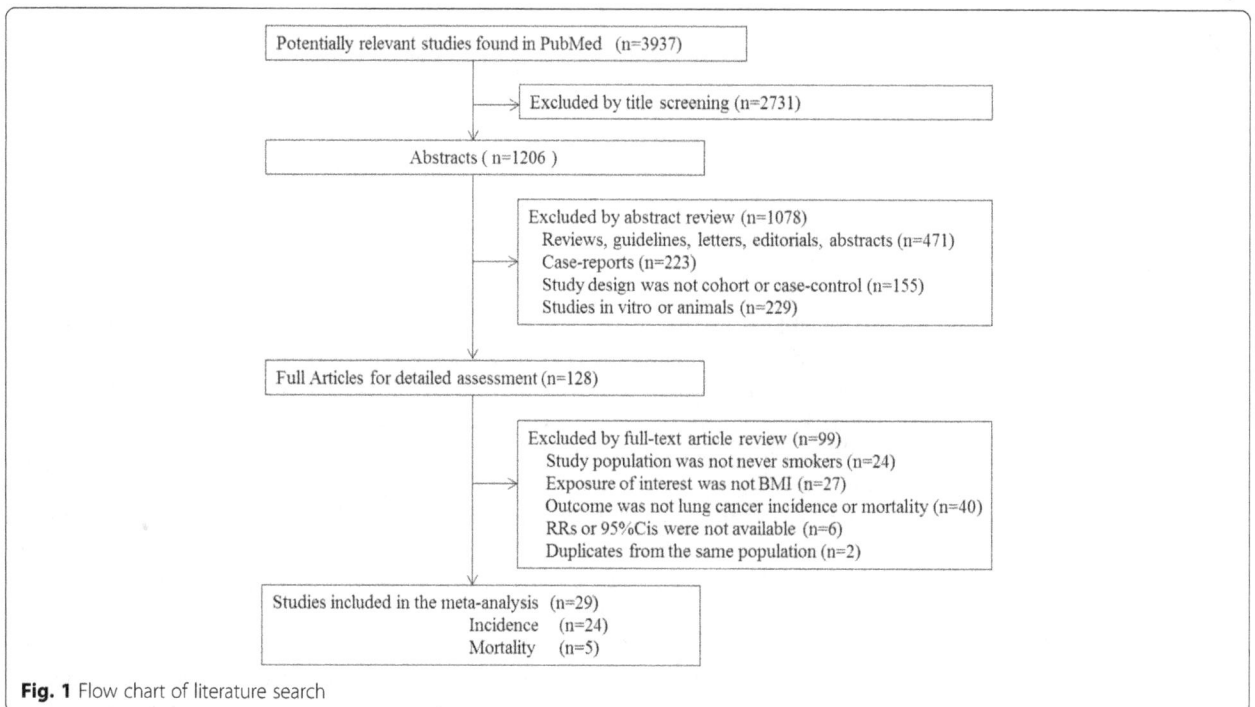

Fig. 1 Flow chart of literature search

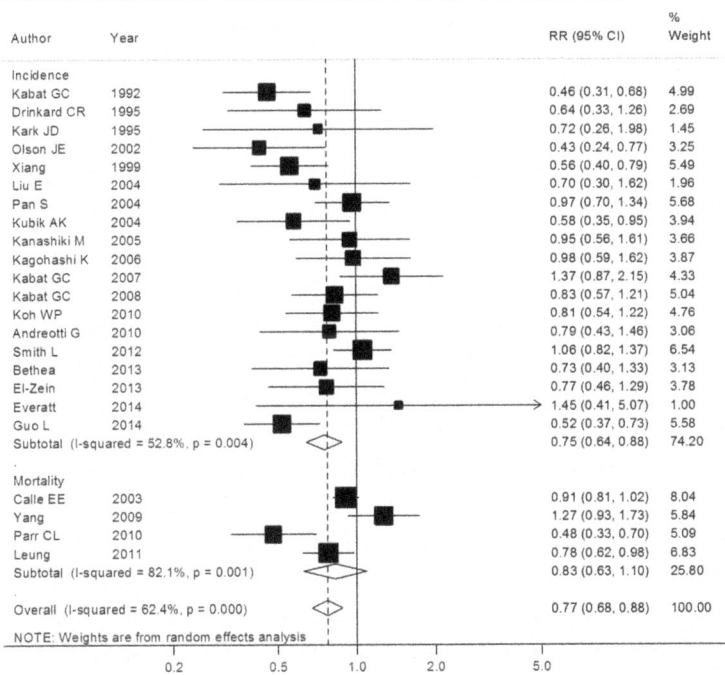

Fig. 2 Excess weight and lung cancer risk in never smokers. Box sizes reflect the weights of studies included in the meta-analysis, horizontal lines are the 95% CIs, and the summary RR is represented by the diamond. RR: relative risk, CI: confidence interval

heterogeneity ($I^2 = 86.44\%$) (Fig. 3).The RRs were 0.89(95% CI: 0.82–0.96, $P < 0.01$) for cohort studies and 0.90(95% CI: 0.79–1.03, $P = 0.13$) for case-control studies (Table 1). No significant differences were observed in subgroup analyses stratified by most confounders. When stratified by sex, the RRs were 0.89(95% CI: 0.81–0.97, $P < 0.01$) and 0.96(95% CI: 0.83–1.11, $P = 0.60$) for women and men, respectively (Fig. 4). The combined analysis of studies in which BMI was measure > 5 years before diagnosis gave an RR of 0.90 (95% CI: 0.84–0.96, $P < 0.01$) per 5 kg/m2 increase in BMI.

No evidence of a nonlinear relationship between BMI and lung cancer risk in never smokers was found (p for nonlinearity = 0.18), and an inverse linear trend was fitted in a random-effects meta-regression model (Fig. 5). Compared with BMI of 20 kg/m^2, the RRs were 1.17(95% CI: 1.02–1.34, $P = 0.02$), 0.87(95% CI: 0.83–0.92, $P < 0.01$), 0.81(95% CI: 0.76–0.87, $P < 0.01$), and 0.80 (95% CI: 0.68–0.94, $P < 0.01$) for BMI of 15, 25, 30, and 35 kg/m^2, respectively. When stratified by sex, the inverse linear trend was still present for women but disappeared for men.

Meta-regression, sensitivity analyses, and publication bias
As described above, substantial heterogeneity was observed across studies, but meta-regression analyses showed that most of the confounders including BMI assessment, ethnicity, design, quality, outcome, and

diagnosis method were not significantly associated with the heterogeneity. After excluding the 2 outlier studies by Kabat, et, al. [29] and Kondo, et, al. [30], the heterogeneity was reduced to some extent, but the results were unchanged. The results were still robust after removing one specific study each time in the sensitivity analysis. A slight publication bias was found in the analysis of the obesity category ($p = 0.046$ by Egger's test, $p = 0.20$ by Begg's test), but no studies were needed to be filled with the use of trim and fill method, suggesting that the influence could be negligible. In fact, the bias might be caused by insufficient data reported in original studies on the category of obesity, since in other category analyses, the funnel plots seemed to be symmetrical, and no significant publication biases were found.

Discussion
In the pooled analysis of 29 observational studies, involving more than 10,000 lung cancer cases in 15 million never smokers, the results suggested that higher BMI was associated with lower lung cancer risk, especially in women. In contrast with previous meta-analyses, our study includes the largest sample up to now, and the results were stable both in the subgroup and dose-response analyses.

Previous studies reported that obesity was associated with a lower risk of certain cancer types, particularly smoking related-cancers [2, 11, 12, 31]. However, the results were less convincing owing to the small sample size

Table 1 Subgroup analyses for the association between BMI and lung cancer risk in never smokers

Categories	Subgroups	Number of studies	RR (95% CI)	P value	Heterogeneity			P-interaction
					chi-squared	I^2	P-heterogeneity	
Obesity		18	0.78(0.65–0.94)	0.01	37.23	54.30%	< 0.01	
Design	Cohort	14	0.74(0.60–0.91)	< 0.01	27.83	53.30%	0.01	0.32
	Case-control	4	0.97(0.58–1.62)	0.90	8.75	65.70%	0.03	
Outcome	Incidence	15	0.79(0.63–0.99)	0.04	30.83	54.60%	< 0.01	0.74
	Mortality	3	0.71(0.45–1.12)	0.14	6.40	68.70%	0.04	
Gender	Male	5	0.69(0.41–1.15)	0.16	16.58	69.80%	< 0.01	0.81
	Female	8	0.86(0.72–1.02)	0.08	7.49	19.90%	0.28	
Ethnicity	Non-Asian	13	0.82(0.64–1.04)	0.10	27.92	57.00%	< 0.01	0.51
	Asian	5	0.70(0.54–0.91)	< 0.01	5.56	28.00%	0.24	
Quality	High	12	0.76(0.61–0.94)	0.01	27.5	60.00%	0.004	0.72
	Low	6	0.84(0.55–1.29)	0.43	9.72	48.60%	0.08	
Diagnosis	Registry	10	0.77(0.59–1.00)	0.05	22.28	59.60%	< 0.01	0.89
	Pathology	8	0.79(0.59–1.06)	0.11	14.16	50.60%	0.05	
Adjustment for confounders								
Alcohol intake	Yes	11	0.83(0.68–1.02)	0.07	18.98	47.30%	0.04	0.49
	No	7	0.68(0.45–1.04)	0.07	16.25	63.10%	0.01	
Vegetable/fruit intake	Yes	6	0.81(0.58–1.13)	0.22	12.80	60.90%	0.02	0.80
	No	12	0.76(0.59–0.97)	0.03	23.41	53.00%	0.02	
Physical activity	Yes	9	0.91(0.75–1.11)	0.34	12.18	34.30%	0.14	0.19
	No	9	0.67(0.49–0.93)	0.02	18.15	55.90%	0.02	
Medical history[a]	Yes	3	0.78(0.58–0.95)	0.24	35.80	60.90%	< 0.01	0.61
	No	15	0.90(0.76–1.07)	0.02	0.78	0.00%	0.68	
Overweight		15	0.76(0.65–0.87)	< 0.01	28.37	50.60%	0.01	
Design	Cohort	12	0.74(0.62–0.88)	< 0.01	27.30	59.70%	< 0.01	0.78
	Case-control	3	0.80(0.63–1.02)	0.08	1.03	0.00%	0.60	
Outcome	Incidence	12	0.76(0.64–0.90)	< 0.01	16.92	35.00%	0.11	0.93
	Mortality	3	0.73(0.53–1.01)	0.06	10.51	81.00%	< 0.01	
Gender	Male	5	0.92(0.62–1.36)	0.68	14.38	72.20%	< 0.01	0.44
	Female	8	0.82(0.72–0.93)	< 0.01	6.52	0.00%	0.48	
Ethnicity	Non-Asian	11	0.87(0.78–0.97)	< 0.01	10.34	3.30%	0.41	0.09
	Asian	4	0.61(0.44–0.86)	< 0.01	10.87	72.40%	0.01	
Quality	High	10	0.85(0.77–0.94)	< 0.01	9.47	4.90%	0.40	0.32
	Low	5	0.70(0.46–1.06)	0.09	13.76	70.90%	< 0.01	
Diagnosis	Registry	8	0.82(0.68–0.98)	0.03	14.38	51.30%	0.04	0.25
	Pathology	7	0.68(0.55–0.84)	< 0.01	8.74	31.40%	0.19	
Adjustment for confounders								
Alcohol intake	Yes	11	0.79(0.68–0.92)	< 0.01	18.32	45.40%	0.05	0.37
	No	4	0.67(0.46–0.97)	0.03	6.36	52.80%	0.10	
Vegetable/fruit intake	Yes	5	0.89(0.79–0.99)	0.03	1.46	0.00%	0.83	0.15
	No	10	0.68(0.54–0.85)	< 0.01	22.26	50.60%	< 0.01	
Physical activity	Yes	9	0.87(0.77–0.97)	0.02	8.86	9.70%	0.35	0.14
	No	6	0.66(0.49–0.88)	< 0.01	12.85	61.10%	0.02	

Table 1 Subgroup analyses for the association between BMI and lung cancer risk in never smokers (Continued)

Categories	Subgroups	Number of studies	RR (95% CI)	P value	Heterogeneity chi-squared	I^2	P-heterogeneity	P-interaction
Medical history[a]	Yes	3	0.89(0.79–1.00)	0.05	24.35	0.00%	0.66	0.42
	No	12	0.72(0.60–0.87)	< 0.01	0.84	50.60%	0.01	
Excess weight		23	0.77(0.68–0.88)	< 0.01	58.46	62.40%	< 0.01	
Design	Cohort	16	0.80(0.69–0.94)	< 0.01	40.07	62.60%	< 0.01	0.47
	Case-control	7	0.71(0.56–0.91)	< 0.01	13.78	56.50%	0.03	
Outcome	Incidence	19	0.75(0.64–0.88)	< 0.01	38.12	52.80%	< 0.01	0.60
	Mortality	4	0.83(0.63–1.10)	0.19	16.73	82.10%	< 0.01	
Gender	Male	8	0.88(0.70–1.11)	0.29	17.94	55.40%	0.02	0.85
	Female	12	0.75(0.62–0.91)	< 0.01	28.89	61.90%	< 0.01	
Ethnicity	Non-Asian	14	0.80(0.68–0.95)	< 0.01	28.25	54.00%	< 0.01	0.66
	Asian	9	0.74(0.59–0.94)	0.01	26.05	69.30%	< 0.01	
Quality	High	16	0.83(0.73–0.95)	< 0.01	30.06	50.10%	0.01	0.18
	Low	7	0.68(0.50–0.90)	< 0.01	17.7	66.10%	< 0.01	
Diagnosis	Registry	11	0.88(0.75–1.05)	0.15	24.27	58.80%	< 0.01	0.06
	Pathology	12	0.68(0.57–0.81)	< 0.01	19.97	44.90%	0.05	
Adjustment for confounders								
Alcohol intake	Yes	12	0.83(0.71–0.97)	0.02	26.74	58.90%	0.01	0.31
	No	11	0.71(0.57–0.89)	< 0.01	22.73	56.00%	< 0.01	
Vegetable/fruit intake	Yes	7	0.85(0.69–1.05)	0.13	17.29	57.10%	< 0.01	0.37
	No	16	0.73(0.62–0.87)	< 0.01	34.93	65.30%	< 0.01	
Physical activity	Yes	9	0.87(0.77–0.99)	0.04	10.14	21.10%	0.26	0.52
	No	14	0.75(0.61–0.92)	< 0.01	41.15	68.40%	< 0.01	
Medical history[a]	Yes	7	0.84(0.68–1.04)	0.11	13.32	55.00%	0.04	0.52
	No	16	0.75(0.63–0.89)	< 0.01	40.57	63.00%	< 0.01	
BMI increase per 5 Kg/m²		28	0.89(0.84–0.95)	< 0.01	86.44	68.80%	< 0.01	
Design	Cohort	20	0.89(0.82–0.96)	< 0.01	58.12	67.30%	< 0.01	0.88
	Case-control	8	0.90(0.79–1.03)	0.13	24.77	71.70%	0.01	
Outcome	Incidence	23	0.89(0.83–0.96)	< 0.01	65.3	66.30%	< 0.01	0.98
	Mortality	5	0.89(0.76–1.04)	0.16	20.98	80.90%	< 0.01	
Gender	Male	12	0.96(0.83–1.11)	0.60	28.43	61.30%	< 0.01	0.42
	Female	13	0.89(0.81–0.97)	< 0.01	34.74	65.50%	< 0.01	
Ethnicity	Non-Asian	18	0.91(0.84–0.98)	0.01	47.23	64.00%	< 0.01	0.66
	Asian	10	0.88(0.78–0.98)	0.03	33.12	72.80%	< 0.01	
Quality	High	20	0.91(0.86–0.98)	< 0.01	51.74	63.30%	< 0.01	0.39
	Low	8	0.85(0.72–1.00)	0.05	26.41	73.50%	< 0.01	
Diagnosis	Registry	15	0.93(0.86–1.00)	0.06	42.41	67.00%	< 0.01	0.35
	Pathology	13	0.86(0.78–0.95)	< 0.01	32.26	62.80%	< 0.01	
Adjustment for confounders								
Alcohol intake	Yes	15	0.89(0.83–0.95)	< 0.01	36.97	62.10%	< 0.01	0.60
	No	13	0.92(0.79–1.07)	0.28	48.42	75.20%	< 0.01	
Vegetable/fruit intake	Yes	7	0.93(0.84–1.02)	0.13	12.57	52.3%	0.05	0.77
	No	21	0.89(0.82–0.96)	< 0.01	72.90	72.6%	< 0.01	

Table 1 Subgroup analyses for the association between BMI and lung cancer risk in never smokers *(Continued)*

Categories	Subgroups	Number of studies	RR (95% CI)	P value	Heterogeneity			P-interaction
					chi-squared	I^2	P-heterogeneity	
Physical activity	Yes	10	0.92(0.86–0.98)	< 0.01	11.33	20.60%	0.25	0.96
	No	18	0.90(0.81–0.99)	< 0.01	86.44	77.3%	< 0.01	
Medical history[a]	Yes	11	0.90(0.83–0.97)	< 0.01	29.05	65.60%	< 0.01	0.84
	No	17	0.88(0.80–0.98)	0.02	56.45	71.70%	< 0.01	

Note: In the subgroup analyses, [a]medical history included history of chronic lung disease, history of family lung cancer, diabetes status, and hormone treatment. Other confounders such as total energy intake, environmental status and concomitant medication (use of aspirin and metformin) were not common in original studies; thus, subgroup analyses stratified by them were not performed

and other confounding factors, especially smoking. Meta-analysis is a quantitative approach that combines the results from multiple studies and increases the statistical power to resolve uncertainty in single studies for a more reliable conclusion. Thus, our study has a number of advantages. We included all the eligible epidemiological studies investigating the association between BMI and lung cancer risk in never smokers and redefined comparable exposure categories, which allowed for better control of confounders, subgroup analyses, and further dose-response analyses.

As we mentioned previously, several hypotheses have been put forward to explain the inverse association between lung cancer risk and BMI. As our study was limited to never smokers, the confounding of smoking, one of the most common arguments for the trend, was avoided as much as possible. A second hypothesis is that the lower BMI might reflect preclinical weight loss caused by early lung cancer itself or other related diseases. To solve this doubt, only studies in which BMI was measured 5 or more years before diagnosis were analyzed, and the inverse association remained unchanged. In fact, the participants with previous clinical weight loss were excluded at recruitment in most studies. It was also speculated that socioeconomic factors might be relevant to the inverse association, such as indoor air pollution in developing countries; however, our results indicated that the inverse association was stable across the strata of ethnicity.

Interestedly, we found a sex difference in the association between BMI and lung cancer risk, although p-interaction for sex is not statistically significant. Previous studies reported paradoxical results concerning the

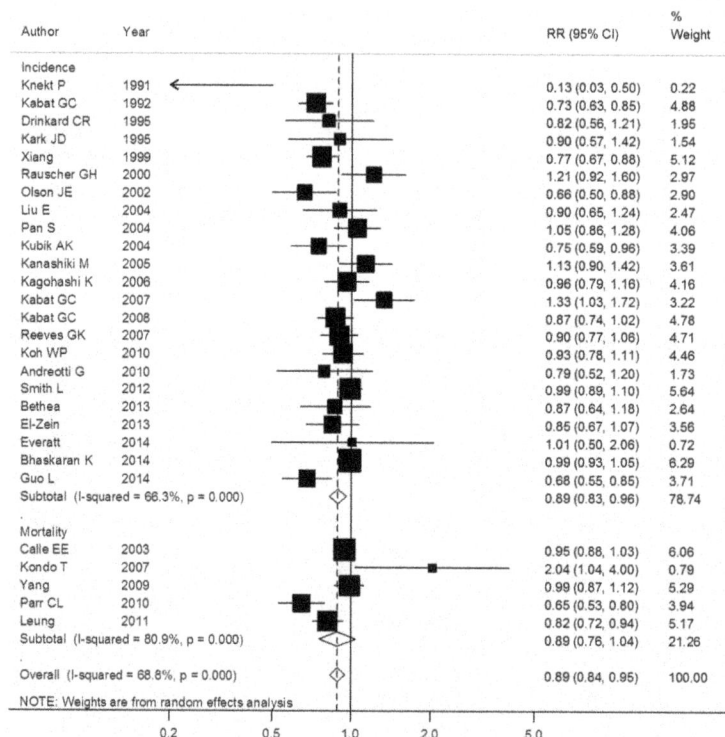

Fig. 3 Association between BMI and lung cancer risk per 5 kg/m² increase. Box sizes reflect the weights of studies included in the meta-analysis, horizontal lines are the 95% CIs, and the summary RR is represented by the diamond. BMI: body mass index, RR: relative risk, CI: confidence interval

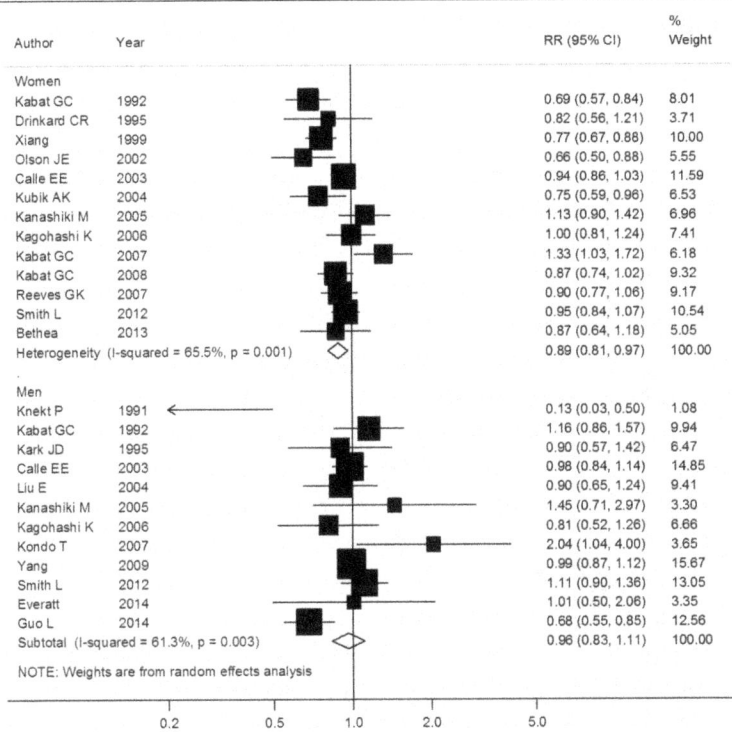

Fig. 4 Association between BMI and lung cancer risk per 5 kg/m² increase, stratified by sex. Box sizes reflect the weights of studies included in the meta-analysis, horizontal lines are the 95% CIs, and the summary RR is represented by the diamond. BMI: body mass index, RR: relative risk, CI: confidence interval

differences between sexes [11, 12], Smith *et al.* found that BMI was more strongly related to lower lung cancer risk in women than in men in a large cohort study [26]. The authors speculated that estrogens might play a protective role in lung cancer development [26], which was in accordance with our results. Notably, since more men than women are smokers, the results for the men in our

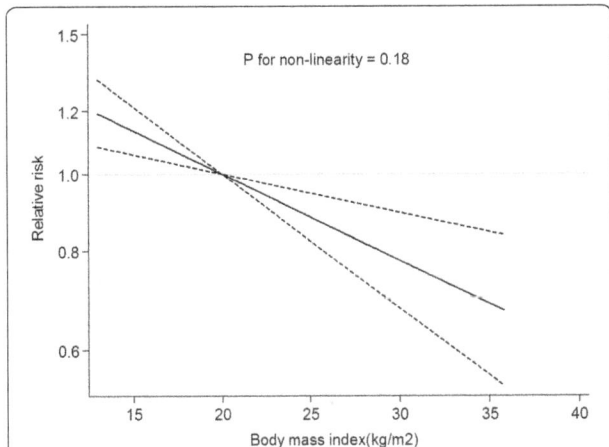

Fig. 5 Dose-response analysis for body mass index and lung cancer risk in never smokers. The solid line represents the trend between BMI and lung cancer risk, and the dashed lines represent the 95% confidence intervals. The displayed *p*-values refer to the test for nonlinearity

meta-analysis might be influenced by the relatively smaller sample size, more studies are warranted to explore the sex difference.

Not only epidemiological studies revealed the possibility that obesity might lower lung cancer risk, but some biological discoveries also provided useful hints. It has long been noted that lower BMI might increase the susceptibility of DNA to chemical carcinogens in cigarettes [27], and excess weight was associated with decreased chromosome damage [28]. Some studies also suggested that adipose tissue was helpful to keep the memory of $CD8^+$ T cells to maintain normal immune functions [32]. In addition, increased insulin-like growth factor-1 level which might explain the obesity-carcinogenesis connection was found not to be associated with lung cancer [33]. Paradoxically, systemic inflammation, which might increase lung cancer risk [33], is also closely associated with obesity [34]. These studies provide possible direction for more in-depth research in this field to better clarify the obesity paradox in lung cancer development.

The results of our study should be interpreted with caution, as associations found in a meta-analysis of observational studies do not reveal causation. Several other limitations should also be considered. First, concerning the outcomes of interest, both the incidence and mortality of lung cancer were included. It is reasonable to do this since lung cancer is relatively rare in the overall population, and previous studies reported that the incidence and mortality of lung cancer almost coincided with each other [35]. Second, inherent limitations in original studies were inevitable, especially for the case-control studies, which were prone to recall and selection bias, inconsistencies in baseline characteristics of original studies including different study populations, pathology type, ethnicity, ages, and duration all contributed to heterogeneity across studies. However, no individual confounder significantly influenced the heterogeneity by meta-regression, and subgroup analyses by these confounders were almost the same, indicating the stability of our results. Third, in some studies, BMI was calculated by self-reported weight and height, and different exposure ranges were adopted across different studies, which might lead to some incomparability of results. To solve the problem, we conducted different category comparisons and dose-response analyses as well as subgroup analyses stratified by BMI assessment, and the results were consistently stable to support our conclusion, which was further validated by the sensitivity analyses In addition, although no significant differences were found between studies whether they were adjusted for common confounders or not, insufficient adjustment of other potential confounders, including secondhand smoking, occupational exposure to lung carcinogens (e.g., radon), concomitant medication (e.g., using of aspirin and metformin) might distort our results, and we also had insufficient data on different histological types of lung cancer for further subgroup analyses. Lastly, only articles in full-text were included in our analysis, abstracts, trial registries were not retrieved, some studies might be missed. However, no significant publication bias was observed except in the analysis of the obesity category, and no studies were required using the "trim and fill" method, suggesting that the influence was slight.

Every sword has two edges. Obesity has been stereotyped as a risk factor for many chronic diseases including most types of cancer, but our study shows that higher BMI is associated with lower lung cancer risk, especially in women. Our results do not suggest increasing body weight to decrease the risk of lung cancer; however, underweight is also inadvisable, and maintaining a proper weight is the best choice. The results of our study are helpful to explain the J-shaped association between BMI and total mortality [1]. Further studies should be focused on the mechanisms underlying the phenomena, and extra efforts are needed to reduce the unfavorable effects of obesity on most cancer types and other chronic diseases.

Conclusions

In conclusion, the results of our meta-analysis indicate that higher BMI is associated with lower lung cancer risk, especially in women, which alter our common understanding of the relationship between obesity and cancer, although the causal relationship between these two factors cannot be determined from this analysis. Additional studies are required to validate these findings and to better understand the biologic rationale for this observation.

Additional files

Additional file 1: Table S1. Characteristics of studies included in the meta-analysis of obesity and lung cancer risk in non-smokers. (DOCX 88 kb)

Additional file 2: Table S2. Quality scores of the cohort studies included in the meta-analysis, assessed by the Newcastle-Ottawa scale. (DOCX 20 kb)

Additional file 3: Table S3. Quality scores of the case-control studies included in the meta-analysis, assessed by the Newcastle-Ottawa scale. (DOCX 18 kb)

Abbreviations
BMI: body mass index; CI: confidence interval; FTO: fat mass- and obesity-associated gene; RR: relative risk

Authors' contributions
HZ and SZ conceived and drafted the study; HZ and SZ conducted the literature research and collected all data; HZ and SZ analyzed and interpreted data; All authors commented on drafts of the paper and approved the final manuscript.

Competing interests
The authors declare that they have no competing interests.

Author details
[1]Department of thoracic surgery, Shangqiu First People's Hospital, Shangqiu 476100, Henan, China. [2]Department of Thoracic and Cardiovascular Surgery, the First Affiliated Hospital of Henan University, No. 357 Ximen Street, Kaifeng City 475000, Henan Province, China.

References
1. Whitlock G, Lewington S, Sherliker P, Clarke R, Emberson J, Halsey J, Qizilbash N, Collins R, Peto R. Body-mass index and cause-specific mortality in 900 000 adults: collaborative analyses of 57 prospective studies. Lancet. 2009;373(9669):1083–96.
2. Bhaskaran K, Douglas I, Forbes H, dos-Santos-Silva I, Leon DA, Smeeth L. Body-mass index and risk of 22 specific cancers: a population-based cohort study of 5.24 million UK adults. Lancet. 2014;384(9945):755–65.
3. Parr CL, Batty GD, Lam TH, Barzi F, Fang X, Ho SC, Jee SH, Ansary-Moghaddam A, Jamrozik K, Ueshima H, et al. Body-mass index and cancer mortality in the Asia-Pacific cohort studies collaboration: pooled analyses of 424,519 participants. Lancet Oncol. 2010;11(8):741–52.
4. Ligibel JA, Alfano CM, Courneya KS, Demark-Wahnefried W, Burger RA, Chlebowski RT, Fabian CJ, Gucalp A, Hershman DL, Hudson MM, et al. American Society of Clinical Oncology position statement on obesity and cancer. J Clin Oncol. 2014;32(31):3568–74.
5. Siegel RL, Miller KD, Jemal A. Cancer statistics, 2016. CA Cancer J Clin. 2016; 66(1):7–30.

6. Knekt P, Heliovaara M, Rissanen A, Aromaa A, Seppanen R, Teppo L, Pukkala E. Leanness and lung-cancer risk. Int J Cancer. 1991;49(2):208–13.

7. Henley SJ, Flanders WD, Manatunga A, Thun MJ. Leanness and lung cancer risk: fact or artifact? Epidemiology. 2002;13(3):268–76.

8. El-Zein M, Parent ME, Rousseau MC. Comments on a recent meta-analysis: obesity and lung cancer. Int J Cancer. 2013;132(8):1962–3.

9. Yang Y, Jiao Y. Authors' reply to comments on a recent meta-analysis: obesity and lung cancer. Int J Cancer. 2013;132(8):1964–5.

10. Shen N, Fu P, Cui B, Bu C-Y, Bi J-W. Associations between body mass index and the risk of mortality from lung cancer: a dose–response PRISMA-compliant meta-analysis of prospective cohort studies. Med. 2017;96(34):e7721.

11. Yang Y, Dong J, Sun K, Zhao L, Zhao F, Wang L, Jiao Y. Obesity and incidence of lung cancer: a meta-analysis. Int J Cancer. 2013;132(5):1162–9.

12. Duan P, Hu C, Quan C, Yi X, Zhou W, Yuan M, Yu T, Kourouma A, Yang K. Body mass index and risk of lung cancer: systematic review and dose-response meta-analysis. Sci Rep. 2015;5:16938.

13. El-Zein M, Parent ME, Nicolau B, Koushik A, Siemiatycki J, Rousseau MC. Body mass index, lifetime smoking intensity and lung cancer risk. Int J Cancer. 2013;133(7):1721–31.

14. Gupta A, Majumder K, Arora N, Mayo HG, Singh PP, Beg MS, Hughes R, Singh S, Johnson DH. Premorbid body mass index and mortality in patients with lung cancer: a systematic review and meta-analysis. Lung Cancer. 2016; 102:49–59.

15. Zhang X, Liu Y, Shao H, Zheng X. Obesity paradox in lung Cancer prognosis: evolving biological insights and clinical implications. J Thorac Oncol. 2017; 12(10):1478–88.

16. Lam VK, Bentzen SM, Mohindra P, Nichols EM, Bhooshan N, Vyfhuis M, Scilla KA, Feigenberg SJ, Edelman MJ, Feliciano JL. Obesity is associated with long-term improved survival in definitively treated locally advanced non-small cell lung cancer (NSCLC). Lung Cancer. 2017;104:52–7.

17. Gazdar AF, Thun MJ. Lung cancer, smoke exposure, and sex. J Clin Oncol. 2007;25(5):469–71.

18. Gláucia F. Cota, Marcos R. de Sousa, Tatiani Oliveira Fereguetti, Ana Rabello. Efficacy of Anti-Leishmania Therapy in Visceral Leishmaniasis among HIV Infected Patients: A Systematic Review with Indirect Comparison. PLOS Negl Trop Dis. 2013;7(5):e2195.

19. Hamling J, Lee P, Weitkunat R, Ambuhl M. Facilitating meta-analyses by deriving relative effect and precision estimates for alternative comparisons from a set of estimates presented by exposure level or disease category. Stat Med. 2008;27(7):954–70.

20. Higgins JP, Thompson SG, Deeks JJ, Altman DG. Measuring inconsistency in meta-analyses. BMJ. 2003;327(7414):557–60.

21. Greenland S, Longnecker MP. Methods for trend estimation from summarized dose-response data, with applications to meta-analysis. Am J Epidemiol. 1992;135(11):1301–9.

22. Orsini NBR, Greenland S. Generalized least squares for trend estimation of summarized dose-response data. Stata J. 2009;6(1):17.

23. Xiang Y, Gao Y, Zhong L, Jin F, Sun L, Cheng J, Zhai Y. A case-control study on relationship between body mass index and lung cancer in non-smoking women. Zhonghua Yu Fang Yi Xue Za Zhi. 1999;33(1):9–12.

24. Guo L, Li N, Wang G, Su K, Li F, Yang L, Ren J, Chang S, Chen S, Wu S, et al. Body mass index and cancer incidence:a prospective cohort study in northern China. Zhonghua Liu Xing Bing Xue Za Zhi. 2014;35(3):231–6.

25. Song YM, Sung J, Ha M. Obesity and risk of cancer in postmenopausal Korean women. J Clin Oncol. 2008;26(20):3395–402.

26. Smith L, Brinton LA, Spitz MR, Lam TK, Park Y, Hollenbeck AR, Freedman ND, Gierach GL. Body mass index and risk of lung cancer among never, former, and current smokers. J Natl Cancer Inst. 2012;104(10):778–89.

27. Loft S, Vistisen K, Ewertz M, Tjonneland A, Overvad K, Poulsen HE. Oxidative DNA damage estimated by 8-hydroxydeoxyguanosine excretion in humans: influence of smoking, gender and body mass index. Carcinogenesis. 1992; 13(12):2241–7.

28. Li X, Bai Y, Wang S, Nyamathira SM, Zhang X, Zhang W, Wang T, Deng Q, He M, Wu T, et al. Association of body mass index with chromosome damage levels and lung cancer risk among males. Sci Rep. 2015;5:9458.

29. Kabat GC, Wynder EL. Body mass index and lung cancer risk. Am J Epidemiol. 1992;135(7):769–74.

30. Kondo T, Hori Y, Yatsuya H, Tamakoshi K, Toyoshima H, Nishino Y, Seki N, Ito Y, Suzuki K, Ozasa K, et al. Lung cancer mortality and body mass index in a Japanese cohort: findings from the Japan collaborative cohort study (JACC study). Cancer Causes Control. 2007;18(2):229–34.

31. Radoi L, Paget-Bailly S, Cyr D, Papadopoulos A, Guida F, Tarnaud C, Menvielle G, Schmaus A, Cenee S, Carton M, et al. Body mass index, body mass change, and risk of oral cavity cancer: results of a large population-based case-control study, the ICARE study. Cancer Causes Control. 2013; 24(7):1437–48.

32. Cui G, Staron MM, Gray SM, Ho PC, Amezquita RA, Wu J, Kaech SM. IL-7-induced glycerol transport and TAG synthesis promotes memory CD8+ T cell longevity. Cell. 2015;161(4):750–61.

33. Engels EA. Inflammation in the development of lung cancer: epidemiological evidence. Expert Rev Anticancer Ther. 2008;8(4):605–15.

34. Iyengar NM, Gucalp A, Dannenberg AJ, Hudis CA. Obesity and Cancer mechanisms: tumor microenvironment and inflammation. J Clin Oncol. 2016;34(35):4270–6.

35. Reeves GK, Pirie K, Beral V, Green J, Spencer E, Bull D. Cancer incidence and mortality in relation to body mass index in the million women study: cohort study. BMJ. 2007;335(7630):1134.

20

Long non-coding RNA RUNXOR accelerates MDSC-mediated immunosuppression in lung cancer

Xinyu Tian[1,2†], Jie Ma[2†], Ting Wang[3], Jie Tian[2], Yu Zheng[2], Rongrong Peng[2], Yungang Wang[2], Yue Zhang[1], Lingxiang Mao[1*], Huaxi Xu[2] and Shengjun Wang[1,2*]

Abstract

Background: RUNX1 overlapping RNA (RUNXOR) is a long non-coding RNA that has been indicated as a key regulator in the development of myeloid cells by targeting runt-related transcription factor 1 (RUNX1). Myeloid-derived suppressor cells (MDSCs) are a heterogeneous population of cells consisting of immature granulocytes and monocytes with immunosuppression. However, the impact of lncRNA RUNXOR on the development of MDSCs remains unknown.

Methods: Both the expressions of RUNXOR and RUNX1 in the peripheral blood were measured by qRT-PCR. Human MDSCs used in this study were isolated from tumor tissue of patients with lung cancer by FCM or induced from PBMCs of healthy donors with IL-1β + GM-CSF. Specific siRNA was used to knockdown the expression of RUNXOR in MDSCs.

Results: In this study, we found that the lncRNA RUNXOR was upregulated in the peripheral blood of lung cancer patients. In addition, as a target gene of RUNXOR, the expression of RUNX1 was downregulated in lung cancer patients. Finally, the expression of RUNXOR was higher in MDSCs isolated from the tumor tissues of lung cancer patients compared with cells from adjacent tissue. In addition, RUNXOR knockdown decreased Arg1 expression in MDSCs.

Conclusions: Based on our findings, it is illustrated that RUNXOR is significantly associated with the immunosuppression induced by MDSCs in lung cancer patients and may be a target of anti-tumor therapy.

Keywords: lncRNA RUNXOR, MDSCs, RUNX1, Anti-tumor immunity, Lung cancer

Background

Lung cancer has become a leading cause of male cancer-related death worldwide because of its poor outcome and late diagnosis. Despite the development of chemotherapy and the integration of targeted therapy aimed at lung cancer, the overall outcomes are still not ideal [1]. Meanwhile, immunotherapy is becoming increasingly promising in the treatment of lung cancer [2, 3]. Nowadays, the immunosuppression induced by myeloid-derived suppressor cells (MDSCs) has been demonstrated to be a main cause of tumor escape in anti-tumor therapies targeting lung cancer [4–6].

MDSCs are a heterogeneous population of immature myeloid cells consisting of precursors for granulocytes, macrophages or dendritic cells (DCs), which accumulate during tumor progression [7, 8]. MDSCs display a broadly distinct phenotype. In mice, the phenotype of MDSCs is CD11b + Gr1+, which contain two subsets: polymorphonuclear MDSCs (PMN-MDSCs) characterized as CD11b + Ly6G + Ly6Clo and monocytic MDSCs (M-MDSCs) characterized as CD11b + Ly6G-Ly6Chi. In human, MDSCs represent a population of cells with the phenotype of CD11b + CD33 + HLA-DR-CD14-, which are further subdivided into PMN-MDSCs and M-MDSCs based on the differential expression of Lin and CD15 [9, 10]. In cancer progression, MDSCs inhibit the anti-tumor immune responses induced by CD4+ T cells, CD8+ T cells and NK cells by releasing Arg1, ROS and iNOS. In addition, MDSCs can also induce Treg

* Correspondence: maolingxiang@aliyun.com; sjwjs@ujs.edu.cn
†Xinyu Tian and Jie Ma contributed equally to this work.
[1]Department of Laboratory Medicine, The Affiliated People's Hospital, Jiangsu University, Zhenjiang 212012, China
Full list of author information is available at the end of the article

cells and promote IL-10 production [11, 12]. Currently, therapies targeting MDSCs mainly involve eliminating these cells, inhibiting their suppressive effects or promoting their differentiation [13].

Functional genomics studies have revealed that ~ 90% of human genes produce non-coding RNAs (ncRNAs) consisting of long non-coding RNAs (> 200 nt) and microRNAs [14, 15]. Unlike microRNAs, lncRNAs are capable of being capped and polyadenylated. Increasing evidences indicate that lncRNAs are involved in different cellular processes via a variety of mechanisms [16–20]. The lncRNA RUNXOR, which is approximately 216 kb in length, is a long intragenic non-coding RNA. RUNXOR interacts epigenetically with the RUNX1 gene, which normally functions as a tumor suppressor and modulates the expression of a number of important hematopoietic regulator genes. LncRNA RUNXOR is unspliced and overlaps with RUNX1 introns and exons. In AML cells, RUNXOR regulates RUNX1 expression by directly binding to promoters and enhancers via its 3′-end and may be physically involved in chromosomal translocation that occur in malignancies. In addition, by directly binding to chromatin, RUNXOR is involved in the orchestration of a long-range intrachromosomal loop. The formation of intrachromosomal loop is a typical epigenetic mechanism by which a regulatory element can mediate the expression of a gene even when locate far away from the gene. The most remarkable property of RUNXOR is that this lncRNA is able to use its 3′-end to recruit RUNX1 protein to bind RUNX1 promoter and induce epigenetic modulation via a variety of enhancers [21]. In our previous study, we have demonstrated that miR-9 mediates the development of MDSCs by targeting RUNX1 [12]. Thus, in this study, we aimed to determine whether RUNXOR regulates the immunosuppression of MDSCs by targeting RUNX1 in the progression of lung cancer.

Methods

Patients and samples
One hundred peripheral blood samples which contained lung adenocarcinoma ($n = 53$), squamous cell lung cancer ($n = 24$) and small cell lung cancer ($n = 23$) were collected from lung cancer patients. To separate the cells from the plasma, we centrifuged peripheral blood samples at 20 °C and 2000 rpm for 5 min. Then ACK lysing buffer was used to lyse red blood cells, and the remaining cells were used in the subsequent experiments. Paired peripheral blood samples, pre- and post-surgery, were collected from 40 lung cancer patients. Paired lung cancer tissues and adjacent tissues were collected from 9 patients with lung cancer who underwent primary surgical resection. The study was approved by the respective Ethics Committee of the Affiliated

People's Hospital of Jiangsu University. Written informed consent was obtained from all the subjects in accordance with the Declaration of Helsinki.

Isolation of MDSCs from tumor tissue
Collagenase II (Sigma-Aldrich, St. Louis, MO) was used to digest tumor tissue and adjacent tissue derived from patients with lung cancer that had been cut into small pieces (1–2 mm^3) at 37 °C for 2 h on a rotating platform to obtain a single-cell suspension. The cells were collected and stained with human anti-HLA-DR, anti-CD33, anti-CD11b and anti-CD14 mAbs (eBioscience, San Diego, CA) for 30 min. Stained cells were collected and then analyzed via flow cytometry (FACSAria, BD Biosciences).

Induction of human MDSCs
Density-gradient centrifugation over a Ficoll-Hypaque solution (Haoyang Biological Technology Co., Tianjin, China) was used to isolate human peripheral blood mononuclear cells (PBMCs). Then 40 ng/mL IL-1β (Peprotech, NJ) and 40 ng/mL GM-CSF (Peprotech) were used to stimulate PBMCs from healthy donors for 4 days. At day 4, the cells were collected and isolated by using human anti-CD33 beads (Miltenyi Biotec, Auburn, CA).

Flow cytometry
To confirm the percentages of CD4+ and CD8+ T cells, 50 ng/ml phorbol myristate acetate (PMA; Sigma-Aldrich, California) and 1 µg/ml ionomycin (Sigma-Aldrich) were used to stimulate PBMCs from lung cancer patients and healthy donors for 2 h and then cells were incubated in the presence of 1 µg/ml brefeldin-A (eBioscience, San Diego) for another 4 h. Post stimulation, cells were then stained with human anti-CD3 and anti-CD8 mAbs (eBioscience), fixed, permeabilized and stained with a human anti-IFN-γ mAb (eBioscience) following the instructions of the Intracellular Staining Kit (Invitrogen, Carlsbad, CA).

RNA isolation and quantitative real-time PCR
Total RNA was extracted from cells with TRIzol reagent (Invitrogen, California) following the manufacturer's instructions. Random primers and a ReverTra Ace® qPCR RT Kit (Toyobo, Osaka, Japan) were used to synthesize cDNA. Bio-Rad SYBR Green Supermix (Bio-Rad, Hercules) was used to perform quantitative real-time PCR in triplicate. The primer sequences were as follows: human β-actin, sense 5-GAGTGTGGAGACCATCAAG GA-3, antisense 5-TGTATTGCTTTGCGTTGGAC-3; human RUNX1, sense 5-TGATGGCTGGCAATGATGA A-3, antisense 5-TGCGGTGGGTTTGTGAAGAC-3; human 18S, sense 5-CGGACAGGATTGACAGATTG-3, antisense 5- GCCAGAGTCTCGTTCGTTATC-3; human

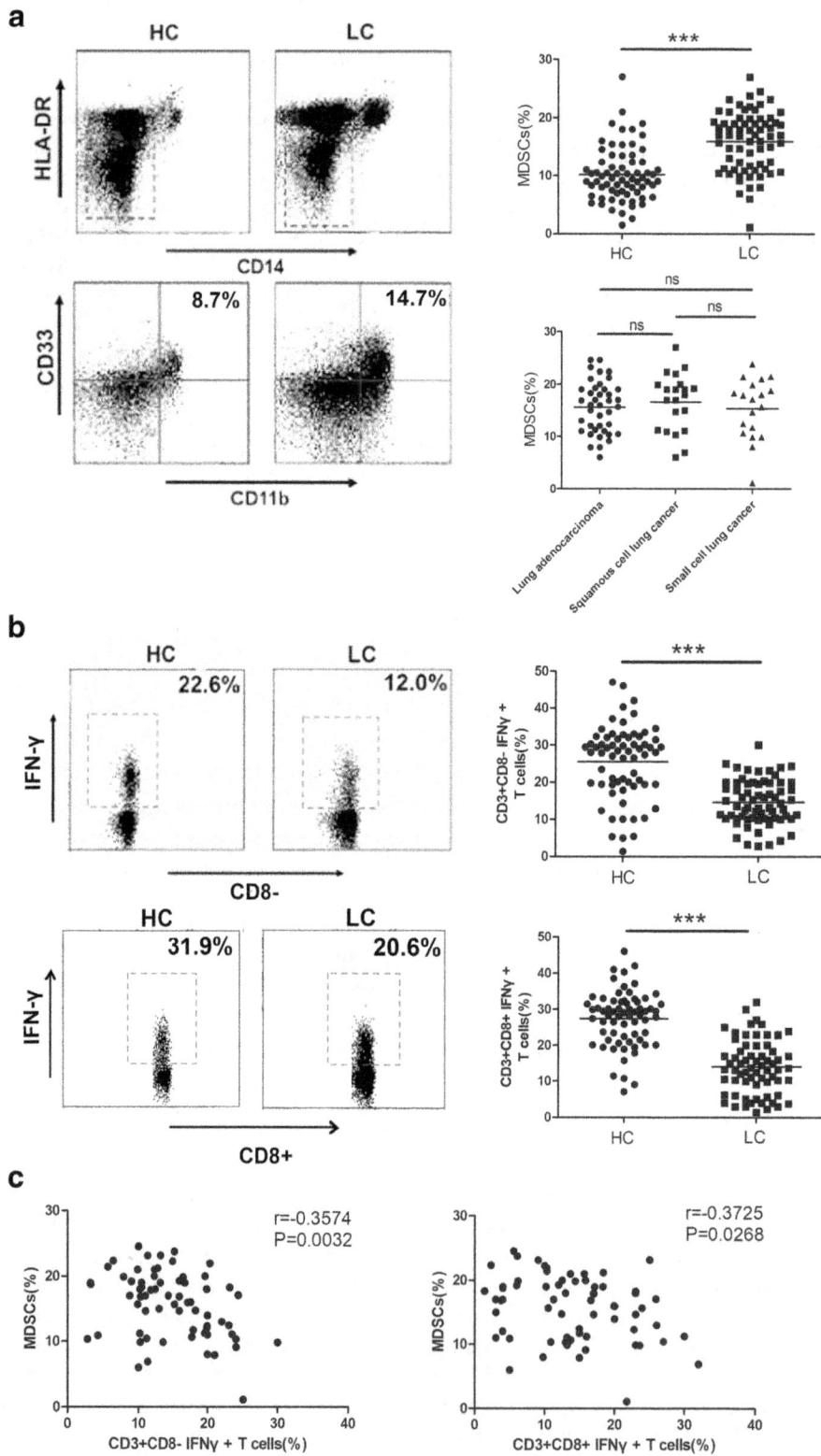

Fig. 1 The percentage of MDSCs in the peripheral blood of lung cancer patients is negatively correlated with the ratio of Th1/CTL cells. **a-b** The proportions of CD11b + CD33 + HLA-DR-CD14- MDSCs (*n* = 61), CD3 + CD8-IFN-γ + Th1 cells and CD3 + CD8 + IFN-γ + CTLs (*n* = 56) in the peripheral blood of lung cancer patients and healthy donors were detected by flow cytometry (FCM). **c** The correlation between the proportion of Th1/CTL cells and the percentage of MDSCs in the peripheral blood of lung cancer patients. ***P < 0.001, **P < 0.01, ns = no significance

ARG1, sense 5-. CCTTTGCTGACATCCCTAAT-3, antisense 5-GATTCTTCCGTTCTTCTTGACT-3; and human RUNXOR, sense 5-CCTGTTCACGGTCCAAACT GG-3, antisense 5-CGGCAAGATCACAGTCCCTAGC-3. The expression level of each gene was expressed as the ratio to the β-actin transcript level. The data were analyzed with Bio-Rad CFX Manager software.

Transfection

50 nM RUNXOR siRNA or its negative control (Ribobio Co., Guangzhou, China) was used to transfect MDSCs plated in 48-well plates according to the manufacturer's protocol.

Graphing and statistical analysis of data

To generate bar graphs or graphs of tumor regression, data from all experiments were entered into GraphPad Prism 5.0 (GraphPad, San Diego, CA). The data are presented as the mean ± SD. Student's t-test was used to determine the statistical significance of differences between groups. And Spearman's correlation coefficient was used to confirm correlations between variables. Differences were considered significant at a p level less than 0.05.

Results
The proportion of MDSCs is negatively correlated with the percentage of Th1/CTL cells in the peripheral blood of lung cancer patients

MDSCs are a population of cells that accumulate during the progression of various cancers. In human, the phenotype of MDSCs is CD11b + CD33 + HLA-DR-CD14-. These cells inhibit the anti-tumor immune response via different mechanisms: MDSCs produce suppressive molecules, such as Arg1, ROS or iNOS, to directly suppress the anti-tumor immune response induced by Th1/CTL cells and promote tumor progression; MDSCs can also promote the production of IL-10 to inhibit the CTL response by inducing Tregs or developing into tumor-associated macrophages (TAMs) [10, 22–25]. To determine whether the MDSCs proportion changes during lung cancer progression, we detected the percentage of MDSCs in the peripheral blood of healthy controls and lung cancer patients. Compared with the healthy controls, the proportion of MDSCs increased in the peripheral blood of lung cancer patients ($P < 0.001$, Fig. 1a). We also compared the proportion of MDSCs in the peripheral blood of lung cancer patients with different histological categories. The results indicated that the proportion of MDSCs in various histological categories showed no significant difference (Fig. 1a). At the same time, the proportions of Th1 cells and CTL cells decreased in lung cancer patients ($P < 0.01$, Fig. 1b). In the subsequent correlation analysis, we found that the proportion of MDSCs was significant negatively correlated with the percentage of Th1 or CTL (Fig. 1c)

cells in the peripheral blood of lung cancer patients. These data suggest that MDSCs are a population of cells that inhibit Th1/CTL cells and induce anti-tumor immunity.

LncRNA RUNXOR level is upregulated in lung cancer

We used real-time fluorescence quantitative PCR (qRT-PCR) to detect the expression of lncRNA RUNXOR in the peripheral blood of lung cancer patients. We found that compared with healthy controls, the RUNXOR level increased in the peripheral blood of lung cancer patients ($P < 0.001$, Fig. 2a). In addition, by analyzing the RUNXOR level in different types of lung cancers, we found that RUNXOR was differently expressed between squamous cell lung cancer and lung adenocarcinoma, which indicated that RUNXOR might be used to distinguish lung cancer types ($P < 0.05$, Fig. 2b). Interestingly, we found that RUNXOR expression was significantly downregulated in the blood of lung cancer patients who have underwent surgery ($P < 0.05$, Fig. 2c). Additionally, the data in Table 1 showed that the RUNXOR level was remarkably correlated with smoking history ($P = 0.039$), TNM stage ($P < 0.0001$), histological tumor type ($P = 0.016$) and lymph node metastasis ($P = 0.0028$) in lung

Table 1 Correlation between RUNXOR expression and the clinicopathological parameters of lung cancer patients

Relative expression of RUNXOR				
Parameter	Number	Low	High	P-value
Age				0.0294
< 60	33	8	25	
≥ 60	67	19	48	
Gender				0.3677
Male	74	22	52	
Female	26	6	20	
Tumor size				0.8746
≤ 3 cm	24	16	8	
> 3 cm	76	9	67	
Smoking history				0.039
Smokers	66	11	55	
Never smokers	34	17	17	
Lymph node metastasis				0.0028
Positive	67	9	58	
Negative	33	15	18	
TNM stage				< 0.0001
I + II	12	7	5	
III + IV	88	14	74	
Histological tumor type				0.016
Squamous cell carcinoma	53	14	39	
Adenocarcinoma	24	6	18	
Small cell lung cancer	23	9	14	

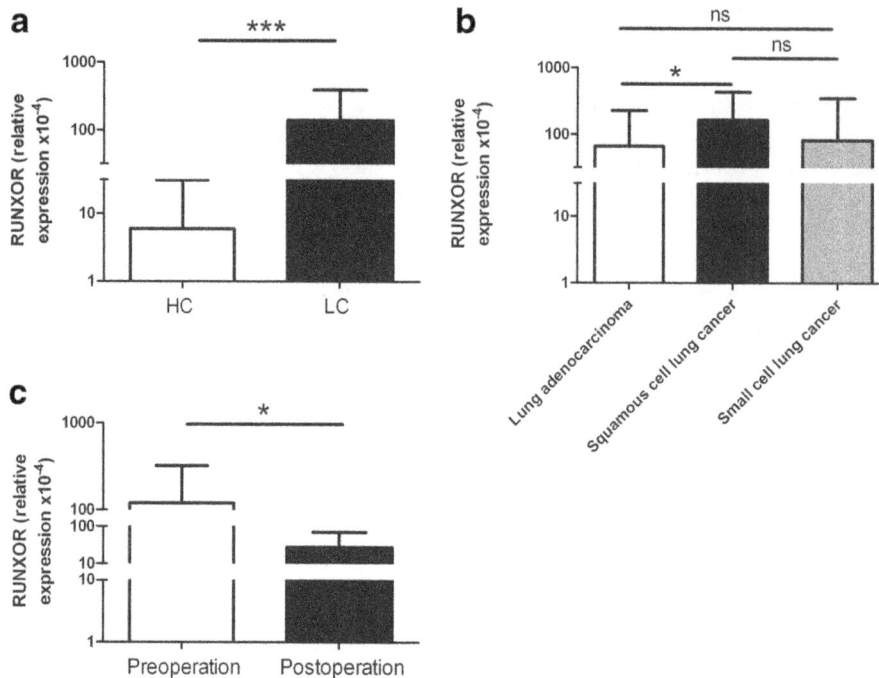

Fig. 2 The level of lncRNA RUNXOR upregulated in lung cancer. **a** Relative expression of the lncRNA RUNXOR in the peripheral blood of lung cancer patients and healthy donors. **b** The relative expression of lncRNA RUNXOR in peripheral blood from different types of lung cancers. **c** The relative expression of lncRNA RUNXOR in the peripheral blood of lung cancer patients pre- and post-operation. ***$P < 0.001$, *$P < 0.05$, ns: no significance

cancer. These results show that the lncRNA RUNXOR level is closely related with lung cancer.

The expression of RUNXOR is associated with the immunosuppression of MDSCs

Previous work has revealed that RUNXOR is significantly up-regulated in AML which is characterized by the proliferation of immature myeloid cells [21]. As described above, RUN-XOR is associated with lung cancer. Based on these findings, we hypothesized that RUNXOR might be involved in MDSC-induced immunosuppression in lung cancer. According to the correlation analysis, RUNXOR expression was positively correlated with the proportion of MDSCs and Arg1 level (Fig. 3a), which is the main suppressive molecule of MDSCs, in the peripheral blood of lung cancer patients. Meanwhile, RUNXOR expression was negatively correlated with the percentage of Th1 and CTL (Fig. 3b) cells in the peripheral blood of lung cancer patients. To further determine whether RUNXOR was expressed by MDSCs, we isolated CD11b + CD33 + HLA-DR-CD14- MDSCs from tumor and adjacent tissues of lung cancer patients and detected the expression of RUNXOR by using qRT-PCR. Compared with cells of the same phenotype from adjacent tissue, RUNXOR expression was increased in MDSCs from tumor tissue ($P < 0.05$, Fig. 3c). We also used a specific siRNA to inhibit the expression of RUNXOR and then detected the Arg1 level in MDSCs from tumor tissue. The production of Arg1 by

MDSCs from tumor tissue was significantly downregulated ($P < 0.01$, Fig. 3d). We also used PBMCs from normal donors to induce MDSCs with GM-CSF + IL-1β and detected the expression of RUNXOR in the induced CD33+ MDSCs. We found that the RUNXOR level was increased in the induced MDSCs compared with PBMCs without stimulation ($P < 0.001$, Fig. 3e). Arg1 expression was clearly decreased in induced CD33+ MDSCs after RUNXOR knockdown (P < 0.01, Fig. 3f). To further verify whether RUNXOR could regulate the development of MDSCs from progenitor cells in the bone marrow, we detected the proportion of induced CD33+ cells in PBMCs post transfection with siRUNXOR, and found that the percentage of MDSCs decreased after knockdown of RUNXOR ($P = 0.065$, Fig. 3g). These data show that the expression of RUNXOR is positively correlated with MDSC-induced immunosuppression in lung cancer.

The expression of RUNX1 is negatively correlated with the immunosuppression of MDSCs

RUNX1 is a critical molecule in the development of myeloid cells [26–28]. In our previous study, we confirmed that miR-9 regulates the immunosuppression and maturation of MDSCs by targeting RUNX1. In addition, RUNX1 is reported to be a target gene of RUNXOR, and RUNXOR is involved in the epigenetic regulation of RUNX1. RUNXOR interacts with the promoters and enhancers of RUNX1 gene via its 3′-terminal fragment.

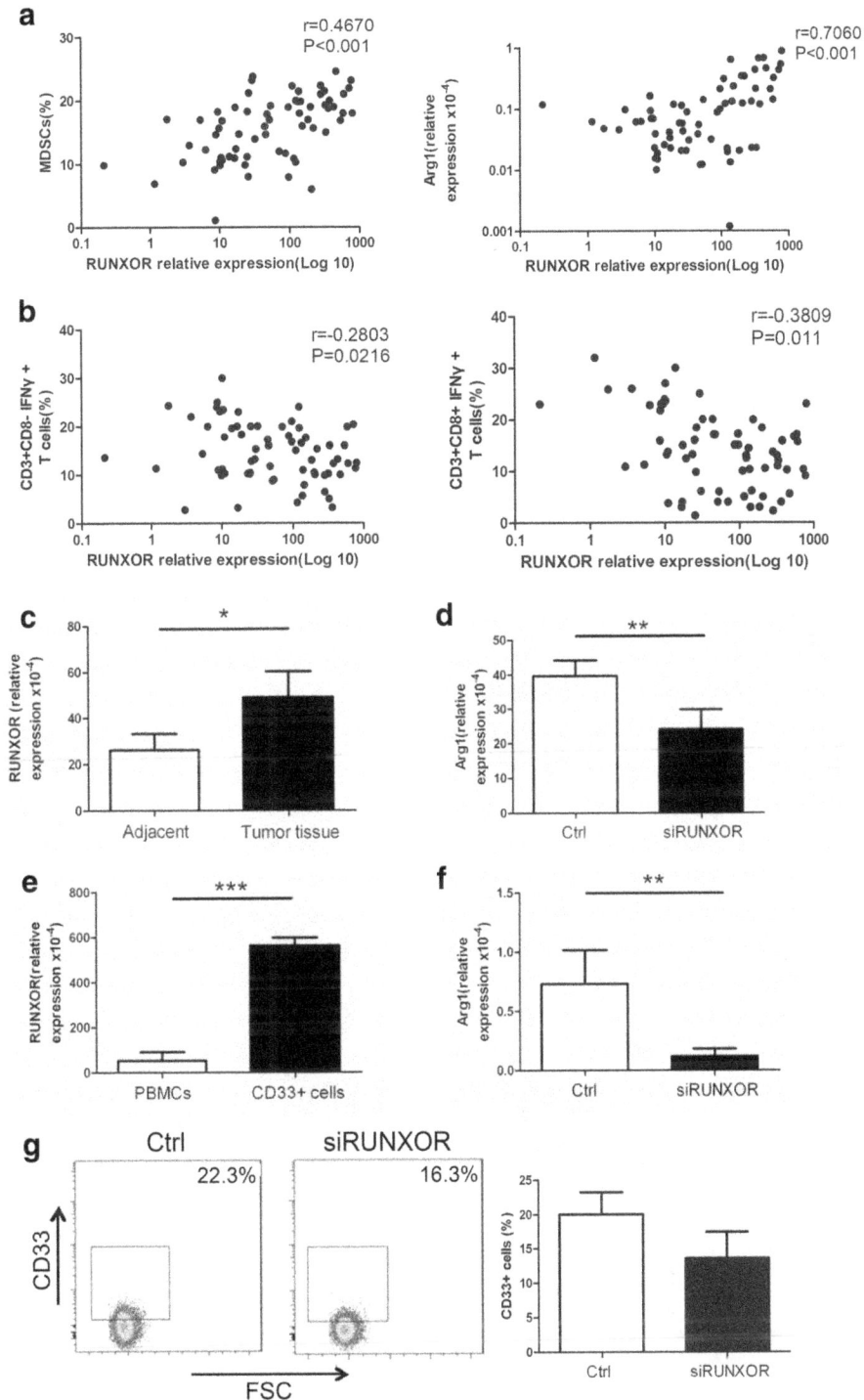

Fig. 3 The expression of RUNXOR is associated with the immunosuppression of MDSCs. **a** The correlation between the expression of the lncRNA RUNXOR and the proportion of MDSCs and the expression of Arg1. **b** The correlation between the expression of lncRNA RUNXOR and the proportion of Th1/CTL cells. **c** The expression of lncRNA RUNXOR in MDSCs from tumor tissues of lung cancer patients. **d** The expression of Arg1 in MDSCs from tumor tissue of lung cancer patients after treatment with siRUNXOR. **e** The expression of lncRNA RUNXOR in CD33+ MDSCs induced from PBMCs of healthy donors. **f** The expression of Arg1 in induced MDSCs after treatment with siRUNXOR. **g** The effect of RUNXOR knockdown on the induction of CD33+ MDSCs. ***$P < 0.001$,**$P < 0.01$, *$P < 0.05$

RUNXOR also participates in the formation of an intra-chromosomal loop and then interacts with the H3-K27 methylase EZH2 and RUNX1 protein, which are known to regulate the gene function of RUNX1 [12, 21]. Here, we detected the expression of RUNX1 in the peripheral blood of lung cancer patients and found that compared with healthy controls, the RUNX1 level was decreased in lung cancer patients ($P < 0.001$, Fig. 4a). And RUNX1 level was the highest in the peripheral blood of patients with lung adenocarcinoma (Fig. 4b). In addition, RUNX1 expression in both the MDSCs from the tumor tissue of lung cancer patients and MDSCs induced with GM-CSF and IL-1β was decreased compared with cells of the same phenotype from adjacent tissue and PBMCs, respectively ($P < 0.05$, Fig. 4c). Meanwhile, we also showed

that RUNX1 expression was negatively correlated with the proportion of MDSCs (Fig. 4d) in the peripheral blood of lung cancer patients. These results demonstrate that RUNX1 is negatively correlated with the immuno-suppression of MDSCs.

RUNXOR knockdown can increase the expression of RUNX1 in MDSCs

To confirm whether RUNXOR regulates the expression of RUNX1 in MDSCs, we firstly analyzed the correlation between RUNXOR and RUNX1 and found that RUN-XOR expression was negatively correlated with RUNX1 expression (Fig. 5a). In addition, the expression of RUNX1 increased after surgery in the peripheral blood of lung cancer patients, while the expression of

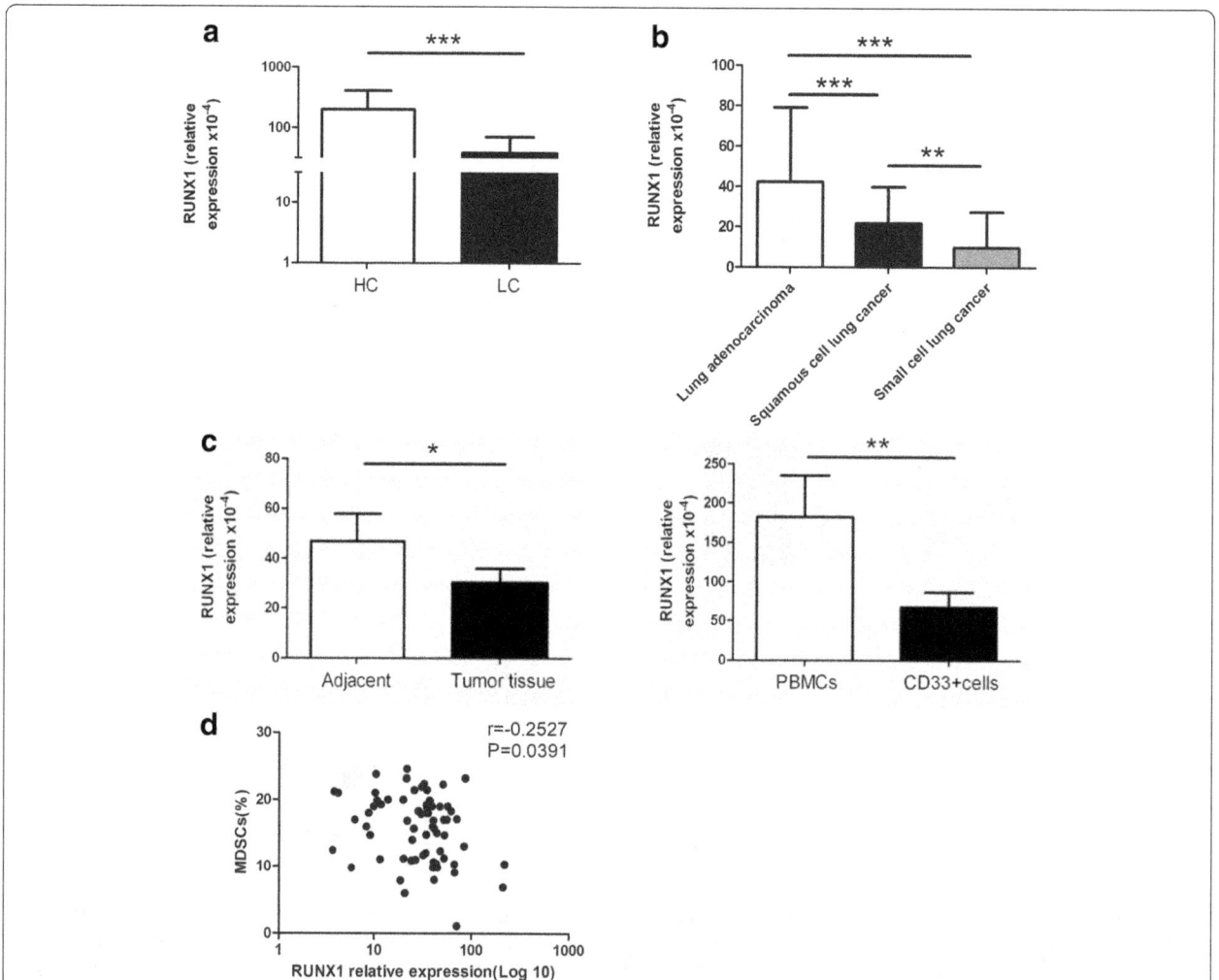

Fig. 4 The expression of RUNX1 is negatively correlated with the immunosuppression of MDSCs. a The expression of RUNX1 in the peripheral blood of lung cancer patients and healthy donors. b The expression of RUNX1 in the peripheral blood of lung cancer patients with different histological categories. c The expression of RUNX1 in MDSCs isolated from the tumor tissues of lung cancer patients or induced from the PBMCs of healthy donors. d The correlation between the expression of the lncRNA RUNXOR and the proportion of MDSCs in the blood of lung cancer patients. (e) The correlation between the expression of the lncRNA RUNXOR and Arg1 in the blood of lung cancer patients. ***$P < 0.001$, **$P < 0.01$, *$P < 0.05$

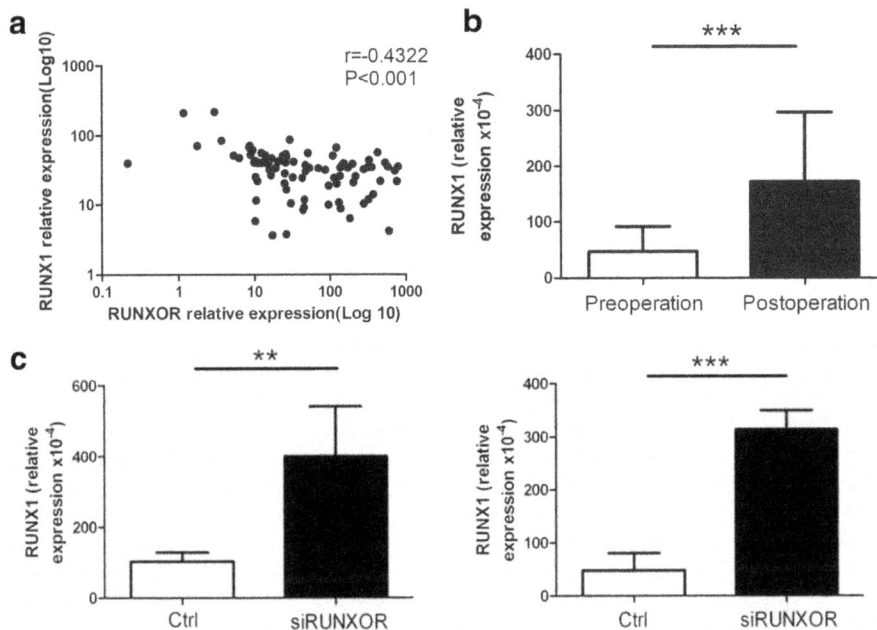

Fig. 5 RUNXOR knockdown can increase the expression of RUNX1 in MDSCs. **a** The correlation between the expression of RUNXOR and RUNX1 in the peripheral blood cells of lung cancer patients. **b** The differential expression of RUNX1 in the blood samples of lung cancer patients pre- and post-operation. **c** The expression of RUNX1 in both MDSCs from the tumor tissue of lung cancer patients and MDSCs induced from PBMCs of healthy donors with RUNXOR knockdown. ***$P < 0.001$, **$P < 0.01$

RUNXOR decreased after surgery in the peripheral blood of lung cancer patients ($P < 0.001$, Fig. 5b). We next used a specific siRNA to interfere with RUNXOR expression and detected the RUNX1 expression in both MDSCs from the tumor tissue of lung cancer patients and MDSCs induced from healthy donor PBMCs with GM-CSF + IL-1β. After knockdown of RUNXOR, the expression of RUNX1 was upregulated in isolated and induced MDSCs (Fig. 5c). Thus, RUNXOR knockdown can increase the expression of RUNX1 in MDSCs.

Discussion

LncRNAs play critical roles in various biological processes and diseases, including tumor progression [29–31]. Previous studies have demonstrated that RUNXOR, which overlaps with RUNX1, is a novel intragenic lncRNA that plays an important role in leukemogenesis [21]. In AML cells, RUNXOR directly binds to promoters and enhancers of the RUNX1 gene and participates in a long distance intrachromosomal interaction between two RUNX1 promoters. RUNXOR is also capable of facilitating the translocation of the RUNX1 gene. In addition, RUNXOR recruits epigenetic regulators, the EZH2 and RUNX1 proteins, to bind the promoter of the RUNX1 gene [21]. In this study, we demonstrated that the lncRNA RUNXOR is associated with the immunosuppression mediated by

MDSCs, which consist of immature myeloid cells, in lung cancer patients.

The expression of lncRNA RUNXOR was detected in peripheral blood samples from lung cancer patients. Compared with healthy controls, RUNXOR expression in the peripheral blood of lung cancer patients was upregulated. In addition, the RUNXOR level was decreased in the blood of lung cancer patients after surgery. Since RUNXOR is found to be expressed in immature myeloid cells, we wondered whether it also exists in the MDSCs of lung cancer patients. We analyzed the correlation between RUNXOR expression and the proportions of MDSCs and Th1/CTL cells in the blood of lung cancer patients. The RUNXOR level was positively correlated with the MDSCs percentage and Arg1 level, while it was negatively correlated with the proportion of Th1/CTL cells, which indicated that RUNXOR expression may be involved in the immunosuppression of MDSCs in lung cancer patients. Thus, to confirm whether RUNXOR was expressed in MDSCs, we not only isolated CD11b + CD33 + HLA-DR-CD14- MDSCs from tumor tissue but also induced CD33+ MDSCs from PBMCs of healthy donors, and then detected the expression of RUNXOR in these MDSCs. We found that the expression of RUNXOR in MDSCs did increase. After RUNXOR knockdown, the expression of Arg1 in MDSCs was downregulated. To elucidate the mechanism by which RUNXOR regulates the immunosuppression of MDSCs, we detected the expression of a potential target gene of RUNXOR, RUNX1, in the blood samples of lung cancer patients and found that the RUNX1 level was downregulated in the peripheral blood of lung cancer patients compared with that of healthy controls. In addition, RUNX1 expression was restored in MDSCs when transfected with siRUNXOR, and RUNX1 was negatively correlated with the proportion of MDSCs from lung cancer patients. These data indicated that RUNXOR may affect the function of MDSCs via modulating RUNX1.

However, the exact regulatory mechanism by which RUNXOR regulates the suppressive function of MDSCs via targeting RUNX1 remains unclear. It has been shown that RUNXOR recruits EZH2 and RUNX1 to regulate the RUNX1 gene epigenetically in AML cells [21]. In addition, we previously demonstrated that miR-9 modulates the function and development of MDSCs by targeting RUNX1 [12]. Thus, we hypothesize that RUNXOR and miR-9 may cooperate to mediate the expression of RUNX1 at both the transcriptional and post-transcriptional level. In addition, we found that RUNXOR knockdown decreased the induction of MDSCs in vitro. These results indicate RUNXOR is associated with the development and immunosuppressive function of MDSCs in lung cancer.

Conclusions
Taken together, our results indicate that RUNXOR is significantly associated with the immunosuppression induced by MDSCs in lung cancer patients and may be a target of anti-tumor immunity therapy.

Abbreviations
AML: Acute myeloid leukemia; Arg1: Arginase 1; CTL: Cytotoxic T lymphocyte; EZH2: Enhancer of zeste homolog 2; GM-CSF: Granulocyte-macrophage colony-stimulating factor; IL-1β: Interleukin-1β; LncRNAs: Long non-coding RNAs; MDSCs: Myeloid-derived suppressor cells; M-MDSCs: Monocytic myeloid-derived suppressor cells; NcRNAs: Non-coding RNAs; PBMCs: Peripheral blood mononuclear cells; PMN-MDSCs: Polymorphonuclear myeloid-derived suppressor cells; RUNX1: Runt-related transcription factor 1; RUNXOR: RUNX1 overlapping RNA; Th1: T helper 1

Funding
This work was supported by the Summit of the Six Top Talents Program of Jiangsu Province (Grant No. 2015-WSN-116), Jiangsu Province's Key Medical Talents Program (Grant No. ZDRCB2016018), Specialized Project for Clinical Medicine of Jiangsu Province (Grant No. BL2014065), Natural Science Foundation of Jiangsu (Grant No. BK20150533), Project funded by the China Postdoctoral Science Foundation (Grant No. 2016 M600382), and Jiangsu Postdoctoral Science Foundation funded project (Grant No.1601082B). The funding body had no role in the design of the study and collection, analysis, and interpretation of data or preparation of the manuscript.

Authors' contributions
XT performed the experiments, analyzed the data, and wrote the paper; MJ, TW, JT, RP, HX and LM analyzed the data; YuZ, YW and YueZ performed the experiments; and SW designed the study and wrote the paper. All authors read and approved the final manuscript.

Competing interests
The authors declare that they have no competing interests.

Author details
[1]Department of Laboratory Medicine, The Affiliated People's Hospital, Jiangsu University, Zhenjiang 212012, China. [2]Institute of Laboratory Medicine, Jiangsu Key Laboratory of Laboratory Medicine, School of Medicine, Jiangsu University, Zhenjiang, China. [3]Department of Laboratory Medicine, Jiangsu Cancer Hospital, Nanjing, China.

References
1. Byron E, Pinder-Schenck M. Systemic and targeted therapies for early-stage lung cancer. Cancer control : journal of the Moffitt Cancer Center. 2014;21: 21–31.
2. Kumar R, Collins D, Dolly S, McDonald F, O'Brien MER, Yap TA. Targeting the PD-1/PD-L1 axis in non-small cell lung cancer. Curr Probl Cancer. 2017;41: 111–24.
3. Rafei H, El-Bahesh E, Finianos A, Nassereddine S, Tabbara I. Immune-based therapies for non-small cell lung cancer. Anticancer Res. 2017;37:377–87.
4. Ma J, Xu H, Wang S. Immunosuppressive role of myeloid-derived suppressor cells and therapeutic targeting in lung cancer. J Immunol Res. 2018;2018 6319649
5. Shi G, Wang H, Zhuang X. Myeloid-derived suppressor cells enhance the expression of melanoma-associated antigen A4 in a Lewis lung cancer murine model. Oncol Lett. 2016;11(1):809–16.
6. Atretkhany KN, Drutskaya MS. Myeloid-derived suppressor cells and Proinflammatory cytokines as targets for Cancer therapy. Biochemistry Biokhimiia. 2016;81:1274–83.
7. Kumar V, Patel S, Tcyganov E, Gabrilovich DI. The nature of myeloid-derived suppressor cells in the tumor microenvironment. Trends Immunol. 2016;37: 208–20.
8. Lin Y, Yang X, Liu W, Li B, Yin W, Shi Y, et al. Chemerin has a protective role in hepatocellular carcinoma by inhibiting the expression of IL-6 and GM-CSF and MDSC accumulation. Oncogene. 2017;36:3599–608.
9. Youn JI, Collazo M, Shalova IN, Biswas SK, Gabrilovich DI. Characterization of the nature of granulocytic myeloid-derived suppressor cells in tumor-bearing mice. J Leukoc Biol. 2012;91:167–81.
10. Gabrilovich DI, Nagaraj S. Myeloid-derived suppressor cells as regulators of the immune system. Nat Rev Immunol. 2009;9:162–74.
11. Tian X, Tian J, Tang X, Rui K, Zhang Y, Ma J, et al. Particulate beta-glucan regulates the immunosuppression of granulocytic myeloid-derived suppressor cells by inhibiting NFIA expression. Oncoimmunology. 2015;4: e1038687.
12. Tian J, Rui K, Tang X, Ma J, Wang Y, Tian X, et al. MicroRNA-9 regulates the differentiation and function of myeloid-derived suppressor cells via targeting Runx1. J Immunol. 2015;195:1301–11.
13. Umansky V, Blattner C, Gebhardt C, Utikal J. The role of myeloid-derived suppressor cells (MDSC) in cancer progression. Vaccine. 2016; https://doi.org/10.3390/vaccines4040036.
14. Zeng C, Guo X, Long J, Kuchenbaecker KB, Droit A, Michailidou K. Identification of independent association signals and putative functional variants for breast cancer risk through fine-scale mapping of the 12p11 locus. Breast cancer research : BCR. 2016;18:64.
15. Heward JA, Lindsay MA. Long non-coding RNAs in the regulation of the immune response. Trends Immunol. 2014;35:408–19.
16. Tian X, Tian J, Tang X, Ma J, Wang S. Long non-coding RNAs in the regulation of myeloid cells. J Hematol Oncol. 2016;9:99.
17. Wu T, Yin X, Zhou Y, Wang Z, Shen S, Qiu Y, et al. Roles of noncoding RNAs in metastasis of nonsmall cell lung cancer: a mini review. J Cancer Res Ther. 2015;11(Suppl 1):C7–10.
18. Wan L, Sun M, Liu GJ, Wei CC, Zhang EB, Kong R, et al. Long noncoding RNA PVT1 promotes non-small cell lung cancer cell proliferation through epigenetically regulating LATS2 expression. Mol Cancer Ther. 2016;15:1082–94.
19. Peng H, Liu Y, Tian J, Ma J, Tang X, Rui K, et al. The long noncoding RNA IFNG-AS1 promotes T helper type 1 cells response in patients with Hashimoto's thyroiditis. Sci Rep. 2015;5:17702.
20. Reddy MA, Chen Z, Park JT, Wang M, Lanting L, Zhang Q, et al. Regulation of inflammatory phenotype in macrophages by a diabetes-induced long noncoding RNA. Diabetes. 2014;63:4249–61.

21. Wang H, Li W, Guo R, Sun J, Cui J, Wang G, et al. An intragenic long noncoding RNA interacts epigenetically with the RUNX1 promoter and enhancer chromatin DNA in hematopoietic malignancies. Int J Cancer. 2014; 135:2783–94.
22. Pan T, Liu Y, Zhong LM, et al. Myeloid-derived suppressor cells are essential for maintaining feto-maternal immunotolerance via STAT3 signaling in mice. J Leukoc Biol. 2016;100:499–511.
23. Muthuswamy R, Corman JM, Dahl K, Chatta GS, Kalinski P. Functional reprogramming of human prostate cancer to promote local attraction of effector CD8(+) T cells. Prostate. 2016;76:1095–105.
24. Movahedi K, Guilliams M, Van den Bossche J, Van den Bergh R, Gysemans C, Beschin A, et al. Identification of discrete tumor-induced myeloid-derived suppressor cell subpopulations with distinct T cell-suppressive activity. Blood. 2008;111:4233–44.
25. Rodriguez PC, Ochoa AC. Arginine regulation by myeloid derived suppressor cells and tolerance in cancer: mechanisms and therapeutic perspectives. Immunol Rev. 2008;222:180–91.
26. Sood R, Kamikubo Y, Liu P. Role of RUNX1 in hematological malignancies. Blood. 2017;129:2070–82.
27. Mandoli A, Singh AA, Prange KH, Tijchon E, Oerlemans M, Dirks R, et al. The hematopoietic transcription factors RUNX1 and ERG prevent AML1-ETO oncogene overexpression and onset of the apoptosis program in t(8;21) AMLs. Cell Rep. 2016;17:2087–100.
28. Paglia DN, Yang X, Kalinowski J, Jastrzebski S, Drissi H, Lorenzo J. Runx1 regulates myeloid precursor differentiation into osteoclasts without affecting differentiation into antigen presenting or phagocytic cells in both males and females. Endocrinology. 2016;157:3058–69.
29. Wang J, Peng H, Tian J, Ma J, Tang X, Rui K, et al. Upregulation of long noncoding RNA TMEVPG1 enhances T helper type 1 cell response in patients with Sjögren syndrome. Immunol Res. 2016;64:489–696.
30. Wang Y, Yang T, Zhang Z, Lu M, Zhao W, Zeng X, et al. Long non-coding RNA TUG1 promotes migration and invasion by acting as a ceRNA of miR-335-5p in osteosarcoma cells. Cancer Sci. 2017;108:859–67.
31. Tian X, Ma J, Wang T, Tian J, Zhang Y, Mao L, Xu H, Wang S. LncRNA HOTAIRM1-HOXA1 axis down-regulates the immunosuppressive activity of myeloid-derived suppressor cells in lung cancer. Front Immunol. 2018;9:473.

21

The effect of low insurance reimbursement on quality of care for non-small cell lung cancer in China: a comprehensive study covering diagnosis, treatment, and outcomes

Xi Li[1], Qi Zhou[1], Xinyu Wang[1], Shaofei Su[1], Meiqi Zhang[1], Hao Jiang[1], Jiaying Wang[1] and Meina Liu[1,2]*

Abstract

Background: The insurance reimbursement rate of medical cost affects the quality and quantity of health services provided in China. The nature of this relationship, however, has not been reliably described in the field of non-small cell lung cancer (NSCLC). The objective of the current study was to examine the impact of low reimbursement rates of medical costs on diagnosis, treatment and outcomes among patients with NSCLC.

Methods: We examined care of 2643 NSCLC patients and we divided the study cohort into a high reimbursement rate group and a low reimbursement rate group. The impact of reimbursement rates of medical costs on quality of care of NSCLC patients were examined using logistic regression and generalized linear models.

Results: Compared with patients insured with high reimbursement rate, patients insured through lower reimbursement rate programs were less likely to benefit from early detection and treatment services. Delayed detection was more common in low reimbursement group and they were less likely to be recommended for adjuvant chemotherapy, or to receive adjuvant chemotherapy and postoperative radiation therapy and they had lower odds to receipt chemotherapy response assessment. However, low reimbursement rate group had lower rate of in-hospital mortality and metastases.

Conclusions: Low reimbursement rate mainly negatively influenced the diagnosis and treatment of NSCLC. Reducing the gap in reimbursement rate between the three health insurance schemes should be a focus of equalizing access to care and improving the level of medical compliance and finally improving quality of care of NSCLC.

Keywords: Insurance reimbursement rate, Non-small cell lung cancer, Quality indicators, Diagnosis, treatment, and outcomes

Background

Insurance is a significant determinant of access to health care and, consequently, of high quality of care. The level of insurance reimbursement of medical costs plays a vital role in determining the quality and quantity of health services provided [1–6]. Health insurance, a mutual help and risk-pooling health protection system, generally does not cover health care costs in full. The primary payer status varies, with different insurance types having markedly different deductibles, copays, and reimbursement caps. Insurance and the alleviation of cost-related barriers to health care have achieved tremendous progress in the prevention, early detection, and high-quality treatment of cancer. However, this has not been experienced equally by all segments of the insured population, and individuals insured with lower reimbursement rates may be disadvantaged.

Many developing countries have begun to establish and implement universal health coverage. China essentially

* Correspondence: liumeina369@163.com
[1]Department of Biostatistics, School of Public Health, Harbin Medical University, Harbin, China
[2]School of Public Health, Harbin Medical University, No.157 Baojian Road, Harbin 150081, China

achieved this goal by the end of 2011. China's health insurance system is a combination of compulsory and voluntary insurance types. It primarily consists of three basic social health insurance programs, which are uniformly government-supported and cover more than 95.7% of the Chinese population [7]. The programs have their own defined target populations, premiums, benefit programs, and implementation guidelines [8]. New Rural Cooperative Medical Scheme (NCMS) is designed for the rural population. Its enrollment covers 62% of the Chinese population. Urban Resident Basic Medical Insurance (URBMI) targets the unemployed, children, the disabled, and elderly people in urban areas, and Urban Employed Basic Medical Insurance (UEBMI) is for urban employees. UEBMI covers 19% of the population, and URBMI covers 16% [9]. Insurance mainly pays for in-hospital care. The reimbursement rate for NCMS is 50–65%—much lower than UEBMI's rate of 85–95% but similar to URBMI's rate of 50% [6].

Much attention has been paid to the effect of insurance status on quality of care [10–15], but few studies have focused on the effect of a critical attribute of insurance—reimbursement rate [5, 6]. Past work has analyzed the relationship between insurance status and quality of care for non-small cell lung cancer (NSCLC) [16–18], mostly focusing on limited aspects such as clinical treatment or subsequent progress. For example, Potosky and colleagues examined the impact of insurance status on the initial treatment of NSCLC [19], and Bradley et al. analyzed cancer diagnosis and survival disparities by insurance types [20]. Few studies have investigated the whole process from NSCLC diagnosis, to treatment, to prognosis using process-of-care and outcome indicators, and no studies have evaluated the effect of reimbursement rate on quality of care for NSCLC. Thus, this study aimed to explore the influences of a lower-rate reimbursement program for patients with NSCLC throughout the process, including preoperative diagnosis, treatment, and postoperative outcomes.

Methods
Study cohort
This study was part of research fields of our research group to evaluate the quality of care for breast, colorectal, and lung cancers. After receiving the approval of the medical institutional records directors at each site, we obtained the medical records of all patients meeting the inclusion criteria. Patients who received initial examinations and treatment at other facilities before receiving inpatient treatment at the selected hospitals remained eligible for the study. From the available pool of eligible patients primarily diagnosed with NSCLC, we excluded 57 patients who were unwilling or unable to consent and identified a study cohort of 3075 individuals aged 18–70 with a primary diagnosis of NSCLC made from 6

December 2010 to 17 December 2014 who underwent inpatient treatment for stage I–IV cancer in the selected hospitals. Follow-up was conducted with those patients diagnosed before 2012 through facility visits and telephone calls. This follow-up began two to 4 weeks after the patients left the hospital and was repeated every 3 months for 2 years. Patients outside the age range, those who received only outpatient care, and those who also had other malignant tumors or mixed small-cell lung cancer were excluded from the study. Because this study aimed to analyze the influence of low reimbursement rates on quality of care for NSCLC, patients with obscure primary payer status and those who self-discharged were not included in the study. The final analytical sample comprised 2643 insured patients who received inpatient treatment for stage I–IV NSCLC. Fig. 1 presents the number of study flow diagram of the patient population.

Data collection
A questionnaire for NSCLC cases was drafted by a team of oncology professionals, clinical physicians, and epidemiologists. The questionnaire (see Additional file 2) gathered routinely collected medical information on several domains: patient demographics, tumor characteristics, diagnosis, NSCLC treatment and prognosis, and information necessary for identifying eligible patients for evidence-based care. Data on primary payer status were collected as part of the patient demographics. Before the data collection, data abstractors received 3 weeks of training organized by oncology professors and the principal investigators. Information extraction was performed systematically, following the operations manual. To guarantee the validity and reliability of the questionnaire, we conducted a pilot test. During the data collection process, regular correspondence was maintained with those compiling the data to identify any ambiguities or deficiencies in the information collection to facilitate timely modification and accelerate the process of data extraction. Following the data collection, 5% of the records were randomly selected for a secondary data collection using methods identical to the first data collection, and the test-retest reliability was high (up to 95%).

Patient demographics
Baseline demographic information abstracted from the medical history records included age group (< 50, 50–60, ≥ 60), gender, primary payer status (NCMS, URBMI, or UEBMI), household income, smoking, comorbidities, and postoperative clinical report information. According to the disparities of reimbursement rate among insurance type, we divided the study cohort into two payer groups, including a high reimbursement rate group (UEBMI) and a low reimbursement rate group (URBMI and NCMS). Per capita annual income was derived from the bulletin of social development published by the statistical bureau.

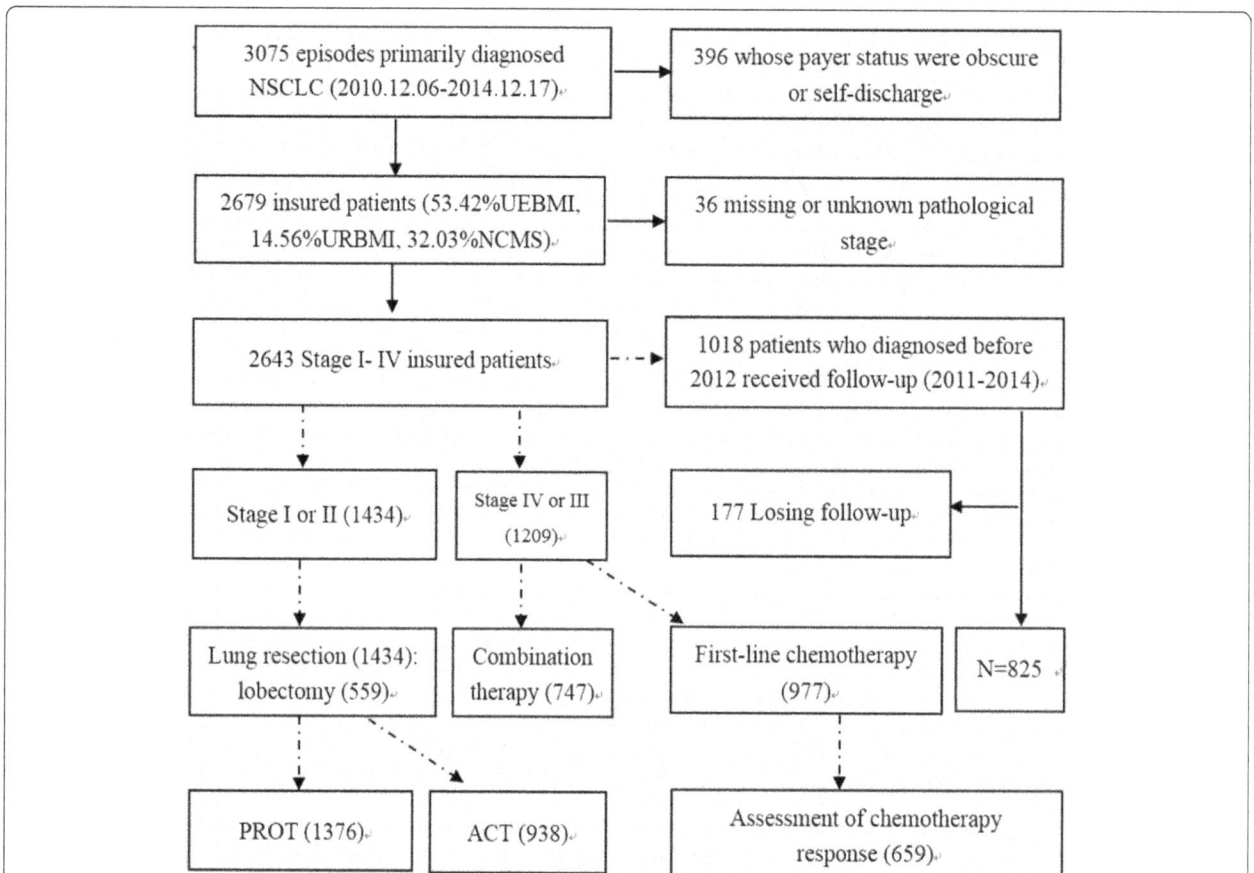

Fig. 1 "Solid line" means study flow diagram of the patient population. "Dotted line" means flowchart for treatments and follow-up group. The number in parentheses represents the sum of patients eligible for the evidence-based care, due to the limited space, we only showed the stage related care and its eligible population size. Abbreviations: NSCLC: non-small cell lung cancer, NCMS: New Rural Cooperative Medical Scheme, URBMI: Urban Resident Basic Medical Insurance, UEBMI: Urban Employed Basic Medical Insurance, ACT: Adjuvant chemotherapy, PORT: postoperative radiation therapy

The national average annual income from 2011 to 2014 was used to divide the patients into two groups (low-income and high-income). We also calculated an Charlson comorbidity index (CCI: 0, 1 to 3, ≥ 4), a weighted index of 16 conditions found to significantly influence prognosis among cancer patients, with scores assessed based on relative mortality risk. Patients were considered to have a comorbid condition if a listed disorder was mentioned in their medical or treatment-related records. Institutional Research Board of Harbin Medical University approved the study and written informed consent was obtained from all individual participants included in the study.

Tumor characteristics

Lung cancer-specific information assessed for each patient included primary lesion site, tumor size, histological grade, histological classification (adenocarcinoma, squamous cell carcinoma, other), tumor stage (I–IV), distant metastases, and bronchial stump. Variables with more than 5% missing data ware regarded as "unknown." Otherwise, missing data were taken as real missing data. However, there were some

deficiencies in the medical records, mainly in tumor stage, which included incorrect or incomplete information. Given the significance of stage information for identifying eligible patients for a certain clinical treatment, we filled in the missing information and corrected errors by consulting oncologists and pathologists and through the joint effort of our team based on the condition of the primary tumor, lymphatic metastasis, and distant metastasis of the patients and using the international Tumor-Node-Metastasis (TNM) classification system [21].

Dependent variables

The research team selected 11 priority process-of care measures based on the evidence-based guidelines of recommended care, established associations between care and outcomes, relatively independent of each indicator, and data integrity. This selection included the diagnostic and treatment process and was developed by our research group through consulting many references and conducting a three-round modified Delphi panel process. The selected measures were skeletal scintigraphy and brain Magnetic

Resonance Imaging (MRI) or Computed Tomography (CT), pulmonary function test (PFT), epidermal growth factor receptor gene mutation test, adjuvant chemotherapy (ACT), recommendation for ACT, postoperative radiation therapy (PORT), radiographic assessment of chemotherapy response, first-line chemotherapy, lobectomy, surgical resection, and combination therapy. Each process-of-care indicator was defined by its inclusion or exclusion criteria according to the standard eligibility definition (see Additional file 1). Considering suspected universal adherence, postoperative pathological report and electrocardiogram were removed. In addition, because of data incompleteness (close to 50% missing) or insufficient eligible patients, performance status assessment and neoadjuvant chemotherapy were excluded from our research. Figure 1 presents the flowchart for the main treatments.

Five quality-of-care measures were also selected as outcomes of interest in this study: postoperative complications, metastases, in-hospital mortality, 2-year fatality rate, and length of hospital stay.

Primary payer status

Primary payer status was routinely recorded in patient discharge records. In cases where payer status information was missing here, the medical records home page could alternatively be reviewed to find the information. In the few cases where payer status was missing from both locations, it was treated as "unknown." Self-discharge patients were excluded because of ambiguity regarding payer status; in these patients' records, uninsured patients, commercially insured patients, and even those with multiple insurance coverage were merged. In addition, other patients with indeterminate payer status information were also excluded from the study.

Statistical analysis

Descriptive statistics were used to compare baseline characteristics and the utilization of the 16 process-of-care and outcome-of-care indicators by primary payer status. We calculated the number of eligible cases for each individual measure in each payer group. Utilization of each indicator was calculated using the sum of patients receiving care as the numerator and the sum of patients eligible for that type of care as the denominator. Composite performance scores were calculated using opportunity-based scores, defined as the sum of eligible patients who actually received care divided by total care opportunities [22]. Simple bivariate comparisons were conducted with Chi-squared or Kruskal–Wallis H tests, depending on the variable type.

Separate regression models were used for each measure. Individual and tumor characteristics, as well as hospital category, were selected as covariates that potentially influence primary care experiences and the incidence of particular outcomes. Multivariate logistic regression models

were used to examine the independent effects of insurance type on treatment and outcome by controlling for these confounding effects. Because the variables were not normally distributed, the association between length of stay and insurance type was analyzed using generalized linear models with a gamma distribution and log link function. The odd ratios (ORs) and their 95% confidence intervals were estimated. Concordance indexes were calculated to determine model diagnostics, providing an estimate of the predictive accuracy of the models. A value of 0.5 demonstrates that outcomes are completely random, whereas a value of 1 demonstrates the perfect predictive accuracy of the model. All data were analyzed anonymously. All analyses were performed using SAS version 9.3.1 (SAS Institute, Cary, NC) and used two-tailed tests of statistical significance, with the significance level set at $P < 0.05$.

Result

Baseline demographic information and tumor characteristics

Of the sample of 2643 patients, 1419 (53.69%) were covered by insurance with high reimbursement rate and 1224 (46.31%) were covered by insurance with low reimbursement rate. Over half of the patients were diagnosed with stage I or II NSCLC, and 56% received treatment at specialized tumor hospitals. Non-squamous cell histology was observed in 63.83% (1687 in 2643) of the patients, and the majority of these cases were adenocarcinoma (1344 in 1687). With respect to socioeconomic status, less than one-fifth of the patients earned over the national average annual income.

There were variations in the baseline demographic data and tumor characteristics of NSCLC patients who were insured with low reimbursement rate versus insured with high reimbursement rate. Of the 12 variables examined, statistically significant variations were observed in 10. In comparison with high reimbursement group, patients insured through low reimbursement rate programs had a similar primary lesion site, similar proportion of smokers and incidence rate of positive bronchial stump. Low reimbursement rate group were less likely to have family history of NSCLC (4.41% vs. 6.69%), to complicate other diseases (CCI = 0, 23.12% vs. 14.59%), but they were younger to suffer from NSCLC (age < 50, 24.67% vs. 15.86%), more likely to be diagnosed in a later stage (stage III- IV, 47.63% vs. 43.11%), to be diagnosed with low differentiated carcinoma (32.43% vs. 26.15%), and to have lower socioeconomic status (high income, 4.00% vs. 29.32%). Details of patients' demographic data and tumor characteristics by primary payer status are listed in Table 1.

Disparities in utilization of NSCLC treatment process and outcomes by primary payer status

Composite performance scores for the NSCLC process of treatment and outcome didn't vary significantly by

Table 1 Baseline demographic and tumor characteristics by primary payer status[a]

Characteristics	Overall n (%)	High reimbursement rate, n (%)	Low reimbursement rate, n (%)	P
CCI				
0	490(18.54)	207(14.59)	283(23.12)	<.0001
1~3	2085(78.89)	1174(82.73)	911(74.43)	
4~	68(2.57)	38(2.68)	30(2.45)	
Gender				
male	1677(63.45)	939(66.17)	738(60.29)	0.0018
female	966(36.55)	480(33.83)	486(39.71)	
Age				
< 40	82(3.10)	33(2.33)	49(4.00)	<.0001
40~	445(16.84)	192(13.53)	253(20.67)	
50~	1083(40.98)	600(42.28)	483(39.46)	
60~	1033(39.08)	594(41.86)	439(35.87)	
Smoking				
no	1174(44.42)	631(44.47)	543(44.36)	0.9567
yes	1469(55.58)	788(55.53)	681(55.64)	
Family history of NSCLC				
none	2494(94.36)	1324(93.31)	1170(95.59)	0.0112
have	149(5.64)	95(6.69)	54(4.41)	
primary lesion site				
left	1051(39.77)	560(39.46)	491(40.11)	0.9437
right	1416(53.58)	764(53.84)	652(53.27)	
other	176(6.66)	95(6.69)	81(6.62)	
Historical stage				
High differential	302(11.27)	189(13.32)	112(9.15)	<.0001
Moderately differential	710(26.50)	412(29.03)	294(24.02)	
Low differential	779(29.08)	371(26.15)	397(32.43)	
unknown	868(32.84)	447(31.50)	421(34.40)	
Histological classification				
Squamous carcinoma	956(36.17)	483(34.04)	437(38.64)	0.0063
adenocarcinoma	1334(50.47)	759(53.35)	577(47.14)	
other	353(13.36)	179(12.61)	174(14.22)	
Procedure class				
lobectomy	1576(59.63)	876(61.73)	210(55.56)	0.0049
wedge resection	67(2.53)	45(3.17)	6(1.59)	
pneumonectomy	229(8.66)	104(7.33)	34(8.99)	
exploratory thoracotomy	771(29.17)	394(27.77)	128(33.86)	
Bronchial stump				
negative	1696(64.17)	923(65.05)	773(63.15)	0.5386
positive	43(1.63)	24(1.69)	19(1.55)	
unknown	904(34.20)	472(33.26)	432(35.29)	
Clinical stages				
IA	559(21.15)	333(23.47)	226(18.46)	0.0065
IB	426(16.12)	213(15.01)	213(17.40)	

Table 1 Baseline demographic and tumor characteristics by primary payer status[a] *(Continued)*

Characteristics	Overall n (%)	High reimbursement rate, n (%)	Low reimbursement rate, n (%)	P
IIA	325(12.30)	183(12.90)	142(11.60)	
IIB	124(4.69)	64(4.51)	60(4.90)	
IIIA	607(22.97)	301(21.21)	309(25.00)	
IIIB	147(5.56)	71(5.00)	76(6.21)	
IV	455(17.22)	254(17.90)	201(16.42)	
Hospital type				
Specialized	1480(56.00)	741(52.22)	739(60.38)	<.0001
General	1163(44.00)	678(47.78)	485(39.62)	
Average per capital income				
High income	465(17.59)	416(29.32)	49(4.00)	<.0001
Low income	2178(82.41)	1003(70.68)	1175(96.00)	

[a]Data are expressed as numbers and percentages of patients. Percentages may not sum up to 100% due to round-off.Abbreviations: *CCI* the Charlson comorbidity index, *NSCLC* non-small cell lung cancer

primary payer status (Table 2). The unadjusted adherence or incidence of each indicator by primary payer status is shown in Table 3. Compared with patients insured with high reimbursement rate, underutilization of process-of-care indicators was found among patients insured with low reimbursement rate, who had comparatively lower probability for being recommended for ACT (37.96% vs. 48.26%, P = 0.0187) or receiving ACT (44.69% vs. 52.24%, P = 0.0484), PORT (0.49% vs. 2.88%, P = 0.0010) or radiographic assessment of chemotherapy response (47.02% vs. 59.41%, P = 0.0014). A high level of PFTs were given to patients insured with low reimbursement rate, with a receipt rate approaching 87.85%. Regarding disparities in outcomes, in-hospital mortality (1.47% vs. 3.66%, P = 0.0005) and metastases rates (8.09% vs. 10.75%, P = 0.0488) were lower in patients insured with low reimbursement rate. Of all surgical patients, 5.53% developed complications and 9.65% of patients had metastases; there were no statistically significant difference in 2-year mortality by payer status (P = 0.2862). The mean total length of hospital stay was 21.11 days (standard deviation [SD] = 16.76) and was similar across payer statuses (P = 0.0672) but the length of preoperative hospital stay varied (P < 0.0001).

Figure 2 present the results for adjusted adherence to quality indicators and incidence of adverse outcomes by payer status. The majority of types of recommended care were underused among patients insured through the lower reimbursement rate program. After adjusting for patients' demographic and tumor characteristics, low reimbursement rate group were less likely to have skeletal scintigraphy and brain MRI or CT (OR = 0.701, 95%CI 0.510–0.962), or to receive ACT (OR = 0.627, 95%CI 0.450–0.873), PORT (OR = 0.129, 95%CI 0.036–0.469) and radiographic assessment of chemotherapy response (OR = 0.627, 95%CI 0.441–0.893) than high reimbursement rate group. As for the outcome, low reimbursement rate group were less likely to die in the hospital (OR = 0.458, 95%CI 0.250–0.837) or have postoperative metastases (OR = 0.635, 95%CI 0.450–0.897) than high reimbursement group, but there was no significant difference of 2-year mortality risk between groups. The comparison of the total and preoperative length of hospital stay by primary payer status is displayed in Table 4. No marked differences were found in the preoperative length of hospital stay by payer status, but the length of total stay did differ significantly after adjusting for confounding variables.

Discussion

The impact of primary payer status on quality of care for NSCLC was comprehensively assessed from diagnosis, to treatment, to outcome, using 11 process-of-care indicators and five outcome indicators. Using public health data, we established an association between primary payer status and quality of care that is of

Table 2 Adherence to composite indicator by payer status[a]

composite indicator	High reimbursement rate		Low reimbursement rate		P
	M	N (%)	M	N (%)	
Process	5463	3226 (59.05)	4611	2714(58.86)	0.8448
Outcome	3881	293(7.55)	3419	243(9.36)	0.4697

[a]"M" means the sum of total patients who were eligible and have none of the contraindications for each indicator, "N" means eligible patients who were actually received the treatment, the percentile in parentheses represents composite score of process-of-care indicators and outcome indicator according to payer status

Table 3 Unadjusted adherence to quality-of-care indicators by payer status (%)[a]

Indicators (No. eligible)	Overall	High reimbursement rate	Low reimbursement rate	P
ECT and brain MRI or CT (752)	57.58	60.92	54.33	0.0677
PFTs (1909)	81.72	76.65	87.85	<.0001
EGFR mutation test (453)	3.31	4.76	1.49	0.0533
ACT (938)	48.84	52.24	44.69	0.0484
Recommended for ACT (533)	44.09	48.26	37.96	0.0187
PORT (1376)	1.82	2.88	0.49	0.0010
ACT response assessment (659)	53.41	59.41	47.02	0.0014
First-line chemotherapy (977)	69.54	68.60	70.56	0.5087
Lobectomy (559)	84.97	83.18	87.61	0.1505
Surgical resection (1434)	96.16	96.85	95.32	0.1342
Combination therapy (747)	61.58	60.87	62.27	0.6942
Complications (1916)	5.53	5.42	5.66	0.8181
Metastases (1916)	9.65	10.75	8.09	0.0488
In-hospital mortality (2643)	2.65	3.66	1.47	0.0005
2-year mortality rate (825)	21.45	19.72	22.80	0.2862
total length of hospital stay (2643)	21.11 ± 16.76	21.30 ± 16.56	20.89 ± 17.00	0.0672
preoperative length of hospital stay (1916)	7.56 ± 6.55	7.84 ± 6.27	7.22 ± 6.86	<.0001

[a]Discrete variables were expressed as counts (%) and continuous variables were expressed as a mean ± range. *Abbreviations: ECT and brain MRI or CT* skeletal scintigraphy and brain magnetic resonance imaging or computed tomography, *PFTS* pulmonary function tests, *EGFR* epidermal growth factor receptor, *ACT* adjuvant chemotherapy, *PORT* postoperative radiation therapy

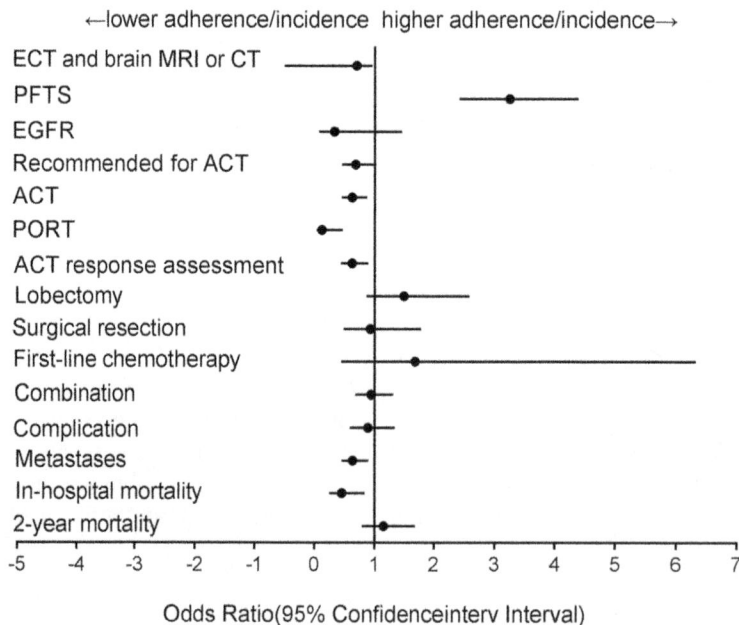

Fig. 2 Adjusted adherence to quality indicators and incidence of adverse outcome in lower reimbursement rate group compare with higher reimbursement rate group (OR, 95%CI). All indicators uniformly adjusted for ACCI, gender, smoking, family history of NSCLC, average per capital income, historical stage, histological classification, pathological stage, hospital type. Outcome indicators additionally adjusted procedure class. Abbreviations: ECT and brain MRI or CT: skeletal scintigraphy and brain Magnetic Resonance Imaging or Computed Tomography, PFTS: pulmonary function tests, EGFR: epidermal growth factor receptor, ACT: Adjuvant chemotherapy, PORT: postoperative radiation therapy

Table 4 Preoperative and total length of hospital stay for NSCLC patients hospitalized for surgical care by payer status[a]

Variables	Coefficient	SE	$wald\chi^2$	P
total length of hospital stay				
High vs Low	−0.1173	0.0335	12.26	0.0005
preoperative length of hospital stay				
High vs Low	−0.0351	0.0584	0.36	0.5475

[a]Adjusted for CCI, age, gender, family history of NSCLC, average per capital income, historical stage, histological classification, pathological stage, hospital type, procedure class. *Abbreviations*: *CCI* the Charlson comorbidity index, *NSCLC* non-small cell lung cancer

importance for both clinical and public health practice. The mean concordance indexes of the models was 0.76, indicating high discriminatory accuracy and the ability to make an accurate prediction. Although the results presented here were based on the insured population aged 18–70 with a primary diagnosis of NSCLC, the relevant population varied by model depending on the eligible population and the missing data or unobtainable values for each indicator. To obtain practical and targeted results, the pool of covariates for diagnosis, treatment, and outcome indicators were not identical across models. The covariates were selected based on clinical evidence-based correlations with each treatment.

After adjusting for patients' demographic and tumor characteristics, clear disparities in NSCLC diagnosis and treatment were found by payer status. Patients insured through lower reimbursement rate programs were less likely to benefit from early detection and treatment services. These findings are in line with prior studies identifying negative effects of low reimbursement rates on diseases detection and treatment [5, 23, 24].

Non-adherence was associated with higher health care expenses [25]. As it is reported that medical expenses could account for non-compliance in 10% of patients [26]. The prepayment structure of health insurance schemes have intended to shift funds from the rich to the poor. But according to our results, patients insured with low reimbursement rate earned less actually paid more. Generally, an underutilization of clinically recommended care was found for patients insured with a low reimbursement rate, who were partly made up of rural-to-urban migrants or those referred from township or county-level hospitals. Lower reimbursement rates of medical costs signified higher out-of-pocket payments for patients, especially for the catastrophic expenditures required in cancer care [27]. This could undermine patients' willingness to seek care. Reimbursement rates for patients covered by different insurance types varied by hospital type. NCMS funding generally requires patients to visit designated hospitals in their county. Although these patients qualify for the reimbursement of medical charges outside of their home counties, the rates are reduced dramatically [6, 28].This may

directly cause a low adherence to treatment regimens and finally leads to interrupted or suspended treatment among this payer status group [29]. However, those covered by insurance with high reimbursement rate had almost equivalent reimbursement rates in all medical institutions, thus they could seek medical care at higher level medical institutions, which helps to ensure a relatively high quality of medical care.

Low incomes and inadequate reimbursement rates led to curtailed access. Many factors other than reimbursement rate are also likely to limit access to care. ACT was generally received by patients on day 30 after curative resection and then repeated at three-week intervals. Likewise, there are intervals in PORT. Under these circumstances, a long distance to the hospital, increased travel burdens, patient or family preferences, a lack of understanding of the importance of appropriate adjuvant therapy, and the unmeasured confounding of performance status may be barriers to adherence to treatment for patients insured with low reimbursement rate [30]. Because radiographic assessment of chemotherapy response is expensive and requires a high-level facility not found in township hospitals and limited reimbursement may undermine care-seeking behavior of patients insured with low reimbursement rate. There is an exception to the trend of underutilization among patients insured with low reimbursement rate: They have the highest adherence of PFTs. Future work should focus on specific aspects of recommendations for care, access to care, and delivery of care, incorporating integrated data. This may contribute to understanding the underlying mechanisms generating treatment disparities among NSCLC patients by primary payer status.

In contrast to previous studies [31, 32], we found that patients insured with low reimbursement rate have a lower rate of in-hospital mortality and metastases, and stayed shorter in the hospital; no significant negative influence of low reimbursement rate was found on 2-year mortality in this payer group. Except for the influences of low reimbursement rate of medical cost, a confounding influence may be found in the convention that "fallen leaves return to their roots—to revert to one's origin", because rural patients may refuse further therapy on their deathbed, choosing to die at home rather than in the hospital. Besides, facilities generally would not collect follow-up data on these patients, and this may have contributed to a low in-hospital mortality rate for patients insured with low reimbursement rate. Our mortality estimate for this group was somewhat lower than that found in prior research [19], because we used a treated and insured population consisting mostly of early stage and surgery (59.43% for lobectomy) patients [33–35]. The fact that insurance mainly reimburses for inpatient care that may contribute to shorter hospital stays among low reimbursement groups.

No marked differences were found in length of preoperative hospital stay, implying similar preoperative waiting times across insurance types.

We provide an integrated appraisal of the effect of low reimbursement rates on the continuum of care for patients with NSCLC, including diagnosis, treatment, and outcome. The results were not perfectly in accordance with our expectations. Further study is required to explore the association between care and outcome. The identified disparities by primary payer status serve as an important proxy for the apparent cost-related barriers to health care among patients insured with low reimbursement rates and other health system-related issues. Non-adherence was associated with higher out-of-pocket expenses. Increased reimbursement rate for medical might be effective in securing good medical compliance. Our findings could provide support for health reforms on equalizing reimbursement rate, aiming at equalizing access to care and improving the level of medical compliance and finally improving quality of care of NSCLC.

Because of several limitations, caution must be exercised in interpreting the results of this study. First, we conducted observational research; therefore, we cannot prove causation between quality-of-care measures and insurance. Second, the hospitals participating in our study were exclusively tertiary teaching facilities located in urban areas, and this limits the generalizability. Future studies should also consider non-teaching, privately owned, community, and other classes of hospitals in a larger regional scope. Third, we did not analyze all established quality-of-care or confounding variables (e.g., distance from residence to hospital), and education levels were not adjusted in the multivariable analysis because of a large number of missing values. This may further limit the interpretation and generalizability of the results. Fourth, the follow-up time was too short to capture more significant differences in mortality. Different results may be obtained through continual tracking.

Conclusion
We conducted univariate and multivariate analyses for a set of 16 quality-of-care indicators for NSCLC. The study found that low reimbursement rates had primarily negative influences on the diagnosis and treatment of NSCLC in patients. Patients insured through lower reimbursement rate programs were less likely to benefit from early detection and treatment services.

Abbreviations
ACCI: Age-adjusted Charlson comorbidity index; ACT: Adjuvant chemotherapy; CT: Computed tomography; MRI: Magnetic resonance imaging; NCMS: New Rural Cooperative Medical Scheme; NSCLC: Non-small cell lung cancer; PFT: Pulmonary function test; PORT: Postoperative radiation therapy; UEBMI: Urban employed basic medical insurance; URBMI: Urban resident basic medical insurance

Funding
This work was supported by National Natural Science Foundation of China 81573255 to Meina Liu, which participated in the design of the study and data collection.

Authors' contributions
XL, XW, SS, MZ, HJ and JW had been involved in data collection and are responsible for the integrity of the data and the accuracy of the data analysis. XL, QZ, and ML participated in designing the study and interpreting the results. XL has been involved in drafting the manuscript and revising it critically. All authors read and approved the final manuscript.

Competing interests
The authors declare that they have no competing interests.

References
1. Hsia J, Kemper E, Kiefe C, Zapka J, Sofaer S, Pettinger M, Bowen D, Limacher M, Lillington L, Mason E: The importance of health insurance as a determinant of cancer screening: evidence from the Women's Health Initiative; 2000.
2. Institute of Medicine (US) Committee on the Consequences of Uninsurance. Care without Coverage: Too Little, Too Late [J]. J Natl Med Assoc. 2002; 97(11):1578.
3. Ward E, Halpern M, Schrag N, Cokkinides V, Desantis C, Bandi P, Siegel R, Stewart A, Jemal A. Association of insurance with cancer care utilization and outcomes. CA Cancer J Clin. 2008;58(1):9–31.
4. Skaggs DL, Lehmann CL, Rice C, Killelea BK, Bauer RM, Kay RM, Vitale MG. Access to orthopaedic care for children with medicaid versus private insurance: results of a national survey. J Pediatr Orthop. 2006;26(3):400–4.
5. Hagihara A, Murakami M, Chishaki A, Nabeshima F, Nobutomo K. Rate of health insurance reimbursement and adherence to anti-hypertensive treatment among Japanese patients. Health Policy. 2001;58(3):231–42.
6. Pan Y, Chen S, Chen M, Zhang P, Qian L, Li X, Lucas H. Disparity in reimbursement for tuberculosis care among different health insurance schemes: evidence from three counties in Central China. Infect Dis Poverty. 2016;5(1):7.
7. Meng Q, Xu L, Zhang Y, Qian J, Cai M, Xin Y, Gao J, Xu K, Boerma JT, Barber SL. Trends in access to health services and financial protection in China between 2003 and 2011: a cross-sectional study. Lancet. 2012;379(9818):805–14.
8. Yip WC, Hsiao WC, Chen W, Hu S, Ma J, Maynard A. Early appraisal of China's huge and complex health-care reforms. Lancet. 2012;379(9818):833–42.
9. Yu H. Universal health insurance coverage for 1.3 billion people: what accounts for China's success? Health Policy. 2015;119(9):1145–52.
10. Bradley CJ, Given CW, Roberts C. Late stage cancers in a Medicaid-insured population. Med Care. 2003;41(6):722–8.
11. Roetzheim RG, Pal N, Tennant C, Voti L, Ayanian JZ, Schwabe A, Krischer JP. Effects of health insurance and race on early detection of Cancer. J Natl Cancer Inst. 1999;91(16):1409.
12. Harlan LC, Greene AL, Clegg LX, Mooney M, Stevens JL, Brown ML. Insurance status and the use of guideline therapy in the treatment of selected cancers. Journal of Clinical Oncology Official Journal of the. Proc Am Soc Clin Oncol. 2005;23(36):9079.
13. Shi L. Type of health insurance and the quality of primary care experience. Am J Public Health. 2001;90(12):1848–55.
14. Bisgaier J, Rhodes KV. Auditing access to specialty care for children with public insurance. N Engl J Med. 2011;364(24):2324–33.
15. Kwok J, Langevin SM, Argiris A, Grandis JR, Gooding WE, Taioli E. The impact of health insurance status on the survival of patients with head and neck cancer. Cancer. 2010;116(2):476.
16. Groth SS, Al-Refaie WB, Zhong W, Vickers SM, Maddaus MA, D'Cunha J, Habermann EB. Effect of insurance status on the surgical treatment of early-stage non-small cell lung cancer. Ann Thorac Surg. 2013;95(4): 1221–6.
17. Bradley CJ, Dahman B, Bear HD. Insurance and inpatient care: differences in length of stay and costs between surgically treated cancer patients. Cancer. 2012;118(20):5084–91.
18. Biswas T, Walker P, Podder T, Efird JT. Effect of race and insurance on the outcome of stage I non-small cell lung Cancer. Anticancer Res. 2015;35(7):4243–9.

19. Potosky AL, Saxman S, Wallace RB, Lynch CF. Population variations in the initial treatment of non-small-cell lung cancer. J Clin Oncol Off J Am Soc Clin Oncol. 2004;22(16):3261–8.
20. Bradley CJ, Given CW, Roberts C. Disparities in cancer diagnosis and survival. Cancer. 2001;91(1):178–88.
21. Sobin L, Gospodarowicz M, Wittekind C, Gospodarowitcz M, Sobin L, Gosporarowicz M: International Union against Cancer (UICC): TNM classification of malignant tumours. 2009.
22. Peterson ED, Delong ER, Masoudi FA, O'Brien SM, Peterson PN, Rumsfeld JS, Shahian DM, Shaw RE. ACCF/AHA 2010 position statement on composite measures for healthcare performance assessment. J Am Coll Cardiol. 2010; 55(16):1755–66.
23. Halpern MT, Ward EM, Pavluck AL, Schrag NM, Bian J, Chen AY. Association of insurance status and ethnicity with cancer stage at diagnosis for 12 cancer sites: a retrospective analysis. Lancet Oncol. 2008;9(3):222.
24. Greenberg ER, Chute CG, Stukel T, Baron JA, Freeman DH, Yates J, Korson R. Social and economic factors in the choice of lung cancer treatment. A population-based study in two rural states. N Engl J Med. 1988;318(10):612–7.
25. Kane S, Shaya F. Medication non-adherence is associated with increased medical health care costs. Dig Dis Sci. 2008;53(4):1020–4.
26. Col N, Fanale JE, Kronholm P. The role of medication noncompliance and adverse drug reactions in hospitalizations of the elderly. Arch Intern Med. 1990;150(4):841–5.
27. Li Y, Wu Q, Xu L, Legge D, Hao Y, Gao L, Ning N, Wan G. Factors affecting catastrophic health expenditure and impoverishment from medical expenses in China: policy implications of universal health insurance. Bull World Health Organ. 2012;90(9):664.
28. Qiu P, Yang Y, Zhang J, Ma X. Rural-to-urban migration and its implication for new cooperative medical scheme coverage and utilization in China. BMC Public Health. 2011;11(1):520.
29. Lei X, Lin W: The new cooperative medical scheme in rural China: does more coverage mean more service and better health? Health Econ 2009, 18 Suppl 2(Supplement):S25.
30. Ruckdeschel JC, Finkelstein DM, Ettinger DS, Creech RH, Mason BA, Joss RA, Vogl S. A randomized trial of the four most active regimens for metastatic non-small-cell lung cancer. J Clin Oncol. 1986;4(1):14.
31. Lapar DJ, Bhamidipati CM, Mery CM, Stukenborg GJ, Jones DR, Schirmer BD, Kron IL, Ailawadi G. Primary payer status affects mortality for major surgical operations. Ann Surg. 2010;252(252):544–50. discussion 550-541
32. Mcdavid K, Tucker TC, Sloggett A, Coleman MP. Cancer survival in Kentucky and health insurance coverage. Arch Intern Med. 2003;163(18):2135–44.
33. Smith TJ, Penberthy L, Desch CE, Whittemore M, Newschaffer C, Hillner BE, Mcclish D, Retchin SM. Differences in initial treatment patterns and outcomes of lung cancer in the elderly. Lung Cancer. 1995;13(3):235.
34. Mokhles S, Nuyttens JJ, Maat AP, Birim Ö, Aerts JG, Bogers AJ, Takkenberg JJ. Survival and treatment of non-small cell lung Cancer stage I-II treated surgically or with stereotactic body radiotherapy: patient and tumor-specific factors affect the prognosis. Ann Surg Oncol. 2015;22(1):316–23.
35. Billmeier SE, Ayanian JZ, Zaslavsky AM, Nerenz DR, Jaklitsch MT, Rogers SO. Predictors and outcomes of limited resection for early-stage non–small cell lung Cancer. J Natl Cancer Inst. 2011;103(21):1621–9.

Permissions

The contributors of this book come from diverse backgrounds, making this book a truly international effort. This book will bring forth new frontiers with its revolutionizing research information and detailed analysis of the nascent developments around the world.

We would like to thank all the contributing authors for lending their expertise to make the book truly unique. They have played a crucial role in the development of this book. Without their invaluable contributions this book wouldn't have been possible. They have made vital efforts to compile up to date information on the varied aspects of this subject to make this book a valuable addition to the collection of many professionals and students.

This book was conceptualized with the vision of imparting up-to-date information and advanced data in this field. To ensure the same, a matchless editorial board was set up. Every individual on the board went through rigorous rounds of assessment to prove their worth. After which they invested a large part of their time researching and compiling the most relevant data for our readers.

The editorial board has been involved in producing this book since its inception. They have spent rigorous hours researching and exploring the diverse topics which have resulted in the successful publishing of this book. They have passed on their knowledge of decades through this book. To expedite this challenging task, the publisher supported the team at every step. A small team of assistant editors was also appointed to further simplify the editing procedure and attain best results for the readers.

Apart from the editorial board, the designing team has also invested a significant amount of their time in understanding the subject and creating the most relevant covers. They scrutinized every image to scout for the most suitable representation of the subject and create an appropriate cover for the book.

The publishing team has been an ardent support to the editorial, designing and production team. Their endless efforts to recruit the best for this project, has resulted in the accomplishment of this book. They are a veteran in the field of academics and their pool of knowledge is as vast as their experience in printing. Their expertise and guidance has proved useful at every step. Their uncompromising quality standards have made this book an exceptional effort. Their encouragement from time to time has been an inspiration for everyone.

The publisher and the editorial board hope that this book will prove to be a valuable piece of knowledge for researchers, students, practitioners and scholars across the globe.

List of Contributors

Ales Ryska
The Fingerland Department of Pathology, Charles University Faculty of Medicine and University Hospital, Hradec Králové, Czech Republic

Peter Berzinec
Department of Oncology, Specialised Hospital of St Zoerardus Zobor, Nitra, Slovakia.

Luka Brcic
Institute of Pathology, Medical University of Graz, Graz, Austria
Institute of Pathology, University of Zagreb School of Medicine, Zagreb, Croatia

Tanja Cufer
Medical Faculty Ljubljana, University Clinic Golnik, Golnik, Slovenia

Rafal Dziadziuszko
Medical University of Gdansk, Gdansk, Poland

Maya Gottfried
Meir Medical Center, Kfar Saba, Israel

Ilona Kovalszky and Jozsef Timar
1st Institute of Pathology and Experimental Cancer Research, Semmelweis University, Budapest, Hungary

Włodzimierz Olszewski
Institute of Oncology, Warsaw,Poland

Buge Oz
Cerrahpasa Medical Faculty, Istanbul, Turkey

Lukas Plank
Department of Pathology, Comenius University, Jessenius Medical Faculty and University Hospital, Martin, Slovakia

Dhruva K. Mishra
Department of Surgery, Houston Methodist Hospital Research Institute, Houston, TX, USA

Min P. Kim
Department of Surgery, Houston Methodist Hospital Research Institute, Houston, TX, USA

Division of Thoracic Surgery, Department of Surgery, Weill Cornell Medical College, Houston Methodist Hospital, 6550 Fannin Street, Suite 1661, Houston, TX 77030, USA

Ross A. Miller
Department of Pathology and Genomic Medicine, Houston Methodist Hospital, Houston, TX, USA

Kristi A. Pence
Division of Thoracic Surgery, Department of Surgery, Weill Cornell Medical College, Houston Methodist Hospital, 6550 Fannin Street, Suite 1661, Houston, TX 77030, USA

Isa Mambetsariev and Ravi Salgia
Department of Medical Oncology and Therapeutics Research, City of Hope Comprehensive Cancer Center and Beckman Research Institute, 1500 E Duarte Rd, Duarte, CA 91010-3000, USA

Lalit Vora
Department of Diagnostic Radiology, City of Hope Comprehensive Cancer Center and Beckman Research Institute, Duarte, CA 91010, USA

Kim Wai Yu
Department of Pharmacy Services, City of Hope Comprehensive Cancer Center and Beckman Research Institute, Duarte, CA 91010, USA

Yan Wang, Fengying Wu, Jing Zhao, Shengxiang Ren and Caicun Zhou
Department of Medical Oncology, Shanghai Pulmonary Hospital, Tongji University School of Medicine, Tongji University Medical School Cancer Institute, No. 507 Zheng Min Road, Shanghai 200433, People's Republic of China

Shijia Zhang
Department of Medical Oncology, Shanghai Pulmonary Hospital, Tongji University School of Medicine, Tongji University Medical School Cancer Institute, No. 507 Zheng Min Road, Shanghai 200433, People's Republic of China
Department of Respiratory Medicine, Huaihe Hospital, Henan University, Kaifeng, People's Republic of China

Xuefei Li and Chao Zhao
Department of Lung Cancer and Immunology, Shanghai Pulmonary Hospital, Tongji University School of Medicine, Shanghai, People's Republic of China

Gao Xiang, Wang Jiangye, Gao Xueming and Chai Wenxiao
Department of Interventional Medicine, Gansu Provincial Hospital, 204 Dong gang West Road, Lanzhou 730000, China

Li Haiying
First Clinical Medical College, Institute of Hematology, Lanzhou University, Lanzhou, China

Wolfgang M. Brueckl and Joachim H. Ficker
Department of Respiratory Medicine, Allergology and Sleep Medicine, Paracelsus Medical University Nuernberg, General Hospital Nuernberg, Prof.-Ernst-Nathan-Str. 1, Nuremberg, Germany

H. Jost Achenbach
Lung Clinic Lostau, Department of Thoracic Oncology, Lindenstr.2, Lostau, Nuremberg, Germany

Wolfgang Schuette
Hospital Martha-Maria Halle-Doelau, Klinik für Innere Medizin II, Röntgenstr.1, Halle, Germany

Fei He, Tao Lin, Wei-min Xiong, Qiu-ping Xu, Zhi-qiang Liu, Bao-chang He, Zhi-jian Hu and Lin Cai
Department of Epidemiology, School of Public Health, Fujian Medical University, Fuzhou 350108, China
Key Laboratory of Ministry of Education for Gastrointestinal Cancer, Fujian Medical University, Fuzhou 350108, China

Xu Li and Ren-dong Xiao
Department of Thoracic Surgery, The first affiliated hospital of Fujian Medical University, Fuzhou 350005, China

Hui Zhang, Yuefeng Wang, Yongmei Cui, Neng Jiang, Wenting Jiang, Han Wang, Shuhua Li, Zhuo Wang, Yangshan Chen, Yu Sun, Liantang Wang and Zunfu Ke
Department of Pathology, The First Affiliated Hospital, Sun Yat-sen University, No. 58, ZhongShan Second Road, Guangdong 510080, China

Weiling He
Department of Pathology, The First Affiliated Hospital, Sun Yat-sen University, No. 58, ZhongShan Second Road, Guangdong 510080, China
Department of Gastrointestinal Surgery, The First Affiliated Hospital, Sun Yat-sen University, No. 58, ZhongShan Second Road, Guangdong 510080, China

Yanbin Zhou and Yifeng Luo
Department of Respiratory Medicine, The First Affiliated Hospital, Sun Yat-sen University, No. 58, ZhongShan Second Road, Guangdong 510080, China

Di Xu
Department of Thoracic Surgery, The Central Hospital of Wuhan, No.26 Shenli Street, Jiang'an District, Wuhan 430014, Hubei Province, China

Yang Zhang
Biomedical Engineering, The University of Texas at El Paso, El Paso, TX, USA

Hsian-Rong Tseng
Department of Molecular and Medical Pharmacology, Crump Institute for Molecular Imaging (CIMI), California NanoSystems Institute (CNSI), University of California, Los Angeles, 570 Westwood Plaza, California, Los Angeles 90095-1770, USA

Xuenong Zou
Guangdong Provincial Key Laboratory of Orthopedics and Traumatology, The First Affiliated Hospital, Sun Yat-sen University, No. 58, ZhongShan Second Road, Guangdong 510080, China

Samantha L. Quaife, Charlotte Vrinten, Jo Waller and Andy McEwen
Department of Behavioural Science and Health, University College London, Gower Street, London WC1E 6BT, UK

Rebecca J. Beeken
Department of Behavioural Science and Health, University College London, Gower Street, London WC1E 6BT, UK
Leeds Institute of Health Sciences, University of Leeds, Worsley Building, Clarendon Way, Leeds LS2 9NL, UK

Mamta Ruparel and Samuel M. Janes
Lungs for Living Research Centre, UCL Respiratory, Division of Medicine, Rayne Building, University College London 5 University Street, London WC1E 6JF, UK

Jiejun Wang
Department of Medical Oncology, Changzheng Hospital, The Second Military Medical University, Shanghai 200433, China

Xinghao Ai
Department of Medical Oncology, Changzheng Hospital, The Second Military Medical University, Shanghai 200433, China
Lung Tumor Clinical Medical Center, Shanghai Chest Hospital, Shanghai Jiao Tong University, Shanghai 200030, China

Feng Mao, Shengping Shen, Yang Shentu and Shun Lu
Lung Tumor Clinical Medical Center, Shanghai Chest Hospital, Shanghai Jiao Tong University, Shanghai 200030, China

Bao-Feng Jin, Lin Gong, Qing Zhao,Teng Li, Yan Huang, Xiao-Yan Zhan, Xuan-He Qin, Jin Wu, Shuai Chen, Sai-Sai Guo, Yu-Cheng Zhang, Jing Chen, Wei-Hua Li, Ai-Ling Li, Na Wang, Qing Xia and Tao Zhou
State Key Laboratory of Proteomics, Institute of Basic Medical Sciences, China National Center of Biomedical Analysis, Beijing 100850, China

Fan Yang, Yi-Da Liao, Ke-Zhong Chen, Xiao Li and Jun Wang
Department of Thoracic Surgery, People's Hospital, Peking University, Beijing 100044, China

Xiao-Min Ying and Shuo-Feng Hu
Computational Medicine Laboratory, Beijing Institute of Basic Medical Sciences, Beijing 100850, China

Yuan Cao
The 90th Hospital of Jinan, Jinan 250031, China

Yan-Hong Tai
The 90th Hospital of Jinan, Jinan 250031, China
Department of Pathology, The 307th Hospital of Chinese PLA, Beijing 100071, China

Dan-Hua Shen and Kun-Kun Sun
Department of Pathology, People's Hospital, Peking University, Beijing 100044, China

Lu Chen
Institute of Pathology, Southwest Cancer Center, Southwest Hospital, Chongqing 400038, China

Juan Zeng, Heying Zhang, Yonggang Tan, Cheng Sun, Yusi Liang, Jinyang Yu and Huawei Zou
The First Oncology Department, Shengjing Hospital affiliated with China Medical University, Shenyang 110004, China

Reena Thriumani, Ammar Zakaria, Amanina Iymia Jeffree, Latifah Munirah Kamarudin, Mohammad Iqbal Omar, Ali Yeon Md Shakaff and Abdul Hamid Adom
Centre of Excellence for Advanced Sensor Technology, Universiti Malaysia Perlis, Arau, Perlis, Malaysia

Yumi Zuhanis Has-Yun Hashim
Cell and Tissue Engineering Lab (CTEL), Department of Biotechnology Engineering, Kulliyyah of Engineering, International Islamic University Malaysia (IIUM), Kuala Lumpur, Malaysia
International Institute for Halal Research and Training (INHART), International Islamic University Malaysia (IIUM), Kuala Lumpur, Malaysia

Khaled Mohamed Helmy
Department of Respiratory, Hospital Tuanku Fauziah, Jalan Kolam, Kangar, Perlis, Malaysia

Krishna C. Persaud
School of Chemical Engineering and Analytical Science, University of Manchester, Oxford Road, Manchester, United Kingdom

Taiki Hakozaki and Yusuke Okuma
Department of Thoracic Oncology and Respiratory Medicine, Tokyo Metropolitan Cancer and Infectious Diseases Center Komagome Hospital, 3-18-22 Honkomagome, Bunkyo, Tokyo 113-8677, Japan

Jumpei Kashima
Department of Pathology, Tokyo Metropolitan Cancer and Infectious Diseases Center Komagome Hospital, Tokyo 113-8677, Japan

Nada Ezzeldin
Chest Diseases, National Research Center, Cairo, Egypt

Ahmed El Bastawisy
Medical Oncology, National Cancer Institute, Cairo University, Cairo, Egypt

Amira Darwish
Medical Oncology, National Cancer Institute, Cairo University, Cairo, Egypt
National Cancer Institute (NCI), Fom-Elkhalig Square, Cairo, Egypt

Dalia El-Lebedy, Shereen Hamdy Abd Elaziz and Mirhane Mohamed Hassan
Clinical Pathology, National Research Center, Cairo, Egypt

Amal Saad-Hussein
Environmental Health & Preventive Medicine, National Research Center, Cairo, Egypt

Alexandra Belayew
Laboratory of Molecular Biology, Research Institute for Health Sciences and Technology, Université de Mons, Mons, Belgium

Ludovic Dhont
Laboratory of Molecular Biology, Research Institute for Health Sciences and Technology, Université de Mons, Mons, Belgium
Princess Margaret Research Institute, Princess Margaret Cancer Centre, University Health Network, Toronto, Canada
Cellular and Molecular Epigenetics, Université de Liège-GIGA, Liège, Belgium

Ethan Kaufman, Roya Navab and Shirley Tam
Princess Margaret Research Institute, Princess Margaret Cancer Centre, University Health Network, Toronto, Canada

Ming-Sound Tsao
Princess Margaret Research Institute, Princess Margaret Cancer Centre, University Health Network, Toronto, Canada
Division of Medical Oncology and Hematology, Princess Margaret Cancer Centre, University Health Network, Toronto, Canada
Laboratory of Medicine and Pathobiology, University of Toronto, Toronto, Canada

Melania Pintilie
Biostatistics Department, University of Toronto, Toronto, Canada

Arsène Burny
Université Libre de Bruxelles (ULB), Bruxelles, Belgium

Frances Shepherd
Division of Medical Oncology and Hematology, Princess Margaret Cancer Centre, University Health Network, Toronto, Canada

Céline Mascaux
Department of Muldisciplinary Oncology and Therapeutic Innovations, Assistance Publique des Hôpitaux de Marseille (AP-HM), Aix-Marseille University, Chemin des Bourrely, 13195 Marseille, Cedex 20, France
Centre de Recherche en Cancérologie de Marseille (CRCM, Cancer Research Center of Marseille), Inserm UMR1068, CNRS UMR7258 and Aix-Marseille University UM105, Marseille, France

Xiao Qu, Kai Wang and Qi Liu
Institute of Oncology, Shandong Provincial Hospital Affiliated to Shandong University, 324 Jingwu Road, Jinan 250021, People's Republic of China

Jiajun Du
Institute of Oncology, Shandong Provincial Hospital Affiliated to Shandong University, 324 Jingwu Road, Jinan 250021, People's Republic of China
Department of Thoracic Surgery, Shandong Provincial Hospital Affiliated to Shandong University, 324 Jingwu Road, Jinan 250021, People's Republic of China

Ying Wang
Institute of Oncology, Shandong Provincial Hospital Affiliated to Shandong University, 324 Jingwu Road, Jinan 250021, People's Republic of China
Department of Clinical Oncology, The University of Hong Kong, Laboratory block, 21 Sassoon, Pokfulam, Hong Kong, People's Republic of China

Hongchang Shen
Department of Oncology, Shandong Provincial Hospital Affiliated to Shandong University, 324 Jingwu Road, Jinan 250021, People's Republic of China

Ngar-Woon Kam
Department of Clinical Oncology, The University of Hong Kong, Laboratory block, 21 Sassoon, Pokfulam, Hong Kong, People's Republic of China

Wenxiong Zhang, Yiping Wei, Dongliang Yu, Jianjun Xu and Jinhua Peng
Department of thoracic surgery, The second affiliated hospital of Nanchang University, 1 Min De Road, Nanchang 330006, China

Hongjun Zhu
Department of thoracic surgery, Shangqiu First People's Hospital, Shangqiu 476100, Henan, China

Shuanglin Zhang
Department of Thoracic and Cardiovascular Surgery,the First Affiliated Hospital of Henan University, No. 357 Ximen Street, Kaifeng City 475000, Henan Province, China

Yue Zhang and Lingxiang Mao
Department of Laboratory Medicine, The Affiliated People's Hospital, Jiangsu University, Zhenjiang 212012, China

Xinyu Tian and Shengjun Wang
Department of Laboratory Medicine, The Affiliated People's Hospital, Jiangsu University, Zhenjiang 212012, China

Institute of Laboratory Medicine, Jiangsu Key Laboratory of Laboratory Medicine, School of Medicine, Jiangsu University, Zhenjiang, China

Jie Ma, Jie Tian, Yu Zheng, Rongrong Peng, Yungang Wang and Huaxi Xu
Institute of Laboratory Medicine, Jiangsu Key Laboratory of Laboratory Medicine, School of Medicine, Jiangsu University, Zhenjiang, China

Ting Wang
Department of Laboratory Medicine, Jiangsu Cancer Hospital, Nanjing, China

Xi Li, Qi Zhou, Xinyu Wang, Shaofei Su, Meiqi Zhang, Hao Jiang and Jiaying Wang
Department of Biostatistics, School of Public Health, Harbin Medical University, Harbin, China

Meina Liu
Department of Biostatistics, School of Public Health, Harbin Medical University, Harbin, China
School of Public Health, Harbin Medical University, No.157 Baojian Road, Harbin 150081, China

Index

www.ingramcontent.com/pod-product-compliance
Lightning Source LLC
Chambersburg PA
CBHW082052190326
41458CB00010B/3510